THE FINANCIAL MANAGEMENT OF HOSPITALS AND HEALTHCARE ORGANIZATIONS

Third Edition

THE FINANCIAL MANAGEMENT OF HOSPITALS AND HEALTCARE ORGANIZATIONS

Third Edition

Michael Nowicki

Health Administration Press, Chicago, IL

AUPHA Press, Washington, DC

AUPHA

———

HAP

08   07   06   05   04   5   4   3   2   1

Library of Congress Cataloging-in-Publication Data

Nowicki, Michael, 1952–
    The financial management of hospitals and healthcare organizations / Michael
    Nowicki.— 3rd ed.
        p.   cm.
    Includes bibliographical references and index.
    ISBN 1-56793-226-6
    1. Hospitals—Business management.   2. Hospitals—Finance.   3. Health
facilities—Business management.   4. Health facilities—Finance.   I. Title.
    RA971.3.N69   2004
    362.1'1'0681—dc22   2004047290

The paper used in this publication meets the minimum requirements of American National Standard for Information Sciences—Permanence of Paper for Printed Library Materials, ANSI Z39.48-1984. ⊗™

Acquisitions Editor: Janet Davis; Project manager: Cami Cacciatore; Cover design: Amanda Karvelaitis.

Health Administration Press
A division of the Foundation
   of the American College of
   Healthcare Executives
One North Franklin Street
Suite 1700
Chicago, IL 60606
(312) 424-2800

Association of University Programs
   in Health Administration
730 11th Street, NW
4th Floor
Washington, DC 20001
(202) 638-1448

Healthcare Financial
   Management Association
Two Westbrook Corporate
   Center, Suite 700
Westchester, IL 60154
(708) 531-9600

I dedicate this book to my parents who, by their actions more than their words, instilled in me the value for life-long learning. From my mother, I learned that effort is a reward in itself. From my father, I learned that correct answers count, always.

CONTENTS

FOREWORD

"No margin—no mission" is a quote often attributed to the late Sister Irene Krause, a Healthcare Hall of Fame inductee and a missed colleague. She felt, as do I, that without effective financial management (margin), hospitals and other healthcare organizations cannot fulfill their mission of providing needed medical and healthcare services to their communities. Although healthcare organizations serve as community resources, they also are complex businesses, and like any business, their success depends on the leadership of managers and executives who understand and can apply key financial principles to fulfill their roles.

Healthcare is unique in the way it is financed. It is characterized by a pluralistic system of public and private financing, and public and private delivery of services, that is unmatched in other industries. Depending on their ownership (public or private), healthcare organizations adhere to accounting standards promulgated by either the Government Accounting Standards Board or by the Financial Accounting Standards Board. An understanding of the issues surrounding third-party payment and payment methodologies, government healthcare programs, complex receivables management, managed care requirements, corporate compliance programs, and so on requires special effort and special resources. This book is one of those resources.

Like so many who have worked in the field of hospital administration, my career was influenced by the predecessor to this book, *The Financial Management of Hospitals*. Since 1971, that text, first written by Howard Berman and Lewis Weeks, who were in later editions joined by Steve Kukla, has served as the primary finance textbook for students in hospital administration and as a key reference book on finance for practitioners. When I started in hospital finance in the early 1970s, it was known by most people in the field simply as "Berman and Weeks." As the field of healthcare evolved, as health administration education broadened beyond hospitals, as payment methodologies grew more complex, and as the distinction among the various healthcare settings blurred, it became apparent that a new book was needed. This book, *The Financial Management of Hospitals and Healthcare Organizations*, now in its third edition, reflects that natural evolution. This third edition includes important new information on the financial impact of patient safety, the public's concern about accounting integrity and our industry's response to that concern, and the historic Medicare Prescription Drug, Improvement and Modernization Act of 2003 passed and signed in late 2003.

Michael Nowicki is well qualified to write this text. As a teacher and scholar, he has taught numerous courses on, and has written numerous papers about, hospital and healthcare accounting and finance. During his career, he has worked for not-for-profit, investor-owned, and public healthcare facilities. As a Fellow in the Healthcare Financial Management Association (HFMA), Michael has and continues to serve HFMA in many volunteer capacities—most recently as a member of both the National HFMA Board of Directors and the National HFMA Board of Examiners. In this latter role, Michael worked with other volunteers nationally to oversee HFMA's certification program, which defines the body of knowledge for healthcare finance. Michael also is a Fellow in the American College of Healthcare Executives which, along with his broad-based experiences, helps him take a view of finance from the nonfinancial manager's perspective.

This book follows a rich tradition of providing an important instructional resource to students and practitioners alike. It is my hope that as the field continues to evolve and as healthcare managers and executives face new challenges, this book will continue to serve as that resource.

Richard L. Clarke, FHFMA
President
Healthcare Financial Management Association

PREFACE

The *Financial Management of Hospitals and Healthcare Organizations* is intended to be the primary textbook of choice in introductory courses in healthcare financial management at both the undergraduate and graduate levels, as well as a reference book for program graduates and other practicing healthcare managers. The purpose of this book is to introduce nonfinancial students and managers to the fundamental concepts and skills necessary to succeed as managers in an increasingly competitive employment environment.

For instance, program graduates find employment in a variety of healthcare settings. Therefore, the focus of this book—as well as the title of the book—extends beyond the hospital. Program graduates consistently report a deficiency in quantitative skills; this book includes problems representing key concepts. Traditional-age students report a need to apply the quantitative skills introduced in financial management. To address both these concerns, a contemporary, comprehensive casebook with practice problems is available in the companion book, *Practice Problems and Case Study to Accompany The Financial Management of Hospitals and Healthcare Organizations, Third Edition.*

In this edition, Part I includes an overview of financial management, the organization of financial management, and the tax status of healthcare organizations. Part II includes third-party payers and payment methodologies, Medicare and Medicaid, cost accounting and analysis, and rate setting. Part III includes the management and financing of working capital, materials management, and accounts receivable management. Part IV includes strategic and operational planning, budgeting, and capital budgeting. Part V includes financial analyses and management reporting. Finally, Part VI includes an analysis of trends that will affect healthcare organizations in the future including healthcare cost projections and the need for entitlement reform

This book is intended for students and managers with prerequisite knowledge in economics, accounting, and statistics; however, in the event that students and managers lack that prerequisite knowledge, the first chapter includes appendices that review the important concepts in those areas.

Each part of the book includes its own recommended readings list. A glossary of important terms and a list of acronyms used in the text are included at the end of the book. The chapters are modular to allow readers to either delete specific chapters or read the chapters in an order based on individual preference or classroom requirements. I hope you find *The Financial Management of Hospitals and Healthcare Organizations* relevant and current.

ACKNOWLEDGMENTS

I would like to gratefully acknowledge the help of those who assisted me in this endeavor: my wife Tracey and our children Hannah and David who have always supported my research; and my many students over the years who have challenged me to find a better way to explain difficult concepts. A special thanks goes to one of my students, Jill Cytacki, who put me in contact with her father Fred Cytacki who works for Hewlett-Packard. Mr. Cytacki expedited the Hewlett-Packard approvals that were necessary for me to use the HP 10BII financial calculator key stroke instructions found throughout this edition. And a special thanks to those at Health Administration Press who have made this third edition as easy to publish as the first two editions.

And finally, I would like to acknowledge the work of Russ Coile, the noted author and healthcare futurist who died in November of 2003 of complications related to brain cancer. I have relied on Russ's predictions in the last chapter of all three editions and his contributions will be sorely missed. After I did a small favor for Russ at the 2003 ACHE Congress on Healthcare Management, Russ asked if there was anything he could do for me. I asked Russ to be the keynote speaker at the Texas State University Health Administration Conference scheduled for October. This was not a hard sell for Russ because he loved talking to students. Shortly after Congress Russ was diagnosed and underwent brain surgery in May. He never considered rescinding our agreement and in fact made more than 75 presentations during his last year. His presentation to our conference in Austin was one of his last. Preston Gee, another noted author who spoke to our conference, later told me that we were honored to be among the last to hear Russ speak—Preston was right.

Michael Nowicki

FINANCIAL MANAGEMENT

FINANCIAL MANAGEMENT IN CONTEXT

Introduction

Successful organizations, whether they be for-profit, not-for-profit, or governmental, have two things in common: a congruent and well-understood organizational purpose(s); and a functional management team. The purpose of this introductory chapter is to describe financial management in healthcare organizations within the context of organizational purpose and a competent management team.

Organizational Purpose

Organizational purpose is often determined by the owner. While a community-owned, not-for-profit healthcare organization's purpose is to provide healthcare services to the community, a corporate-owned (via stockholders), for-profit healthcare organization's purpose is to provide profit for the owner. By necessity, most organizations have more than one organizational purpose. For instance, even though a not-for-profit healthcare organization's purpose is to provide healthcare services to the community, the organization must do so within the context of economic survival—meaning that the organization must generate a sufficient amount of revenue to offset expenses and allow for growth. A for-profit healthcare organization's purpose is to provide profit for the owner; however, the organization must do so within the context of meeting the customer's needs—meaning that to generate the business necessary for a profit to result, the organization must keep the physicians, patients, employers, and insurance companies satisfied. Most healthcare organizations also have secondary purposes, for example, many government-owned healthcare organizations provide large-scale medical education programs. To maintain congruence, the management team must communicate the organizational purpose not only to the employees, but also to owners, customers, and other important constituents. When multiple purposes are present, the management team must prioritize the purposes.

Healthcare Management

In its broadest context, the objective of healthcare management is to accomplish the organizational purposes. Doing so is not as simple as it sounds if the healthcare organization's purposes are "to provide the community with the services it needs, at a clinically acceptable level of quality, at a publicly responsive level of amenity, at the least possible cost" (Berman, Kukla, and

Weeks 1994, 5). Healthcare managers must identify, prioritize, and often resolve these sometimes-contradictory purposes in a political environment that involves the organization's governing board and medical staff, in a heavily regulated environment that involves licensing and accrediting agencies, and in an economic environment that involves increasing competition resulting in demands for lower prices and higher quality. Competent healthcare managers attempt to accomplish the organizational purposes by planning, organizing, staffing, directing, and controlling (called the management functions); and by communicating, coordinating, and decision making (called the management connective processes). For more information on the management functions and connective processes, see Dunn's *Haimann's Healthcare Management* (2002).

With the exception of nursing home administrators, no licensure requirements are needed to be a practicing healthcare manager. However, facility accrediting organizations such as the Joint Commission on Accreditation of Healthcare Organizations (Joint Commission) require healthcare managers to possess such education and experience as required by the position. Moreover, formal educational programs for healthcare management do exist at both the undergraduate and graduate level. Programs at the undergraduate level can seek program review and approval from the Association of University Programs in Health Administration (AUPHA). Programs at the graduate level can seek program review and accreditation from the Accrediting Commission on Education for Health Services Administration (ACEHSA). Furthermore, healthcare managers can seek membership and certification in professional associations including the American College of Healthcare Executives (ACHE), which has 32,589 affiliates including 5,704 certified as Diplomates and 3,259 certified as Fellows (FACHEs) (ACHE 2004).

Purpose of Healthcare Financial Management

The purpose of healthcare financial management is to provide both accounting and finance information that assists healthcare managers in accomplishing the organization's purposes. No licensure requirements are needed to be a practicing healthcare financial manager. Facility accrediting organizations such as the Joint Commission rarely provide requirements for healthcare financial managers, but prefer to hold the organization's chief executive officer (CEO) responsible for financial management. Formal educational programs for healthcare financial management are not common and usually exist as postgraduate certificate programs. The chief financial officers (CFOs) of most large healthcare organizations possess a master's degree in business administration, a bachelor's degree in accounting, a certificate in public accounting (CPA), and have healthcare experience. For formal continuing education and certification in healthcare financial management, healthcare financial managers can seek membership and certification in healthcare professional associations including the Healthcare Financial Management Association (HFMA). The HFMA has 30,469 affiliates including 513 certified as Certified Healthcare Financial Professionals (CHFPs) and 1,678 certified as Fellows (FHFMAs) (Etheridge 2004).

Accounting

Accounting is generally divided into two major areas: financial accounting and managerial accounting. The purpose of financial accounting is to provide accounting information, generally historic in nature, to external users including owners, lenders, suppliers, and to the government and other insurers. Accounting information prepared for external use must follow formats established by the American Institute of Certified Public Accountants (AICPA) and other similar organizations and must follow generally accepted accounting principles (GAAP) used for standardization. The 1996 *AICPA Audit and Accounting Guide for Health Care Organizations* (AICPA 1996) established four basic financial statements that hospitals should prepare for external users: a consolidated balance sheet; a statement of operations; a statement of changes in equity; and a statement of cash flows.

The purpose of managerial accounting is to provide accounting information, generally current or prospective in nature, to internal users, including managers. Such accounting information supports the planning and control management functions. In this way, managerial accounting is the link between financial accounting and the manager and therefore relies on the information provided by financial accounting. Managerial accounting, or accounting information prepared for internal use, requires no prescribed format and therefore varies greatly among organizations. Managerial accounting topics like budgeting and inventory control require knowledge of economics, statistics, and operations research.

Many managerial accountants believe that cost accounting, which is the study of costs including methods for classifying, allocating, and identifying costs, is either synonymous with or a subset of managerial accounting. However, Finkler, in *Essentials of Cost Accounting for Health Care Organizations* (1994), argues that cost accounting includes all managerial accounting and also requires some financial accounting. Cost accounting and managerial accounting also include topics that could be considered finance.

Finance

Historically, the purpose of finance has been to borrow and invest the funds necessary for the organization to accomplish its purpose. Today, the purpose of finance is to analyze the information provided by managerial accounting to evaluate past decisions and make sound decisions regarding the future of the organization (Finkler 1992). Finance uses techniques like ratio analysis and capital analysis, and requires knowledge of financial and managerial accounting (see Appendix 1.1); economics (see Appendix 1.2); statistics (see

FIGURE 1.1
Financial
Management
Relationships

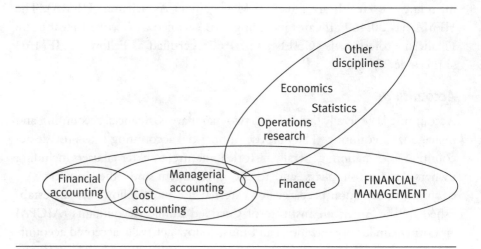

FIGURE 1.1
Financial
Management
Relationships

Appendix 1.3); and operations research. Figure 1.1 shows the relationship of finance to the above-referenced supporting disciplines.

Major Objectives of Healthcare Financial Management

Generate Income

While the purpose of healthcare financial management is to provide accounting and finance information that assists healthcare management in accomplishing the organization's objectives, all organizations have at least one objective in common: to survive and grow. Organizations in other industries might refer to this as maximizing owners' wealth; healthcare organizations typically refer to this as maintaining community services. In either event, the organization will be of little use if it cannot afford to continue to operate.

Therefore, the most important objective of healthcare financial management is to generate a reasonable net income (i.e., the difference between collected revenue and expenses) by investing in assets and putting the assets to work.

Respond to Regulations

Although financial management in healthcare organizations has similar objectives to that of organizations in other industries, different objectives also exist. The federal, state, and local governments regulate healthcare to a significant degree because healthcare organizations are in a position to take advantage of the sick and the elderly, and regulation protects individuals that cannot protect themselves. Federal, state, and local governments pay over 45 percent of all healthcare bills and therefore have a vested interest to ensure that government money is well spent (Levit et al. 2004). Healthcare organizations must also meet quasi-regulations in the form of accreditation or certification standards to qualify for reimbursement from many third-party payers and to qualify for loans from certain lenders. Therefore, the second objective of healthcare financial management is to respond to the myriad of regulations in a timely and cost-effective manner.

Facilitate Relationship with Third-Party Payers

The third objective of healthcare financial management is to facilitate the organization's relationship with third-party payers, who are agents of the patient who have agreed to pay all or a portion of the bill. Third-party payers account for over 75 percent of a healthcare organization's operating revenues (Levit et al. 2004). Financial management must be responsive to third-party payers and in many ways must treat third-party payers as customers in the economic sense of the word, because the third party is the payer of the bill. At the same time, financial management must be attentive to the patient as the customer in the service sense of the word, because the patient has influence over the third-party payer, and in some cases may be partially responsible for the bill.

Influence Method and Amount of Payment

The fourth objective of healthcare financial management is to influence the method and amount of payment chosen by third-party payers. Third-party payers are becoming increasingly aggressive in asking healthcare organizations for discounts in exchange for large numbers of patients. In certain cases, healthcare organizations are discounting prices below costs to maintain market share. Some third-party payers, like Medicare, are asking healthcare organizations to assume part of the financial risk for the patient by agreeing to a prospective payment or, in other words, agreeing in advance to a price for providing care to the patient. Healthcare organizations lose money if they provide care that costs more than the prospective payment. Some third-party payers are asking healthcare organizations to assume substantial risk by agreeing to a capitated price (i.e., a price per head or subscriber) before the subscriber actually needs care. Capitated prices put healthcare organizations at risk for the cost of care if needed, and the utilization of care by the subscriber.

Monitor Physicians

The fifth objective of healthcare financial management is to monitor physicians and their potential financial liability to the organization in terms of their ordering patterns and their possible negligence. Physicians and other professionals account for 32.3 percent of all healthcare spending; 31.3 percent of all healthcare spending goes to hospitals; and 9.0 percent of all healthcare spending goes to nursing homes (Levit et al. 2004). However, physicians influence much of the healthcare spending attributable to hospitals and nursing homes. For example, physicians order the patient admission, the diagnostic testing and treatment for the patient, and the patient discharge. Healthcare financial management must ensure through the utilization review process that physician ordering patterns are consistent with what the patient needs. Regarding the possibility of physician negligence, healthcare financial management must ensure through the credentialing process and the risk management process that the healthcare organization has minimized its exposure to legal liability for the physician's possible negligent actions.

Protect Tax Status

The sixth major objective of healthcare financial management is to protect the organization's tax status. For-profit healthcare organizations seek ways of reducing their tax liability, and not-for-profit healthcare organizations seek ways of protecting their tax-exempt status from the attempts of state and local governments to find new revenue sources. The more difficult objective to accomplish rests with the not-for-profit healthcare organizations, because most healthcare organizations are not-for-profit, and because corporate tax-exempt status has come under judicial and public scrutiny (see Chapter 3).

Quality Assessment and Healthcare Financial Management

> Quality . . . you know what it is, yet you don't know what it is. But that's self-contradictory. But some things are better than others. That is they have more quality. But when you try to say what that quality is, apart from the things that have it, it all goes poof! There's nothing to talk about. But if you can't say what quality is, then for all practical purposes, it doesn't exist at all. But for all practical purposes it does exist. What else are the grades based upon? Why else would people pay fortunes for some things and throw others in the trash pile? Obviously, some things are better than others . . . but what's the "betterness?" . . . So round and round you go, spinning mental wheels and nowhere finding any place to get traction (Pirsig 1974, 179).

During the last 25 years, healthcare organizations have responded to serious pressure to define quality. In the early 1970s, accrediting agencies and third-party payers applied this pressure. In the late 1970s and early 1980s, the consumer movement added pressure. In the late 1980s through the present, competition has added pressure. Economists predict that the pressure will continue as competition drives prices to their lowest, and relatively equal, point, and the market will force healthcare organizations that survive to compete on quality in addition to price. Healthcare organizations have responded to this pressure with two different strategies: a proactive strategy that attempts to adopt a comprehensive view of quality and a reactive strategy that attempts to limit views of quality to those views developed by others.

Proactive Strategy

Healthcare organizations that have adopted a proactive strategy have developed multiple measures of quality, including both direct and indirect measures (Conrad and Blackburn 1985) that go well beyond the minimum measures required by accrediting organizations. Direct measures of quality assume that the organization can define and measure quality itself.

1. *Goal-based measures* assume that progress toward the goals of the strategic and operating plans is quality. The key advantage of goal-based measures is that they focus attention on success or failure.
2. *Responsive measures* assume that customer opinion is quality. The key advantage of responsive measures is that they understand quality from the customer's point of view.
3. *Decision-making measures* assume that decisions are quality. The key advantage of decision-making measures is that they direct accountability to the decision maker.
4. *Connoisseurship measures* assume that expert opinion, like accreditation, is quality. The key advantage of connoisseurship measures is they that inspire high credibility.

Indirect measures of quality assume that the organization cannot define and measure quality itself, but can define and measure the results of quality.

1. *Resource measures* assume that price reflects quality. The key advantage of resource measures is that they provide quantitative data that is readily available.
2. *Outcome measures* assume that results reflect quality. The key advantage of outcome measures is the emphasis on results.
3. *Reputational measures* assume that public perception reflects quality. The key advantage of reputational measures is that they produce ratings for a ratings-conscious public.
4. *Value-added measures* assume that process reflects quality. The key advantage of value-added measures is that, after adjusting for input and output, they focus on process, which the organization can control.

Reactive Strategy

Healthcare organizations that have adopted a reactive strategy have responded only to accrediting agencies and quality consultants. These responses have included:

• Ensuring quality by first centralizing quality efforts in a quality assurance department, then by decentralizing quality efforts to clinical departments, and then further decentralizing quality efforts to all departments;

- Ensuring quality first by studying clinical outcomes, then by studying clinical processes, then by studying all outcomes and all processes, and finally by studying key outcomes and key processes;
- Improving quality first by continuous attention and then by total management; and
- Assessing quality by identifying key processes and desired outcomes.

In defense of accrediting agencies, particularly the Joint Commission, since 1986 the agencies have been relatively consistent in their direction to healthcare organizations. For the Joint Commission, this date corresponds with the hiring of a new president, Dr. Dennis O'Leary, and the introduction of his "Agenda for Change," a strategic direction for the Joint Commission. The philosophic basis for the Joint Commission since 1986 has been to focus on quality, the customer, work processes, measurements, and improvements. To their primary goal of accrediting healthcare organizations, the Joint Commission has added the goal of developing and implementing a national performance measurement database, consistent with the new direction accreditation standards have taken. The standards published in 1995 seem to be standards that will remain relatively constant for at least a few years. The standard related to quality reads, "the [healthcare organization] has a planned, systematic, [organization]-wide approach to process design and performance measurement, assessment, and improvement" (JCAHO 1996a, 134).

Many healthcare organizations are having trouble meeting the new standard; the following is a simplified but instructive summary. Starting with each department's goals and objectives, the manager and employees should discuss desired outcomes and their indicators. Desired indicators should be both sentinel and rate-based. Sentinel indicators measure a process so important that every time the indicators occur, the manager initiates an individual case review. Rate-based indicators measure a process of lesser importance and allow for an error rate; the manager initiates case reviews only if the error rate is exceeded. For instance, an objective of a patient accounts department may be to collect patient bills as rapidly as possible. Desired outcomes may be no lost bills and no more than 5 percent of the total bills going to a collection agency. A sentinel indicator would be a lost bill, initiating a case review on why the bill was lost. The rate-based indicator would be the percentage of total bills going to a collection agency. Reviews would be necessary only if the rate exceeded a predetermined rate, in this example, 5 percent. Reviews should result in recommendations to improve the key processes necessary to meet the desired outcomes. Figure 1.2 reflects these steps.

In response to the Institute of Medicine's (IOM) 1999 report that as many as 98,000 Americans die each year as a result of errors in hospitals, the Joint Commission announced a new set of patient safety and medical error reduction standards to take effect July 1, 2001 (JCAHO 2001). The new standards require accredited hospitals (Lovern 2001)

FIGURE 1.2
Simplified
Quality
Improvement
Process

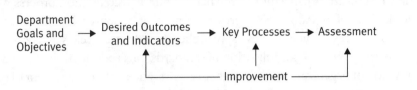

- To make their doctors tell patients when they receive substandard care, or care that differs significantly from anticipated outcomes;
- To implement an organization-wide patient safety program with procedures for immediate response to medical errors;
- To report to the hospital's governing body at least once annually on the occurrence of medical errors; and
- To revise patient satisfaction surveys to ask patients how the organization can improve patient safety.

In July of 2002, the Joint Commission approved the first National Patient Safety Goals (NPSGs) to be effective on surveys after January 1, 2003. NPSG's help accredited organizations address specific areas of concern regarding patient safety. Each goal includes no more than two evidence- or expert-based requirements. Each year the goals are reevaluated and the goals may be continued or replaced based on new patient safety priorities. The Joint Commission announces new NPSGs in July of each year to be effective for survey the following January. The 2003 NPSGs included the following goals (JCAHO 2002a):

- To improve the accuracy of patient identification.
- To improve the effectiveness of communication among caregivers.
- To improve the safety of using high-alert medications.
- To eliminate wrong-site, wrong-patient, wrong-procedure surgery.
- To improve the safety of using infusion pumps.
- To improve the effectiveness of clinical alarm systems.

In July of 2003, the Joint Commission continued the above-referenced goals and added the following goal to make seven 2004 National Patient Safety Goals (NPSGs) to be effective on surveys after January 1, 2004 (JCAHO 2003a).

- To reduce the risk of healthcare-acquired infections.

In October of 2002, the Joint Commission announced "Shared Visions —New Pathways," a program of significant changes to the accreditation process. "Shared Visions" represents agreements between the Joint Commission and healthcare organizations on what a modern accreditation process would look like. "New Pathways" represents a new set of approaches to the accreditation process. Some of these approaches include mid-cycle self-assessments, pre-survey reviews, consolidation of standards, onsite evaluation of standards, revision of organization performance reviews, and active engagement of physicians in the survey process (JCAHO 2002b).

In response to legal concerns regarding the admissability in malpractice actions against the healthcare organization of any form of self-assessments submitted to Joint Commission, the Joint Commission recently announced alternatives to the self-assessment process. One alternative acceptable to the Joint Commission was the performance and attestation that the self-assessment took place, but no submission of the self-assessment to the Joint Commission. The other acceptable alternative was the substitution of a one-day survey in lieu of a self-assessment (Morrissey 2003).

In April of 2003, the Joint Commission announced its intent to make all accreditation visits on an unannounced basis beginning in 2006 in response to criticism that healthcare organizations were not always complying with standards, but were only complying with standards during the scheduled accreditation visits (JCAHO 2003b).

Effects of Quality on Profitability

Deming and others have argued that quality improvements lead to higher profitability. In Deming's case in particular, he introduced the following chain reaction analogy: improvements in quality led to improvements in productivity that led to lower costs that led to lower prices that led to improved market position that led to increased volumes that led to increased profitability (Deming 1982).

There is significant evidence that improved quality has led to improved profitability in healthcare. Solucient, a healthcare information company, and *Modern Healthcare*, each year rank the nation's top 100 hospitals using both clinical and financial measures. The top 100 hospitals consistently outperform their peer group hospitals on both the clinical and financial measures as indicated on Table 1.1

Organizational Ethics and Healthcare Financial Management

The Joint Commission and healthcare professional associations like the ACHE and the HFMA have emphasized organizational ethics in the last several years. Several Joint Commission standards require healthcare organizations to have mechanisms in place to address ethical issues related to such topics as patient rights and management responsibilities. Ethical issues concerning

Hospitals	100 Top Hospitals	Peer Hospitals	100 Top to Peer Hospitals
Mortality Index	0.82	0.97	15.5% lower mortality
Complications Index	0.84	0.94	10.6% fewer complications
Average LOS	3.60	3.94	8.6% shorter ALOS
Average Expense/Discharge	$3,795	$4,677	18.9% lower expenses
Profitability (margin)	6.90%	2.13%	223.9% higher margins

TABLE 1.1
National Performance Comparisons

Source: *Modern Healthcare*. 2003. "They 'Just Do It Better'." *Solucient 100 Top Hospitals.* Supplement to *Modern Healthcare*, 33 (39): 6–12.

patient rights include informed consent, do-not-resuscitate orders, and patient confidentiality. Ethical issues concerning management responsibilities include resource allocation, conflicts of interest, and patient billing practices.

Resource allocation decisions by managers often conflict with the decisions made by physicians and other clinicians regarding patient care. Managers typically represent a utilitarian view of ethics, best represented by the phrase, "the greatest good for the greatest number." This view allows managers to sacrifice the use of resources for one patient to maintain resources for other patients, given the assumption that resources for the healthcare organization are limited. Clinicians typically represent a deontologic view of ethics, best represented by the idea that decisions are governed by duties to patients that take precedence over the ends-based decision making of the manager. This continuous conflict seems to keep resource allocation decisions somewhat balanced. One can only guess what would happen if the manager—or the clinician—always prevailed in this conflict (Summers 1984).

Conflicts of interest occur when an individual owes duties to two or more persons or organizations and when meeting a duty to one somehow harms the other (Darr 1991). The most insidious examples of conflict of interest involve the conflict between a manager's duties to the organization and a manager's duties to self, especially when managers use their positions of authority for personal gain. Although the ACHE Code of Ethics states that the conflict of interest may be merely a matter of degree, even the perception of impropriety may cause a loss of credibility (Nowicki and Summers 2001). This is especially true in financial management, where contracts for services and products are awarded to vendors who may attempt to buy influence with a lunch or a gift (Nowicki 1995).

For the most part, patient billing practices are covered by law; however even certain legal practices have ethical ramifications. For instance, how long should a healthcare organization hold a patient's deposit after the insurance company pays in full? While a healthcare organization may be under no legal obligation to refund overpayments by insurance companies (see Sturn 1995), is keeping someone else's money ethical? What is the organization's obligation to generate a bill free of errors? Many healthcare organizations use ethics committees to provide answers to these and other billing questions. Although healthcare organizations are not required to organize ethics committees, committees are a useful way to solicit community input on billing issues.

Value of Healthcare Financial Management

Healthcare financial management provides accounting information and financial techniques that allow managers to perform the management functions and the management connective processes and therefore accomplish the organizational objectives. In addition to this important indirect value, healthcare financial management has a direct value in the performance of the management functions and management connective processes as explained by Dunn (2002).

Management Functions

- *Planning*: Upon the completion of the strategic plan by the governing body and the operating plan by senior management, financial management is often responsible for the completion of the operating budget and capital budget. The operating budget often provides the incentives to plan properly.
- *Organizing*: Financial management provides a chart of accounts based on the organizational chart that identifies revenue centers and cost centers. Together with the organizational chart, this provides the basis for responsibility accounting, which is the ability to hold department managers responsible for their revenues and expenses.
- *Staffing*: Financial management often staffs a variety of departments and processes important to the healthcare organization. Departments like medical records and information systems are currently being placed under the supervision of financial management, in addition to departments like accounting, admitting, and materials management that have been traditionally under financial management. The increasing importance of nontraditional departments in the billing process appears to justify this trend.
- *Directing*: Also known as motivating and influencing, directing provides financial management the opportunity to use both rewards and penalties to accomplish the organization's purposes.
- *Controlling*: Perhaps the responsibility closest to the overall function of financial management, the control of the budget, financial reports, financial policies and procedures, and financial audits allows financial management to monitor performance and take the appropriate corrective action when performance is unsatisfactory.

These management functions mean little without the management connective processes to integrate the functions.

Management Connective Processes

Communicating is important to financial management for both reporting and advising. Also important is coordinating the relationships between, for example, revenue and expenses; capital budgets and operating budgets; and volumes and prices and collected revenues.

Coordinating is important to financial management as it relates to several relationships: revenue to expenses, capital budgets to operating budgets, volumes to prices to collected revenues, and so forth.

Decision making is important to financial management as a direct measure of quality. Governing boards, chief executive officers, and outside sources like the independent auditors often judge the quality of financial management based on the decisions and recommendations made by financial management. The advantage of this view of quality is that it holds the decision maker accountable. The disadvantage of this view of quality is that it assumes rational decision making. Decisions made in healthcare financial management are often made based on politics or other criteria that are unknown to the evaluator of the decision. Therefore, a decision may be evaluated as bad based on the known facts, but may be evaluated as good based on other criteria unknown to the evaluator.

Effect of Financial Management on the Changing Face of Healthcare

Many say that financial management is the most important predictor of whether healthcare organizations will survive in the current competitive climate and beyond. According to Hodge (1996), the healthcare industry entered an economic depression in the early 1990s that will last through 2005. Like all depressions, the healthcare depression is characterized by rapidly falling prices; restriction of credit including downgrading credit ratings; reduced production; numerous bankruptcies, mergers, and acquisitions; and high unemployment. While his conclusion is not comforting, Hodge points out that healthcare is one of several industries that society has allowed to grow beyond the industry's ability to produce efficiently. The same type of growth followed by depression occurred in agriculture during the 1970s and in oil and financial services during the 1980s, and Hodge predicts that depressions in government and education will follow the depression in the healthcare industry.

Regarding bankruptcies, the most notorious bankruptcy in not-for-profit healthcare history occurred in 1998 with the bankruptcy of the Allegheny Health, Education and Research Foundation (AHERF), a 14-hospital system in Pennsylvania. The AHERF bankruptcy has had a "chilling effect" on bond ratings for most not-for-profit healthcare organizations.

There is significant evidence that the peak of the economic depression was the late-1990s and the healthcare industry is on the upside of economic recovery. The percent increase in hospital prices has risen steadily since its low in 1997: 1.7 percent increase in 1997; 1.9 percent increase in 1998; 2.5 percent increase in 1999; 3.3 percent increase in 2000; 3.6 percent increase in 2001; and 5.1 percent increase in 2002 (Strunk and Ginsberg 2003). Another indication of economic recovery is hospital merger activity which was down for the fourth year in a row with 142 deals reported in 1999 compared to 60 merger deals reported in 2002. Most of the mergers were driven by a desire to consolidate operations, thus improving efficiency (Reilly 2003). Physician medical group mergers were also down from 310 in 1999 to 39 in 2001 (Nowicki 2002).

Clearly, only the well-managed healthcare organizations will survive this depression; financial management will be instrumental in their survival.

Appendix 1.1
Financial Accounting Outline

I. Financial accounting is the science of preparing financial statements for use by individuals and organizations external to the organization.

II. Accounting Equation

Total assets = liabilities + net assets

III. Objectives of Financial Accounting

A. To provide information that is useful to present and potential investors, creditors, and other decision makers

B. To provide information about the economic resources of the healthcare organization, the claims to those resources, and the effects of transactions, events, and circumstances that change those resources

C. To provide information about a healthcare organization's performance

D. To provide information about how a healthcare organization generates and expends cash, about its loans and repayment of loans, and about its capital expenditures

E. To provide information about how a healthcare organization has discharged its stewardship duties to its owners

IV. Accounting Concepts

A. Entity—The healthcare organization stands apart from all other organizations and is capable of taking on economic transactions.

B. Reliability—Accounting records must be based on information that is verifiable from an independent source.

C. Cost valuation—Assets and services are recorded at actual, historic cost.

D. Going concern—The entity will operate long enough to recover the cost of its assets.

E. Stable monetary unit—This is the basis for ignoring the effects of inflation in short-term transactions.

V. Accounting Principles

  A. Accrual accounting—Revenue is recorded when realized (i.e., billed) and expense is recorded when it contributes to operations.

  B. Cash accounting—Revenue and expenses are recorded when cash is actually received or paid.

  C. Accounting period—This is a defined fiscal year or month.

  D. Matching—Related revenue and expense should be reported in the same accounting period.

  E. Conservatism—Uncertainty dictates understating revenues and volumes that lead to revenues, and overstating expenses.

  F. Full disclosure—All economic transactions should be recorded.

  G. Industry practices—Accounting principles are relatively unique to the healthcare industry.

    1. Fund accounting—This allows not-for-profit and governmental healthcare organizations to establish separate entities for specified activities. Typical funds include operating or general funds, specific-purpose funds, plant replacement funds, and endowment funds. Each fund is self-balancing in that assets equal liabilities added to net fund balance.

    2. Contractual allowances—This is the revenue account that records the difference between billed charges and the price a customer has agreed in advance to pay via contract.

    3. Depreciation—This is the expense account that records the estimated cost of an expiring asset.

    4. Funded depreciation—This is the amount saved to replace assets at the end of their useful life.

    5. AICPA Audit Guide for Health Services (1990)

      a. There were major changes in the 1990 edition.

        1) On the statement of revenues and expenses, operating revenue is reported net of contractual allowances.

        2) On the statement of revenues and expenses, operating revenue is reported net of charity care; however, the healthcare organization's policy for charity care, in addition to the level of charity care, must be in the footnotes.

        3) On the statement of revenues and expenses, bad debt expense is reported as an expense based on price.

        4) On the statement of revenues and expenses, donated assets are reported at fair market value as of the date of the gift.

        5) On the statement of revenues and expenses, donated services are reported as an expense, and a corresponding

amount is reported as a contribution, but only if the services are significant and measurable.

    b. There were major changes in the 1996 edition.

        1) Changes were made to the basic financial statements in the:

           a) balance sheet (consolidated)

           b) statement of operations

           c) statement of changes in equity

           d) statement of cash flows

        2) The balance sheet reports net assets

           a) unrestricted

           b) temporarily restricted

           c) permanently restricted

        3) Statement of operations reports performance indicator

           a) revenues over expenses, or

           b) earned income, or

           c) performance earnings

VI. Sarbanes-Oxley Act of 2002

    A. Federal corporate accountability legislation passed in the aftermath of Enron and intended to improve governance and corporate practices. The legislation includes the following standards.

        1. Prohibits accounting firms from providing certain nonaudit services to a client contemporaneously with an audit.

        2. Requires accounting firms to "timely report" to the board's audit committee material communications between the auditor and management.

        3. Requires principal executive and financial officers to certify financial reports, subject to civil and criminal penalties.

        4. Establishes eligibility for audit committee membership, including no affiliation with the company or its subsidiaries, and specific duties of the audit committee.

        5. Directs the Securities and Exchange Commission (SEC) to establish "minimum standards of professional conduct" for lawyers whose practice includes SEC matters.

        6. Prohibits personal loans to directors and executive officers.

        7. Requires companies to maintain an internal control structure and procedures for financial reporting.

        8. Requires companies to disclose whether they have a code of ethics for senior financial officers.

        9. Requires disclosure of off-balance sheet transactions.

        10. Establishes new record retention rules and penalties.

    B. Applies only to public companies; though many states are considering adopting similar legislation for non-profits (i.e., New York).

    C. Some non-profits are holding themselves voluntarily to Sarbanes-Oxley standards.

Appendix 1.2
Economics Outline

I. Economics is the science of producing, distributing, and consuming material goods and services to make better decisions in a world of limited resources.

II. Economic Systems

    A. Capitalism is based on private property rights emphasizing distribution decisions made by the free market based on ability.

        1. Adam Smith's theory was that an "invisible hand" guides the free market economy. Individuals who pursue their own self-interests actually produce economic results beneficial to society as a whole (Smith 1766).

        2. The government's role

            a. national defense

            b. administration of justice

            c. facilitation of commerce

            d. provision of certain public works

    B. Socialism is based on private and government property rights emphasizing distribution decisions made by the government based on effort.

        1. Karl Marx defined socialism as a transitory stage between capitalism and communism. Socialism is classified by government ownership of all important property, and means of distribution of surplus by the government based on the formula: "from each according to ability, to each according to labor" (Marx 1848).

        2. The government's role—"dictatorship of the proletariat" during an economic class struggle

    C. Communism is based on public property rights emphasizing distribution decisions made by the public based on need.

        1. Karl Marx classified communism as the final and perfect goal of historic development characterized by (1) a classless society in which all people live by earning and no person lives by owning; and (2) the abolition of the wage system so that all citizens live and work based on the formula: "from each according to ability, to each according to need."

        2. The government's role: no government

III. Free Markets Under Capitalism

    A. Characteristics of free market

        1. A large number of buyers and sellers, each with a small share of the total business so that no single participant can affect market price

        2. Buyers and sellers are unencumbered by economic or institutional restrictions, and they possess full knowledge of market prices and

alternatives. As a result, they enter or leave markets whenever they wish

B. Functions of free market
1. Establishes competitive prices through the law of supply and demand
2. Encourages efficient use of resources

C. Theories of free market
1. Classical—At market equilibrium (supply equals demand therefore price remains constant); the economy attains full employment; supply creates its own demand; flexibility exists in wages, prices, and interest rates; and savings are invested.
2. Demand side—At market equilibrium the economy does not attain full employment*; demand creates its own supply; wages and prices are "sticky"; and savers and investors are different people with different motivations.
   *The Phillips Curve is the relationship, thought to be inverse, between unemployment and inflation.
3. Supply side—At market equilibrium, the economy does not attain full employment; supply creates its own demand; flexibility exists in wages, prices, and interest rates; and savings are invested.

D. Policy implications of free market theories
1. Classical—Market is self-correcting, no policies are needed.
2. Demand side—Market self-correction is possible; however, it may take a long time. Therefore, government intervention is necessary to stimulate the economy by regulating demand through large-scale government spending programs supported by increased taxes or increased money supply.
3. Supply side—Market self-correction is possible; however, it may take a long time. Therefore, government intervention is necessary to stimulate the economy by stimulating supply (production) through tax reductions*, nonmonetization of government deficits, and deregulation of certain industries.
   *The Laffer Curve is the hypothetical relationship between tax revenues or tax receipts by the government and individual marginal tax rates.

E. Supply side economics—did it work during the 1980s?
1. Efficiency
   a. The inflation rate fell from an annual average of 10.3 percent under Carter to 3.9 percent under Reagan.
   b. The unemployment rate fell from an annual average of 7.5 percent under Carter to 5.3 percent under Reagan.
   c. Per capita disposable income rose from $9,800 under Carter to $11,000 under Reagan.

      d. Interest rates declined from 12.5 percent under Carter to 8.5 percent under Reagan.

  2. Growth—The gross national product (GNP) rose from an annual average of 2.7 percent under Carter to 3.0 percent under Reagan.

  3. Deregulation—Modest gains were achieved under Reagan, most notable was the airline industry.

  4. Equity—Families living in poverty increased from 11.9 percent under Carter to 13.7 percent under Reagan.

  5. Stability—Deficits increased from an annual average of $60 billion under Carter to $190 billion under Reagan.

F. Regulation in the free market

  1. Costs of regulation (Weidenbaum and DeFina 1981)

    a. Direct costs = $10 billion per year

    b. Indirect costs, or compliance costs = $200 billion per year

  2. Economic justifications for regulation

    a. Public interest theory—to protect the public

    b. Industry interest theory—to protect the industry

    c. Public choice theory—to protect government

IV. Healthcare Economics

A. External effects on healthcare economics

  1. Federal debt (in billions)

    1965 = $322.2
    1975 = $541.9
    1985 = $1,817.0
    1995 = $5,001.0
    2000 = $5,674.2
    2001 = $5,807.4
    2002 = $6,228.2
    2003 = $6,872.6
    2004* = $7,528.0
    2005* = $8,142.0
    2006* = $8,679.0
    2007* = $9,222.0
    2008* = $9,782.0
    2009* = $10,335.0
    2010* = $10,884.0
    2011* = $11,316.0
    2012* = $11,598.0
    2013* = $11,842.0

  2. Federal Budget Surpluses (in billions)

    1965 = ($1.4)
    1975 = ($53.2)
    1985 = ($212.3)

1995 = ($163.9)
2000 = $236.4
2001 = $127.3
2002 = ($158.1)
2003 = ($401.1)
2004* = ($480.0)
2005* = ($341.0)
2006* = ($225.0)
2007* = ($203.0)
2008* = ($197.0)
2009* = ($170.0)
2010* = ($145.0)
2011* = ($9.0)
2012* = ($161.0)
2013* = ($211.0)

3. Aging population
  1960 = 9.3 percent over 65 years of age
  1995 = 13.0 percent over 65 years of age
  2030* = 20.7 percent over 65 years of age

B. Internal effects on healthcare economics
  1. Health expenditures by over 65 population
    1960 = 23.6 percent
    1995 = 33.0 percent
    2030* = 52.5 percent
  2. Health expenditures as a percentage of GNP
    1960 = 5.3 percent
    1970 = 7.1 percent
    1980 = 8.9 percent
    1990 = 12.2 percent
    1998 = 13.0 percent
    1999 = 13.0 percent
    2000 = 13.3 percent
    2001 = 14.1 percent
    2002 = 14.9 percent
    2003* = 15.2 percent
    2004* = 15.4 percent
    2005* = 15.6 percent
    2006* = 15.8 percent
    2007* = 16.0 percent
    2008* = 16.2 percent
  3. Health expenditures per person
    1960 = $146
    1970 = $341
    1980 = $1,052

1990 = $2,689
1999 = $4,340
2000 = $4,670
2001 = $5,021
2002 = $5,440
2003* = $5,439
2004* = $5,737
2005* = $6,061
2006* = $6,409
2007* = $6,780
2008* = $7,170

4. Health expenditures by type of service, 2002
   Professional services = 32.3 percent
   Hospital care = 31.3 percent
   Retail outlet sales of medical products = 13.7 percent
   Nursing homes and home health = 9.0 percent
   Program administration = 6.7 percent
   Government public health = 3.3 percent
   Investment (research & construction) = 3.7 percent

5. Health expenditures by funding source, 2002
   Private health insurance = 35.4 percent
   Private out-of-pocket = 13.7 percent
   Other private = 5.0 percent
   Federal Medicare = 17.2 percent
   Federal Medicaid = 9.5 percent
   Other Federal = 5.8 percent
   State and local Medicaid = 6.6 percent
   State and local other = 6.8 percent
   Out-of-pocket = 13.7 percent

6. Health expenditures by percentage increase from previous year
   1990 = 11.7 percent
   1991 = 9.5 percent
   1992 = 8.6 percent
   1993 = 7.3 percent
   1994 = 5.5 percent
   1995 = 5.4 percent
   1996 = 5.2 percent
   1997 = 5.4 percent
   1998 = 4.8 percent
   1999 = 5.6 percent
   2000 = 6.2 percent
   2001 = 8.5 percent
   2002 = 9.3 percent

*projections based on federal government actual data through 2001

Appendix 1.3
Statistics Outline

I. Statistics is the science of collecting, organizing, presenting, analyzing, and interpreting numbers to make better decisions in a world of uncertainty.

II. Descriptive Statistics

    A. Descriptive statistics are used to describe various features of a data set.

    B. Measures of central tendency

        1. Mean, or average, is derived by summing the observations and dividing by the number of observations.

        2. Median is derived by arranging the observations from smallest to largest and selecting the midpoint observation.

        3. Mode is derived by selecting the observation that occurs most often.

        4. Modified mean is derived by deleting the smallest and the largest observations.

        5. Weighted mean is derived by multiplying each observation by a volume, summing the results, and then dividing by the total volume.

    C. Measures of dispersion and shape

        1. Range is the difference between the largest and smallest observation.

        2. Variance is the average of the squared differences between each observation and the mean.

        3. Standard deviation is the square root of the variance.

        4. Shape

            a. Symmetrical—Mean and median are the same.

            b. Right or positive skewed—Mean exceeds the median.

            c. Left or negative skewed—Median exceeds the mean.

    D. The index number is derived by calculating the number in current year divided by the number in base year times 100.

III. Inferential Statistics

    A. Inferential statistics are used to infer the characteristics of a sample to the characteristics of the population.

    B. Probability

    C. Hypothesis testing

    D. Linear regression and correlation are used to predict future events and the strength of the association between variables.

    E. Tests of significance

        1. The t-test is used to determine how likely it is that two mean scores differ by chance.

        2. Analysis of variance is used to determine whether a significant difference exists between two or more means.

3. Analysis of covariance is used to determine whether there is a significant difference between two or more means for groups that are initially unequal.

IV. Healthcare Statistics

A. Adjusted average daily census is derived by dividing the number of inpatient day equivalents (also called adjusted inpatient days) by the number of days in the reporting period.

B. Adjusted expenses per admission is derived by removing expenses incurred for the provision of outpatient care from total expenses and then dividing by the total admissions in the reporting period.

C. Adjusted expenses per inpatient day is derived by dividing total expenses by inpatient day equivalents (also called adjusted inpatient days).

D. Adjusted inpatient days—see inpatient day equivalents

E. Admissions include number of patients, excluding newborns, accepted for inpatient service.

F. Average daily census is the average number of inpatients, excluding newborns, receiving care each day during the reporting period.

G. Average length of stay is derived by dividing the number of inpatient days by the number of admissions.

H. Expenses includes all expenses for the reporting period.

Payroll expenses includes all salaries and wages.

All professional fees and those salary expenditures excluded from payroll are defined as nonpayroll expenses and are included in total expenses. Labor-related expenses is defined as payroll expenses plus employee benefits. Non-labor-related expenses is all other nonpayroll expenses. In accordance with the AICPA Audit Guide (AICPA 1996), bad debt has been reclassified from a "deduction from revenue" to an expense. However, for historic consistency purposes, expense totals may not actually include bad debt expense.

I. FTE is full-time equivalent personnel, derived by adding the number of full-time personnel to one-half the number of part-time personnel.

J. Inpatient day equivalents is derived by multiplying the number of outpatient visits by the ratio of outpatient revenue per outpatient visit to inpatient revenue per inpatient day, and adding the product (which represents the number of patient days attributable to outpatient services) to the number of inpatient days (can also be used to adjust patient days for skilled nursing facilities, rehab, home care, etc.).

K. Occupancy rate is the ratio of average daily census to the average number of statistical (set up and staffed for use) beds (AHA 1985).

L. Revenue—Gross patient revenue (inpatient and outpatient) is revenue from services rendered to patients, including payments received from or on behalf of individual patients. Net patient revenue is derived by subtracting contractual adjustments and charity care from gross patient revenue. Net patient revenue represents what the organization actually intends to collect. Net total revenue is net patient revenue plus all other revenue, including contributions, endowment revenue, government grants, and all other revenue not made on behalf of patients.

References

American College of Healthcare Executives. 2004. [Online retrieval, 2/23/04]. http://www.ache.org/abt_ache/facts.cfm.

American Hospital Association. 1985. *American Hospital Association Hospital Statistics: 1985 Edition.* Chicago: AHA.

American Institute of Certified Public Accountants. 1996. *AICPA Audit and Accounting Guide for Health Care Organizations.* New York: AICPA.

———. 1990. *AICPA Audit and Accounting Guide for Health Care Organizations.* New York: AICPA.

Berman, H. J., S. F. Kukla, and L. E. Weeks. 1994. *The Financial Management of Hospitals, 8th ed.* Chicago: Health Administration Press.

Conrad, C. F., and R. T. Blackburn. 1985. "Program Quality in Higher Education: A Review and Critique of Literature and Research." In *Higher Education: Handbook of Theory and Research*, volume 1, edited by J. Smart. New York: Agathon Press, Inc.

Darr, K. 1991. *Ethics in Health Services Management, 2nd ed.* Baltimore, MD: Health Professions Press.

Deming, W.E. 1982. *Out of the Crisis.* Cambridge, MA: MIT Press.

Dunn, R. 2002. *Haimann's Healthcare Management, 7th ed.* Chicago: Health Administration Press.

Etheridge, H. 2004. Email correspondence to author, January 5.

Finkler, S. A. 1994. *Essentials of Cost Accounting for Health Care Organizations.* Gaithersburg, MD: Aspen Publishers.

Finkler, S. A. 1992. *Finance and Accounting for Nonfinancial Managers.* Englewood Cliffs, NJ: Prentice Hall.

Hodge, M. H. 1996. "Health Care and America's Rolling Depression." *Health Care Management Review* 21 (3): 7–12.

Joint Commission on Accreditation of Healthcare Organizations. 2003a. *Facts About the 2004 National Patient Safety Goals.* [Online retrieval, 01/01/04]. http://www.jcaho.org/accredited+organizations/patient+safety/04+npsg/npsg04.htm.

———. 2003b. *JCAHO to Shift to Unannounced Surveys by 2006.* [Online retrieval, 12/26/03]. http://www.jcaho.org/news+room/news+release+archives/unannounced+surveys.htm.

———. 2002a. *Facts About the 2003 National Patient Safety Goals.* [Online retrieval, 01/01/04]. http://www.jcaho.org/accredited+organizations/patient+safety/03+npsg/npsg03.htm.

———. 2002b. *Joint Commission Debuts New Accreditation Process: Shared Visions—New Pathways.* [Online retrieval, 12/26/03]. http://www.jcaho.org/news+room/news+release+archives/svnp_nr.htm.

———. 2001. [Online retrieval, 01/21/01]. http://www.jcaho.org/news/nb300.html.

———. 1996. *1997 Hospital Accreditation Standards.* Chicago: JCAHO.

Levit, K., C. Smith, C. Cowan, A. Sensenig, and A. Catlin. 2004. "Health Spending Rebound Continues in 2003." *Health Affairs* 23 (1): 147–159.

Lovern, E. 2001. "JCAHO's New Tell-all." *Modern Healthcare* 31 (1): 2, 15.

Marx, K. 1848. *Communist Manifesto.* Reprinted in 1998. New York: Signet Classic Books.

Modern Healthcare. 2003. "They 'Just Do It Better'." *Solucient 100 Top Hospitals.* Supplement to *Modern Healthcare,* 33 (39): 6–12.

Morrissey, J. 2003. "Legal Hangups: JCAHO Offers Self-assessment Options to Avoid Lawsuits." *Modern Healthcare* 33 (36): 8–9.

Nowicki, M. (moderator). 2002. "Surviving Mergers and Sales: Managing Change." *HealthLeaders* 5 (11): RT1–RT15.

Nowicki, M. 1995. "Conflicts of Interest." *Journal of Healthcare Resource Management* 13 (10): 34–35.

Nowicki, M., and J. Summers. 2001. "Managing Impossible Missions: Ethical Quandries and Ethical Solutions." *Healthcare Financial Management* 55 (6): 62–67.

Pirsig, R. 1974. *Zen and the Art of Motorcycle Maintenance.* New York: William Morrow.

Reilly, P. 2003. "Mergers Minus the Mania." *Modern Healthcare* 33 (3): 36–38.

Smith, A. 1766. *Wealth of Nations.* Reprinted in 2000. New York: Modern Library.

Strunk, B. C., and P. B. Ginsburg. 2003. "Tracking Health Care Costs: Trends Stabilize But Remain High in 2002." *Health Affairs* Jan–Jun; Suppl: W3-266–74.

Sturn, W. C. 1995. "Must Insurance Payment Made in Error Be Returned?" *Healthcare Financial Management* 49 (5): 27–30.

Summers, J. 1984. "Doing Good and Doing Well: Ethics, Professionalism, and Success." *Hospital & Health Services Administration* 29 (2): 84–100.

Weidenbaum, M. L., and R. DeFina. 1981. *The Rising Cost of Government Regulations.* St. Louis, MO: Center for the Study of American Business.

ORGANIZATION OF FINANCIAL MANAGEMENT

T he successful accomplishment of organizational purposes requires a sound organizational structure. After the governing body has established a healthcare organization's purposes, management must determine the best way to accomplish them. To do this, management must identify and assign tasks to employees, departments, and divisions, or management must organize. According to Dunn (2002), organizing includes:

- *Specialization*: dividing tasks into manageable categories and assigning the categories to employees with the appropriate skills.
- *Departmentalization*: dividing employees into groups or teams that have similar responsibilities.
- *Defining the span of management*: determining the optimum number of employees that a manager can manage based on the nature of the tasks and the background of the employees.
- *Defining authority*: determining the amount of authority to delegate to employees so that they can perform their assigned tasks.
- *Defining responsibility*: determining the obligation necessary to perform assigned tasks.
- *Establishing a unity of command*: appointing one manager to be responsible for a group of employees.
- *Defining the nature of relationships*: determining whether managers and employees have a line or staff relationship in the organization. In a line relationship, the manager or employee is directly responsible for resources such as employees and supplies. In a staff relationship, the manager or employee acts in an advisory capacity without direct control over resources.

Most healthcare organizations are organized as legal entities called corporations. Corporate status is granted by the state and provides advantages for the healthcare organization. Corporate status provides limited liability, meaning that the owners of the corporation are seldom found to be personally liable for the contracts or negligence of the corporation. Another advantage of corporate status is its continuity of existence, meaning that the corporation continues even after the death of an owner. The third advantage of corporate status is the increased ability to raise capital because investors share only limited risks, but have a proportionately greater opportunity for reward. In the case of for-profit corporations, free transferal of risk is a fourth advantage of corporate status. This means that shareholders of a for-profit healthcare organization are free to sell their shares at any time. For further discussion of these advantages, refer to *Southwick's The Law of Hospital and Health Care Administration* (Showalter 2003).

The purpose of this chapter is to provide a comprehensive description of the organization of financial management in healthcare organizations.

Governing Body

The governing bodies of healthcare organizations with corporate status cannot be held personally liable for either the contracts of the corporation or the negligence of the corporation's employees or agents (i.e., physicians). However, the governing body can be held collectively liable for a breach of its duty to act as a fiduciary, which means its duty to act as a person in a position of great trust and confidence. The legal duties of a fiduciary include loyalty and responsibility. Loyalty requires fiduciaries to act in the best interests of the healthcare organization and to subordinate their personal interests to those of the organization. Responsibility requires fiduciaries to act with reasonable care, skill, and diligence in accomplishing their duties as members of the governing body (Showalter 2003).

In addition to several other duties, the governing body of a healthcare organization is responsible for the proper development, utilization, and maintenance of all resources in the healthcare organization (AHA 1990). The governing body typically delegates the authority for accomplishing this duty to the organization's CEO and maintains the responsibility by monitoring performance through committees. Although the governing body delegates a great deal of authority to the CEO for this and other duties, the governing body maintains legal responsibility. Because of this fact, courts continue to stress the importance of the governing body's duty of responsibility in selecting a competent CEO. In *Reserve Life Insurance Company v. Salter* (1957), one of the first cases establishing this duty, the court was severe in its finding:

> Failing to appreciate their duties and responsibilities led these Trustees to feel, according to their testimony, that they had discharged their duties by picking as Administrator, Salter, a former school teacher, apparently as ignorant of operating a hospital as they themselves were.

The governing body uses organized committees to monitor the CEO's performance. Although committee structures vary from organization to organization, an executive committee of the governing body is typically responsible for routine monitoring of all committees and includes the chairs of all the committees as members. For financial management, the governing body uses a finance committee responsible for monitoring the CEO's performance

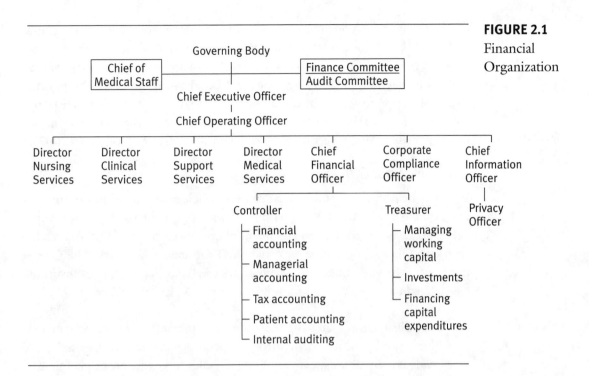

FIGURE 2.1
Financial
Organization

in financial affairs. The finance committee includes governing body members with a financial interest or occupation. In smaller organizations, the duties of the finance committee also include audit responsibilities; in larger organizations, audit responsibilities may be monitored by an audit committee. Generally, the CEO and/or the chief operating officer (COO) and chief financial officer (CFO) attend finance committee meetings ex officio, and also serve as staff support to those committees. Figure 2.1 identifies these relationships.

After the Enron bankruptcy, the federal government passed strict corporate accountability standards known as the Sarbanes-Oxley Act of 2002 (see Appendix 1.1 in Chapter 1). While the standards only apply to for-profit organizations, many not-for-profit organizations are attempting to comply with the standards. Some states like New York are considering passing Sarbanes-Oxley–like state legislation that also applies to not-for-profits.

In November of 2003, Richard Scrushy, founder and former chairman of for-profit HealthSouth, was indicted for 85 counts on conspiracy, fraud and money laundering. The indictment alleges that Scrushy was the mastermind of a wide-ranging scheme to inflate the rehabilitation and outpatient-care company's earnings in order to meet Wall Street expectations. The indictment further alleges that Scrushy added at least $2.7 billion in fictitious income to HealthSouth's books during a multiyear conspiracy dating back to 1996. Scrushy becomes the first CEO (and as a result, healthcare becomes the first industry) indicted under Sarbanes-Oxley which holds the CEO personally liable for financial misreporting. If convicted, Scrushy faces a possible maximum sentence of 650 years in prison, the forfeiture of $279 million in ill-gotten gains, and more than $36 million in fines. While the impact of the Scrushy indictment on the healthcare industry is not yet clear, it seems reasonable to assume that both federal regulatory agencies and bond rating firms will be paying special attention to the healthcare industry in the future. It also seems reasonable to assume that the governing bodies of healthcare organizations will be holding the CEO more accountable for financial reporting (Piotrowski 2003).

Chief Financial Officer

In larger healthcare organizations, the CEO delegates the authority for accomplishing the duties related to financial management to the COO, who delegates authority for day-to-day financial operations to the CFO. In certain cases, the CFO reports directly to the CEO for financial matters. The Committee on Ethics and Eligibility Standards of the Financial Executives Institute has defined the CFO duties as follows (Berman, Kukla, and Weeks 1994):

1. To establish, coordinate, and maintain, through authorized management, an integrated plan for the control of operations. Such a plan would provide cost standards, expense budgets, sales forecasts, profit planning, and programs for capital investments/financing to the extent required in the business.
2. To measure performance against approved operating plans and standards, and to report and interpret the results of operations to all levels of management. This function includes the design, installation, and maintenance of accounting policy, and the compilation of statistical records as required.
3. To measure and report on the validity of the objectives of the business and on the effectiveness of its policies, organization structure, and procedures in attaining those objectives. This includes consulting with all segments of management responsible for policy or action concerning any phase of the operation of the business as it relates to the performance of this function.
4. To report to government agencies, as required, and to supervise all matters relating to taxes.
5. To interpret and report on the effect of external influences on the attainment of the objectives of the business. This function includes the continuous appraisal of economic and social forces and of government influences as they affect the operations of the business.
6. To provide protection for the assets of the business. This function includes establishing and maintaining adequate internal control and auditing, and ensuring proper insurance coverage.

A profile of the average hospital and system CFO in 2003, compared to a profile of the average hospital CFO in 2001 and 1995, according to information provided by the Healthcare Financial Management Association

	1995	2001	2003
Annual compensation	$99,900	$127,000	$151,000
Average age	42	46	47
Percent male	84	76	83
Percent with master's degree	53	49	45
Percent with CPA	83	45	45
Percent with HFMA certification	25	17	20

TABLE 2.1

Hospital CFO Profile

Sources: Healthcare Financial Management Association. 1995. "CFO Compensation by Organizational Size, Ownership." *Healthcare Financial Management* 49 (10): 40–50. Healthcare Financial Management Association. 2001. "CFO Compensation Reaches Record Levels." *Healthcare Financial Management* 55 (6): 68–70. Healthcare Financial Management Association. 2003. "2003 HFMA Compensation Survey." *Healthcare Financial Management* 57 (7): 3–14 (special supplement).

(HFMA), is shown in Table 2.1. The 1995 profile also included personal strengths, personal weaknesses, and future concerns about healthcare.

CFOs reported their strengths as attention to the bottom line and planning. Reported weaknesses included personnel matters and hospital politics. CFOs reported that their greatest future concerns included, in order of importance, capitation, managed care, integrated systems, and information systems. The 2001 and 2003 profiles include a comparison by gender. In 2003, the percentage of women CFOs responding to the survey was down from 24 percent in 2001 to 17 percent in 2003. These results were unexpected and may have more to do with the sample than with practices in the industry. In 2003, women earned an average of $56,700 less then men, up from a difference of $36,800 reported in 2001. However, after adjusting for other determining factors such as job tenure, total number of reporting employees, net patient revenue of the organization, the area's wage index, CPA attainment, eligibility for bonus or profit sharing, and bed count, regression analysis finds that gender is still a significant determinant of compensation, accounting for $15,000 of the reported difference in 2003 and $14,000 of the reported difference in 2001.

At an average age of 47, hospital and system CFOs are relatively young. This means that organizations and associations like HFMA will need to find new ways to motivate CFOs who have reached the top of their career ladder at a young age (the 1995 CFO profile reported that only 8 percent of the surveyed CFOs aspired to be the CEO). Although only 16 percent of the CFOs were women in 1995, that percentage has increased steadily over the years and will continue to increase as women who graduated from business schools in the 1970s and 1980s gain the prerequisite experience to be CFOs. Forty-five percent of the CFOs have advanced degrees, usually in business administration. Most CFOs have undergraduate degrees in accounting and 45 percent are certified in public accounting.

Many CFOs with multiple certifications would argue that certification in HFMA is the most meaningful certification for CFOs in the healthcare industry. However, many CFOs received their public accounting certification shortly after graduation and feel additional certification in HFMA is unnecessary. Currently only 20 percent of the CFOs in the 2003 survey are HFMA certified. Certification in HFMA requires the following:

- Be a member of HFMA for two years;
- Complete 60 college semester hours or the equivalent;
- Earn 60 Founders Awards points by participating in HFMA service opportunities or continuing education (40 of the 60 required points can be earned through participating in education opportunities in societies and organizations other than HFMA);
- Provide a reference from an immediate supervisor and from an HFMA chapter officer or director; and
- Pass a written core exam on the healthcare industry and pass one of four specialty exams in accounting and finance, financial management of physician practices, managed care, or patient financial services. (Exams are Internet-based and must be taken with an HFMA chapter proctor present.)

Several surveys conducted between 1996 and 2001 have identified expanded roles for CFOs requiring a broad range of new traits and skills. Surveys of healthcare CFOs conducted by Witt/Kieffer (Doody 2000) have identified five intrinsic traits possessed by born leaders that CFOs must nurture:

1. Strategic thinking
2. Ability to adjust to change
3. Personal integrity
4. Vision
5. Ability to be a team player

The CFOs also identified six acquired leadership skills (Doody 2000):

1. *Communicate clearly*—the vast majority of the CFOs identified good communication as the most important leadership skill for CFOs;
2. *Provide leadership in day-to-day operations*—the CFOs recognized the importance of providing leadership in a practical, daily manner;
3. *Manage resources and finances*—the CFOs remembered the importance of this very traditional skill that includes planning, organizing, staffing, directing, and controlling;
4. *Build coalitions*—the CFOs recognized that cooperating with others and building coalitions will be imperative to success in the future;
5. *Create a positive organizational culture*—the CFOs realized that as they build coalitions, they must use their political skills to maintain and promote a positive organizational culture; and

6. *Maintain strong physician relationships*—the CFOs report that they are rapidly becoming key players in relationships between organizational providers and physicians due to the increasing importance of financial and regulatory expertise.

At the 2003 CFO Exchange sponsored by HFMA's CFO Forum, HFMA President Dick Clarke introduced a healthcare financial competency model that demands new, more complex roles for healthcare CFOs in addition to more traditional roles as identified in Figure 2.2

In addition to CFO's, certified public accountants (CPAs) are being asked to take on additional roles by the American Institute of Certified Public Accountants in their 1997 publication, *CPA Vision Project—2011 and Beyond*, which identifies needed changes in the nature of being an accountant: greater emphasis on professional demeanor, leadership, and interpersonal communications.

Do CFOs and accountants have the personalities conducive to these expanded roles demanding new competencies? Using Myers-Briggs personality typing, several studies have identified that the predominant personality types of accountants are introversion (I) (versus extroversion), sensing (S) (versus intuitive), thinking (T) (versus feeling), and judging (J) (versus perceiving). Larabee (1994) reported that 37.3 percent of the study sample were STJs (significant compared to 20.5 percent found in the general population) and 56.0 percent were Is (significant compared to 40.1 percent found in the general population). The consistency among the findings of the personality studies on accountants is remarkable considering when the studies were conducted (from 1980 to 1997) and where the studies were conducted (United States, United Kingdom, and the Netherlands).

ISTJs represent 7 to 10 percent of the American population and are serious, responsible, sensible, trustworthy, and honor their commitments. Practical and realistic, they are matter-of-fact and thorough. They are painstakingly accurate and methodical, with great powers of concentration. They value and use logical and impersonal analysis and are organized and systematic in getting things done on time (Tieger and Barron-Tieger 2001).

Time Frame	Past		
	Present ————————→		
	Future —————————————————————→		
Roles	Financial Expert	Business Advisor	Enterprise Leader
Competencies	technical expertise	decision support	strategic leadership
	results oriented	compliance oversight	system influence
	supervisor	coach/teacher	mentor
	internal focus	internal/external	external focus
	risk minimizer	risk quantifier	risk accepter

FIGURE 2.2
Healthcare Financial Competency Model

Do CFOs have the same personalities as accountants, or do only the extroverted accountants become CFOs? In a survey of healthcare senior financial executives (which includes not only CFOs but also vice presidents of finance) conducted by the Healthcare Financial Management Association and Texas State University, it was reported that 37.8 percent of the sample was STJs (compared to 37.3 percent found in the accountant sample and 20.5 percent found in the general population) and 57.0 were Is (compared to 56.0 found in the accountant sample and 20.5 percent found in the general population), confirming that healthcare CFOs have personalities similar to accountants (Nowicki 2003).

Controller and Treasurer

Reporting to the CFO are the controller and the treasurer. The controller is the chief accounting officer of the healthcare organization and is usually responsible for financial accounting, managerial accounting, tax accounting, patient accounting, and internal auditing. The treasurer is responsible for managing working capital, the healthcare organization's investment portfolio, and the financing of capital expenditures. In smaller organizations, the controller function and the treasurer function may be combined into one position, or may be integrated with the CFO's responsibilities.

Corporate Compliance Officer

Many organizations are adding a corporate compliance officer (CCO) to their senior management teams in response to industrywide fraud and abuse concerns. The final compliance program guidelines for hospitals recently issued by the Department of Health and Human Services (HHS) Office of Inspector General (OIG) list the appointment of a CCO as a critical element of any corporate compliance plan (HHS 2000). A 1998 national survey by Witt/Kieffer (Doody 1998) reported that healthcare compliance officers usually report directly to the CEO or board and are seen as peers of the CFO. CCOs are typically responsible for conducting compliance reviews (to assess how well the organization complies with fraud and abuse laws), investigating potential fraud and abuse problems, and examining relationships and contracts for possible illegal provisions. In organizations that have not added a CCO, COOs, staff or retained attorneys, or CFOs are performing these functions. Because no education, certification, or licensure is required for CCOs, CEOs seek individuals that understand the legal issues involved with compliance and exhibit the following personal characteristics that might support the compliance functions (Doody 1998):

- Analytical, inquisitive, persistent;
- Detail-minded;
- Skilled in dealing with people;

- Dispassionate, objective;
- Courageous;
- Discreet; and
- A strong moral sense.

The Health Care Compliance Association (HCCA) surveyed healthcare organizations in 2000 and found the results recorded in Table 2.2 (HCCA 2000). See Table 2.3 for recent compensation trends.

Chief Information Officer

Historically, managing information resources in healthcare organizations has been the responsibility of the CFO, a practice that reflected the need for accurate and timely financial information. However, given the increasing importance of clinical information systems like medical records as well as the

TABLE 2.2

Hospital CCO Profile, 2000

	2000
Maturity of Compliance Programs	
Organizations with active compliance programs	71%
Organizations with appointed CCO	98%
Reporting Relationships	
To board of directors	15%
To CEO/president	58%
Executive vice president	6%
Chief financial officer (CFO)	5%
Legal counsel	4%
Chief operating officer (COO)	4%
Compliance committee	3%
Other	5%
CCO Demographics	
Age	46 years
Female	56%
Highest degree/certification received	
Bachelor's	26%
Master's	40%
Ph.D.	4%
J.D.	15%
CPA	11%
Health Care Certification	6%
Nursing	10%
Average salary	$90,000
Preferred background in order of preference	
1. Hospital administration	
2. Auditing	
3. Law	
4. Regulatory affairs	

TABLE 2.3
Healthcare
Middle
Manager
Compensation
Trends

	1999	2001	2003
Director/Manager of Finance	$78,800	$83,900	$91,700
Director/Manager of Managed Care	$73,700	$80,000	$87,800
Controller	$72,600	$78,300	$85,600
Compliance Officer	$70,400	$79,000	$89,300
Director/Manager of Patient Accounting	$60,800	$71,200	$77,000
Director/Manager of Accounting	$55,800	$62,500	$70,800

Source: Healthcare Financial Management Association. 2003. "2003 HFMA Compensation Survey." *hfm* 57 (7): 3–14 (special supplement).

Y2K scare, many healthcare organizations have assigned the responsibilities for managing information resources to a chief information officer (CIO). Typically reporting directly to the CEO, the CIO is responsible for not only providing management oversight to all information processing and telecommunications systems in the organization, but also for assisting senior management in using information in management decision making (Austin and Boxerman 1998). The responsibilities of CIOs are rapidly evolving to include e-commerce, e-health and other web-based and multimedia technologies; business-service formats to respond tactically to strategic business initiatives; and outsourcing of all or a portion of the information technology departments. As CIOs become an accepted part of the executive team, leadership skills will become more important and technology skills will become less important. In fact, CIOs will delegate many of their technology responsibilities to chief technology officers (Hagland 2000).

Privacy Officer

The Health Insurance Portability and Accountability Act of 1996 (HIPAA) mandated privacy and security regulations for the healthcare industry. The HHS's final rule on privacy issued in 2002 and effective in 2003 requires that the "entity must designate a privacy official who is responsible for the development and implementation of the privacy policies and procedures of the entity" (CMS 2004). The HHS's final rule on security, issued in 2003 and effective in 2005 requires that the "security responsibility be assigned to a specific individual or organization . . . for the management and supervision of the use of security measures to protect data and of the conduct of personnel in relation to the protection of data" (CMS 2004). It is unclear whether the same position could, or should, be responsible for both privacy and security of information. It is clear that specific education, certification, or licensure does not currently exist. The American Health Information Management Association (AHIMA) makes a good case that HIM professionals should have the training and experience to handle most of the skills required for privacy officers. HIM professionals should have (Dennis 2001)

- HIPAA competency;
- Knowledge of how confidential information is used;
- Knowledge of how confidential information is disclosed;
- Knowledge of information technology;
- Knowledge of state and federal laws on information; and
- The ability to promote unpopular positions.

Internal Auditor

As described in Berman, Kukla, and Weeks (1994), independent auditors are quite different from internal auditors. The independent auditor is typically a large accounting firm with a contract with the healthcare organization. The internal auditor is an employee of the organization who usually reports to the controller. The independent auditor's primary concern is the financial reporting needs of external entities, and the internal auditor's primary concern is protecting the organization's assets from fraud, error, and loss. The independent auditor's responsibilities are limited primarily to financial matters; the internal auditor's responsibilities include both financial and operational matters. The independent auditor is only incidentally concerned with identifying fraud (i.e., the independent auditor is not looking for fraud, but is duty-bound to report any fraud found in the organization to the party that engaged the auditor's services); the internal auditor is directly concerned with identifying fraud.

In a comparison of surveys of directors of internal audit completed in 1990 and 1998, researchers found that internal auditors are spending significantly more time on management and operational improvement activities and less time on traditional accounting and compliance activities (Edwards, Kusel, and Oxner 2000).

Independent Auditor

Independent auditors are typically large accounting firms retained by the healthcare organization to ensure that the financial reports sent to external agencies are correct as to accounting format. Examples of external agencies include the state and federal government, commercial insurance companies, and lenders. Correct as to accounting format means that the healthcare organization used generally accepted accounting principles (GAAP) in preparing the report. This does not guarantee that the healthcare organization is financially sound. The American Institute of Certified Public Accountants (AICPA) recently issued Statement on Auditing Standards (SAS) No. 82, Consideration of Fraud in a Financial Statement Audit, which requires independent auditors to obtain reasonable assurance that financial statements are free of material misstatements caused by error or fraud. While SAS No. 82 provides guidelines for independent auditors to use to help detect and document risk factors related to potential fraud, SAS No. 82 does not expand their detection responsibility. Therefore, healthcare organizations and independent auditors should discuss thoroughly the scope and focus of the audit as it relates to the organization's compliance efforts (Reinstein and Dery 1999).

Independent auditors typically audit the healthcare organization once each year. The duration of the audit is partially dependent on the size of the organization. At the end of the audit, the independent auditor produces an audit report comprised of three paragraphs:

1. The introductory paragraph identifies the financial statements audited; management's responsibilities in preparing the financial statements; and the auditor's responsibilities in expressing the audit opinion.
2. The scope paragraph describes the criteria used in the audit (for instance, GAAP).
3. The opinion paragraph includes the auditor's statement about whether the financial statements are correct as to accounting format.

A fourth paragraph, the explanatory paragraph, is included only if GAAP was not used in preparing the financial statements or if any uncertainty exists regarding how the financial statements were prepared. The *AICPA Audit and Accounting Guide for Health Care Organizations* (1996) provides examples of audit reports, including the four different opinions referenced next.

The opinion paragraph is the heart of the audit report and deserves special emphasis. Independent auditors use four types of opinions in rendering their reports:

1. An unqualified opinion means that, in all material respects, the financial statements fairly present the financial position, results of operations, and cash flows of the organization in conformance with GAAP. An unqualified opinion may have an additional explanatory paragraph, but an explanatory paragraph does not affect the opinion. Auditors use an explanatory paragraph when they are basing their opinion in part on the work of a different external auditor, or when they need additional information to prevent the audit report from being misleading when uncertainties exist that they cannot reasonably resolve by the publication date of the audit report.
2. A qualified opinion means that the financial statements fairly present, in all material respects, the financial position, results of operations, and cash flows of the organization in conformance with GAAP, except for matters identified in additional paragraphs of the report. Auditors use a qualified opinion when there is insufficient evidential matter, when the organization has placed restrictions on the scope of the audit, or when the financial statements depart in a material, though not substantial, manner from GAAP.

3. An adverse opinion means that the financial statements do not fairly present the financial position, results of operations, and/or cash flows of the organization in conformance with GAAP. Auditors use additional paragraphs after the opinion to describe the reasons for an adverse opinion.

4. A disclaimer of opinion means that the auditor does not express an opinion on the financial statements, usually because the scope of the audit was insufficient for the auditor to render an opinion.

Alternative Corporate Structures

As previously mentioned, healthcare organizations are chartered as corporations by the state. Prior to the late 1970s, most healthcare corporations consisted of one corporation or a limited number of corporations. Beginning in the late 1970s, a legal strategy called corporate restructuring became popular in response to increasing economic pressures on healthcare organizations. The purpose of corporate restructuring was to maximize the economic position of the healthcare organization by developing new corporations (see Stromberg 1982). Typically, healthcare organizations restructure for one or more of the following four reasons, which dictate the corporate restructuring model.

Healthcare organizations that need to facilitate the development of a new service may develop a wholly controlled subsidiary corporation. For example, a for-profit healthcare organization may develop a wholly controlled subsidiary not-for-profit corporation called a foundation to facilitate education and research. In addition to facilitating education and research, the for-profit healthcare organization shelters some income from taxes by using the income for purposes that are tax-exempt.

Healthcare organizations that need to protect present and future assets may develop a parent holding corporation. For example, for-profit healthcare organizations may develop several parent corporations to layer their liability in the event of malpractice suits. Courts allow only the assets of the organization, and not the assets of the parent corporation, to be introduced during deliberations regarding damage awards.

Healthcare organizations that need to maximize patient care and other operating revenues and even nonoperating revenues may develop a quasi-independent sister corporation. In this model, the healthcare organization can control no more than 49 percent of the governing body of the sister corporation. For example, a healthcare organization, either for-profit or not-for-profit, may develop a gift shop whose governing body usually uses the income to benefit the healthcare organization. The healthcare organization believes that the perception of independence on the part of customers, both in terms of who controls the governing body and who controls the employees or volunteers, gives the gift shop an additional advantage in generating revenue.

Customers are more likely to donate funds to an "independent" corporation than to the healthcare organization that sends them a bill.

Healthcare organizations that need to attract additional funds through philanthropy may develop a wholly independent corporation. In this model, the healthcare organization cannot control any of the governing body. For example, a healthcare organization may develop a foundation whose governing body raises money using relationships established by the healthcare organization. The governing body of the foundation usually uses the income to benefit the healthcare organization, much in the same way that university alumni associations, which are independent from the universities, use their income to benefit universities.

Although corporate restructuring was popular in the late 1970s and 1980s, both Medicare and the Internal Revenue Service (IRS) have increased their interest in the resulting corporations (see Squiers 1986). Medicare's position has been that a portion of the income generated by quasi-independent corporations like gift shops should be deducted from the amount Medicare owes the healthcare organization under cost-based reimbursement. Medicare reasons that a portion of the gift shop sales are attributable to Medicare patients and their visitors.

The IRS's position is that corporate restructuring that allows a corporation to avoid paying taxes should be reviewed to ensure that the primary purpose of the corporate restructuring is legitimate. Areas of concern include the unrelated business income (UBI) generated by not-for-profit healthcare organizations through the formations of their wholly controlled subsidiary corporations (e.g., parking garages, adjacent hotels, catering services, and so on). Healthcare organizations that have restructured their corporations are encouraged to seek specialized legal and tax advice (see the recommended reading list for more information), and organizations contemplating such corporate restructuring are also encouraged to seek such advice. Chapter 3 will provide an overview of the tax status of corporations and review in detail the tax-exempt organization.

References

American Hospital Association. 1990. *Role and Functions of the Hospital Governing Board*. Chicago: AHA.

American Institute of Certified Public Accountants. 1997. *CPA Vision Project—2011 and Beyond*. New York: AICPA.

———. 1996. *AICPA Audit and Accounting Guide for Health Care Organizations*. New York: AICPA.

Austin, C. J., and S. B. Boxerman. 1998. *Information Systems for Health Services Administration, 5th ed*. Chicago: Health Administration Press/AUPHA.

Berman, H. J., S. F. Kukla, and L. E. Weeks. 1994. *The Financial Management of Hospitals, 8th ed*. Chicago: Health Administration Press.

Centers for Medicare and Medicaid Services. 2004. "The Health Insurance Portability and Accountability Act (HIPAA) of 1996." [Online information; retrieved 2/5/04]. http://www.cms.gov/hipaa/.

Clarke, D. 2003. "Healthcare Financial Competency Model." Paper presented at HFMA's 2003 CFO Exchange, San Francisco.

Dennis, J. C. 2001. "The New Privacy Officer's Game Plan." *Journal of AHIMA* 72 (2): 33–37.

Doody, M. F. 2000. "Broader Range of Skills Distinguishes Successful CFOs." *Healthcare Financial Management* 54 (9): 52–57.

Doody, M. F. 1998. "Corporate Compliance Officer Role Is Emerging." *Healthcare Financial Management* 52 (5): 78.

Dunn, R. 2002. *Haimann's Healthcare Management, 7th ed.* Chicago: Health Administration Press.

Edwards, E. D., J. Kusel, and T. H. Oxner. 2000. "The Changing Role of Internal Auditors in Health Care." *Healthcare Financial Management* 54 (8): 62–64.

Hagland, M. 2000. "The Many Hats of a CIO." *Healthcare Informatics* 17 (5): 69–76.

Health Care Compliance Association. 2000. *2000 Profile of Health Care Compliance Officers.* Philadelphia, PA: HCCA.

Healthcare Financial Management Association. 2003. "2003 HFMA Compensation Survey." *hfm* 57 (7): 3–14 (special supplement).

———. 2001. "CFO Compensation Reaches Record Levels." *Healthcare Financial Management* 55 (6): 68–70.

———. 1995. "CFO Compensation Influenced by Organizational Size, Ownership." *Healthcare Financial Management* 49 (10): 40–50.

Larrabe, S. 1994. "The Psychology Types of College Accounting Students." *Journal of Psychology Type* 28: 37–42.

Nowicki, M. 2003. "Evolving Role of the Healthcare CFO." Paper presented at HFMA's 2003 CFO Exchange, San Francisco.

Piotrowski, J. 2003. "HealthSouth's Most Wanted." *Modern Healthcare* 33 (45): 6–7, 16.

Reserve Life Insurance Company v. Salter. 1957. 152 F. Supp. 868.

Reinstein, A., and R. J. Dery. 1999. "AICPA Standard Aids in Detecting Risk Factors for Fraud." *Healthcare Financial Management* 53 (10): 48–50.

Showalter, J. S. 2003. *Southwick's The Law of Hospital and Health Care Administration, 4th ed.* Chicago: Health Administration Press.

Squiers, M. P. 1986. "Corporate Restructuring of Tax-Exempt Hospitals: The Bastardization of the Tax-Exempt Concept." *Law, Medicine and Health Care* 14 (2): 66–76.

Stromberg, R. E. 1982. "Legal Issues for Diversification and Divestiture" as cited by Berman and Weeks. *The Financial Management of Hospitals, 5th ed.* Chicago: Health Administration Press.

Tieger, P., and B. Barron-Tieger. 2001. *Do What You Are: Discover the Perfect Career for You Through the Secrets of Personality Type, 3rd ed.* New York: Little, Brown & Company.

U.S. Department of Health and Human Services. 2000. "HHS Recommends Model Compliance Plans." [Online retrieval, 02/13/01]. http://oig.hhs.gov/medadv/snffinal.htm.

TAX STATUS OF HEALTHCARE ORGANIZATIONS

As discussed in Chapter 2, healthcare corporations are granted legal status as corporations by the state. Although the state can allow a variety of tax designations for corporations, only two are discussed in this chapter: for-profit corporations and not-for-profit corporations.

Rationale for Tax-Exempt Status

As a general rule, for-profit corporations pay taxes: federal and state income taxes on income; state and local sales taxes on purchased goods and, in some states, services; and local real estate and personal property taxes on land, buildings, and major equipment. Not-for-profit corporations pay no taxes and are therefore tax-exempt. To be tax-exempt, corporations must meet certain criteria established by the federal government through the Internal Revenue Service (IRS) and state and local governments (most state and local governments use either the exact or similar criteria to the criteria established by the IRS according to Berman, Kukla, and Weeks (1994).

What is the rationale for the government to grant tax-exempt status to corporations? The first reason is to relieve the government of the burden of providing the services itself. For instance, states grant healthcare organizations tax-exempt status and in exchange the organization provides healthcare services to the state's indigents or to state residents who cannot afford healthcare services. In the absence of this arrangement, the government presumably would provide these healthcare services itself. The second reason that the government grants tax-exempt status to corporations is to reward the corporation for performing services that enhance community values and goals. For instance, governments reward healthcare organizations with tax-exempt status because the organization provides uncompensated health-promotion programs to the community that benefit the overall well-being of the community.

Value of Tax-Exempt Status

Although the potential exposure of a corporation to taxes and fees depends on a variety of variables including accounting practices, Witek, Milligan, and Ryan (1993) made the following general comments regarding valuing tax-exempt status. Federal income tax payments (approximately 34 percent applied to

FIGURE 3.1

Annual Value of Tax-Exempt Status for 122-Bed, Acute Care Hospital

Federal Income Tax	$1,469,000
State Income Tax	$ 334,000
Real Estate	$ 155,000
Personal Property	$ 84,000
City Property Tax	$ 24,000
Total Tax Liability	$2,066,000
Business Licenses and Fees	$ 150,000
Incremental Debt Cost	$ 900,000
Value of Tax-Exempt Status	$3,116,000

Source: Witek, J. E., D. L. Milligan, and J. B. Ryan. 1993. "Managing Charitable Purpose: Issues and Answers." Presented at the American College of Healthcare Executives Annual Administrative Congress on Healthcare Management, Chicago, 4 March.

net income) are generally the largest tax liability. State income tax payments average 6 percent applied to net income in states that have a state income tax. Real estate and personal property taxes are a significant tax liability and are calculated based on a rate per $100 on fair market value for land and appraised value for buildings and major equipment. In addition to exempting tax liabilities, tax-exempt status also exempts the organization from paying most business fees and licenses. One of the most valuable benefits of tax-exempt status is access to tax-exempt bond markets, whose yields are 4 to 5 percent below taxable bond yields.

Therefore, the value of tax-exempt status is the total value of taxes and business licenses and fees exempted, and also the value of access to tax-exempt bond markets. Table 3.1 shows the annual value of tax-exempt status for a 122-bed, acute care hospital in Atlanta, Georgia. Incremental debt cost takes into account the difference between the annual cost of tax-exempt bonds at 3 percent and the annual cost of taxable bonds at 8 percent.

Qualifying for Tax-Exempt Status

As previously mentioned, the IRS has developed the primary criteria for a corporation with tax-exempt status (designated as a 501(c)(3) corporation by the IRS). To qualify for tax-exempt status, corporations must:

1. Operate exclusively for charitable, scientific, or educational reasons;
2. Serve public rather than private interests, in that income may not inure to the benefit of individuals; and
3. Not engage in prohibited transactions including, but not limited to:
   • participating in political campaigns;
   • attempting to influence legislation;

- lending any part of their income without receiving adequate security and interest;
- paying any compensation in excess of reasonable salary levels;
- making any investments for more than adequate consideration;
- selling any asset for less than adequate consideration;
- subverting in any other manner substantial portions of its income or assets; or
- making any part of its services available on a preferential basis.

In 1956, the IRS established that not-for-profit healthcare organizations qualified for tax-exempt status as charitable organizations under Revenue Ruling 56-185. The term charitable organization has never been defined by law but has been interpreted in rulings by the IRS, beginning with ruling 56-185. In effect, this ruling established the financial ability standard in which, to retain tax-exempt status, healthcare organizations are required to provide care to those unable to pay. This ruling was difficult to administer, and charitable organization was redefined in final form in 1959 to include a concept of community benefit or public interest that was broader than just the provision of care to those unable to pay. In 1969, the IRS, in Revenue Ruling 69-545, expanded the financial ability standard to include organizations that promoted health that the IRS "deemed beneficial to the community as a whole even though the class of beneficiaries eligible to receive a direct benefit from its activities does not include all members of the community, such as indigent members of the community, provided that the class is not so small that its relief is not of benefit to the community" (IRS Revenue Ruling 69-545 as cited in Kuchler 1992, 22). This new community benefit standard applied to hospitals that met the following conditions:

- Hospitals must operate a full-time emergency room that accepts all patients regardless of the patient's ability to pay.
- Hospitals must provide care for all patients in the community who are able to pay either with private funds or through public programs like Medicare or Medicaid.

In 1983, the IRS in Revenue Ruling 83-157 again expanded the community benefit standard by exempting the emergency room requirement for hospitals whose state agencies had determined that the hospital's emergency room duplicated existing services in the community (Kuchler 1992). Since 1983, tax-exempt status in general and the community benefit standard specifically have come under scrutiny from research, judicial, congressional, executive, and public sectors. As the next section identifies, the community benefit standard remains the primary IRS test for designating tax-exempt status.

Community Benefits and Tax-Exempt Status

It is difficult to determine who first asked whether a significant difference exists between the amount of community benefits offered by not-for-profit and those offered by for-profit hospitals. Clearly, this question became important to both the legal community and the research community by the mid-1980s. It may well have started with an exchange in the *New England Journal of Medicine* between Arnold Relman, the journal's editor, and Michael Bromberg, president of the American Federation of Hospitals, an association of for-profit hospitals.[1] In 1980, Relman wrote an article warning his readers of the medical-industrial complex—"a large and growing network of private corporations engaged in the business of supplying health-care services [exclusive of supplies and pharmaceuticals] to patients for a profit—services heretofore provided by nonprofit institutions or individual practitioners" (Relman 1980, 963). Relman worried that the medical-industrial complex would put the interests of stockholders before the interests of the community.

Bromberg became the spokesperson for the medical-industrial complex. Answering Relman's claims in the *New England Journal of Medicine*, Bromberg stated that the most important issue regarding the medical-industrial complex was whether for-profit hospitals provided a benefit to the community. Bromberg assured the readers that for-profit hospitals provided much-needed capital that funded a technology boom; that for-profit hospitals provided significant taxes that supported social programs at the local, state, and federal levels; and that for-profit hospitals provided competition that would be good for the community by reducing costs and improving quality. Bromberg also criticized some of the early research that seemed to be supporting Relman's claim. This research found that for-profit hospitals charge more per patient day; perform more ancillary tests per patient day; and "skim the cream," meaning that for-profit hospitals serve only paying patients and provide only profitable services (Bromberg 1983). The question that resulted from the Relman-Bromberg exchange was whether significant differences in community benefits existed between community for-profit hospitals as a group, and community not-for-profit hospitals as a group.

Herzlinger and Krasker addressed that issue in the *Harvard Business Review* in 1987. Using multiple regression, they studied 14 major multihospital systems—six for-profit systems representing 90 percent of all for-profit hospitals in systems, and eight not-for-profit systems representing 68 percent of all not-for-profit hospitals in systems. They found that little difference existed in community benefits provided by hospitals in the for-profit systems and the hospitals in not-for-profit systems.

> For-profits do not deny access to care. In fact, we found the for-profits gave slightly more access to patients who carry little or no health insurance than did the nonprofits. The reasons are straight forward: hospital costs are mostly fixed and the marginal costs of

an additional patient generally are low. Even an indigent patient contributes somewhat to covering the hospital's fixed costs.

For-profits do not "cream" the affluent patients who have insurance coverage. There is no difference in accessibility between for-profits and non-profits to the affluent patient.

While non-profit hospitals receive more social subsidies than for-profits [exemptions from taxes, business fees and licenses, as well as access to tax exempt bonds], they do not achieve better social results. They are not more accessible to the uninsured and medically indigent, nor do they price less aggressively. (Herzlinger and Krasker 1987, 103)[2]

Other studies during the 1980s confirmed that for-profit hospitals provided significant community benefits through the delivery of uncompensated care—both indigent and bad debt—and the delivery of unprofitable services needed by the community. Sloan, Valvona, and Mullner (1986) found that for-profit hospitals deliver approximately 3 to 4 percent of revenues in uncompensated care, and that numerous studies have shown that for-profit hospitals offer a wide scope of services (Gray 1986). In 1993, Witek, Milligan, and Ryan reported that by including taxes as a community benefit, for-profit hospitals in Georgia actually provide substantially more community benefit than not-for-profit hospitals or county hospitals that receive direct tax support (see Table 3.2). A 1992 Government Accounting Office (GAO) study found that community benefits standard results are the same for not-for-profit and for-profit hospitals; therefore, the GAO recommended that the community benefits standard should no longer be used as a distinguishing characteristic. The 1995 *U.S News and World Report* October 2 cover story, "Tax Exempt!" reported that the GAO had found little difference in indigent care between not-for-profit hospitals and for-profit hospitals: not-for-profit hospitals provided indigent care in the amount of 4.8 percent of gross revenues, and for-profit hospitals provided care in the amount of 5.2 percent of gross revenues. Questioning why the nation's 3,100 not-for-profit hospitals, which grossed more than $337 billion in revenues during 1993, were in

Hospital Ownership	Indigent Care	Total Taxes	Total Benefit
County	6.0	(4.0)	2.0
Not-for-profit	4.1	0.0	4.1
For-profit	2.5	3.9	6.4

TABLE 3.2
Community Benefit Comparison in Georgia Hospitals, 1991

Note: Amounts shown as percent of adjusted gross revenue.
Source: Witek, J. E., D. L. Milligan, and J. B. Ryan. 1993. "Managing Charitable Purpose: Issues and Answers." Presented at the American College of Healthcare Executives Annual Administrative Congress on Healthcare Management, Chicago, 4 March.

fact tax-exempt, *U.S. News and World Report* noted that not-for-profit hospitals annually represented approximately $15 billion in lost tax revenue to the government.

In 1996, Morrissey, Wedig, and Hassan published a study of California not-for-profit hospitals with data collected between 1988 and 1991. The study found 80.4 percent of the state's not-for-profit hospitals provided uncompensated care, including both the cost of bad debt and charity care, in excess of their tax subsidies, which averaged $1,579,000 and included income tax subsidies, bond subsidies, and property tax subsidies. However, 19.6 percent of the state's not-for-profit hospitals had not provided uncompensated care in excess of their tax subsidies.

Judicial Challenges to Tax-Exempt Status

The previously mentioned research findings question the community benefits standard; courts have also been reviewing the appropriateness of tax-exempt status. In 1985, the Utah Supreme Court found the state's tax-exemption statutes to be unconstitutional, thus allowing a local taxing authority, the Utah County Tax Commission, to tax Intermountain Health Care, a not-for-profit system of hospitals. The court argued that not-for-profit hospitals had evolved to a position in the marketplace from which distinguishing them from their for-profit counterparts became virtually impossible. Therefore, the court decided that not-for-profit hospitals should be reviewed more rigorously and frequently to ensure that they deserve their tax-exempt status.

> Tax exemptions confer an indirect subsidy and are usually justified as the quid pro quo [consideration] for charitable entities undertaking functions and services that the state would otherwise be required to perform. A concurrent rationale used by some courts is the assertion that the exemptions are granted not only because charitable entities relieve government of a burden, but also because their activities enhance beneficial community values and goals. Under this theory, *the benefits received by the community are believed to offset the revenue lost by reason of the exemption* (emphasis added by author) (Utah 1985).

Under this court's rationale, the amount of community benefits provided by the not-for-profit hospital should equal or exceed the amount of the tax-exemption. In this case, community benefits did not equal the tax-exemption and the court required the not-for-profit hospitals to pay the difference in taxes. Critics of this decision have argued that the community benefit standard is too lenient. The standard defined community benefits as indigent care, community education and service, medical discounts, and donations of time, money, or services made by hospital employees acting as private individuals (Utah State Tax Commission 1990). In 2001 in Salt Lake County, the Board of Equalization voted to maintain tax exemption for four Intermountain

Healthcare facilities, but not before it required the system to once again present its case for exemption (Bellandi 2001).

A similar case in Texas attracted significant, mostly negative, national media attention for not-for-profit hospitals, including a 1993 ABC News *PrimeTime Live* report. In 1988, the Texas Attorney General filed suit against Methodist Hospital in Houston charging that the hospital failed to provide adequate charity care. The Attorney General appointed a statewide task force to address the issues related to uncompensated care. The task force produced a broad definition of uncompensated care that was friendly to the Methodist argument. In early 1993, a district court judge threw out the case against Methodist, ruling that the hospital had broken no current state law and that under current state law only the local appraisal districts could determine whether hospitals qualified for tax-exempt status as charitable organizations. Methodist Hospital, and all other not-for-profit hospitals in Harris County, then received a letter from the local appraisal district asking for data to substantiate claims for property tax exemptions the hospitals had received.

In the meantime, the governor had appointed the Texas Health Policy Task Force to make policy recommendations to the legislature in 1993. After noting several problems with the existing method of providing, financing, and reporting uncompensated care, the task force recommended that not-for-profit hospitals provide amounts of charity care (which excludes bad debt and contractual allowances but includes the cost of charity care and the cost of any Medicaid losses) equal to the value of local and state tax-exempt benefits received by the hospitals. This recommendation was the basis of Texas Senate Bill 427, which is discussed in detail in a following section.[3]

St. Luke's Regional Medical Center in Boise, Idaho, received a $3.4 million property tax bill from the county authorities in 1997. The county based its decision on the fact that the not-for-profit hospital was no longer charitable and therefore should pay taxes based on the following:

- The hospital was not sufficiently supported by donations—donations accounted for less than 2 percent of the hospital's total revenues.
- The recipients of the hospital's services were expected to pay for the services received.
- The hospital did not provide a community benefit because the cost of charity care and bad debt was shifted to other patients through increased charges.
- The hospital was too profitable as evidenced by an 8.9 percent net income.

Harrisburg Hospital has been battling a challenge to its property tax-exempt status since 1993. In 1998, the appeals court in Pennsylvania upheld the revocation of the hospital's tax-exempt status. While the hospital met the first four requirements of a five-requirement test to prove tax-exempt status, the hospital failed to meet the fifth requirement—a requirement that it operate entirely free of the private profit motive. Evidence of the profit motive cited by the court included the following (Thompson Powers 1999):

- The hospital's operating surpluses were routinely passed on to the corporate parent who used the surpluses to fund subsidiary profit-making ventures like the acquisition of physician practices.
- The hospital CEO's compensation, $400,000 in 1994, was excessive compared to the compensation of a peer group of other non-profit executives.
- The hospital's executive bonus plan emphasized financial goals rather than the promotion of charity.
- The hospital required employed physicians to sign non-compete clauses which indicated that the hospital was attempting to protect its market share rather than meet the needs of its community.

Darmouth-Hitchcock Medical Center in Lebanon, New Hampshire, received a $6.5 million property tax bill in 1998 just days after the city tax assessor had revoked the not-for-profit hospital's tax-exempt status based on the following:

- The hospital had the collection policy to receive full payment for services, if at all possible.
- The hospital provided only 2.9 percent of total revenues in charity care—an amount also provided by for-profit hospitals.
- The hospital used surpluses to fund its for-profit subsidiary.

The hospital paid the $6.5 million under protest and paid $7.0 million under protest in 1999. In 2000, the hospital offered the city a $600,000 payment in lieu of taxes (PILOT) with an agreement to increase the $600,000 by 2 percent per year for 20 years. The city rejected the offer, pointing out that the hospital's offer was less than 15 percent of their tax liability, and the case is headed for court (Taylor 2001a).[4]

In 1998, the IRS revoked the tax-exempt status of Great Plains Health Alliance, a not-for-profit hospital management company that leases and manages 25 rural hospitals in Kansas and Nebraska. In announcing the revocation, the IRS said

- Great Plains was a management services company that did little or nothing to deserve its exemption; and
- Leasing and managing hospitals is not an inherently charitable act even if the hospitals are tax exempt.

Great Plains argued that the management services enhanced the charitable missions of its hospitals and were vital not only to the hospitals, but also to the communities they served. The case was scheduled to be heard by the U.S. Tax Court in 2000, but was delayed pending a settlement. In 2001, Great Plains announced a reorganization of its ten leased hospitals that would allow greater local control over decision making. Great Plains paid an unspecified amount of taxes during the three-year period that the IRS had revoked the tax-exempt status. In April of 2001, the IRS approved the reorganization and reinstated the company's tax-exempt status (Taylor 2001b).

In 2003, the Attorney General of Connecticut sued Yale–New Haven Hospital for allegedly hoarding $37 million in charitable funds in order to generate interest income instead of spending the funds to provide indigent care. The attorney general charged the hospital with failing to provide free care to eligible indigent patients while accruing $274,574 in annual interest income and spending only $258,143 on free care. In testimony before the state legislature, the attorney general promised to investigate the state's 500 or so charitable funds designed to provide free care to determine whether the funds deserved their tax-exempt status (Piotrowski 2003).

Also in 2003, the Third District Court of Appeals in Wausau, Wisconsin, upheld a 2002 Circuit Court summary judgment against the 728-physician Marshfield Clinic, Wisconsin's largest physician group with 39 clinics and an annual operating budget of $498 million. In the ruling, the court determined that the clinic was not entitled to property tax exemptions originally granted in 1988 to three clinics in Eau Claire because the clinics had not shown that they used the property exclusively for "benevolent" purposes as defined by state law. The court said that medical care is not always "benevolent" pointing to the fact that 97 percent of Marshfield's patients paid for care either themselves or through insurance. "Marshfield provided absolutely no itemized documentation of how much of the property's use is dedicated to research, education, patient care for destitute patients and [how much of the property's use is dedicated] to paying patients." (Taylor 2003a).

In late 2003, the 5th U.S. Circuit Court of Appeals overruled an Austin, Texas, federal judge who ruled in 2002 in summary judgment that St. David's HealthCare System was tax-exempt. The six-hospital system is a whole-hospital joint venture between for-profit HCA and not-for-profit St. David's. In 1996, HCA and St. David's each contributed three hospitals to form the St. David's HealthCare Partnership after signing a 54-year partnership agreement. After a 1998 audit, the IRS ruled that St. David's, the not-for-profit half of the joint venture, no longer operated exclusively for charitable purposes and in 2000 the IRS revoked St. David's tax-exempt status. The IRS ordered St. David's to pay 1996 taxes for its share of the partnership profits, which St. David's did under protest. St. David's challenged the IRS ruling and won at the trial court level in 2003. The trial court judge ordered the IRS to restore St. David's tax exempt status and said St. David's had operated as a charitable entity since its founding in 1925 and has been granted tax-exempt status since 1938. The judge further stated that while St. David's shares an equal number of partnership board members with for-profit HCA, the partnership protects St. David's charitable, and therefore tax-exempt, mission by the partnership requiring all six hospitals to comply with community benefits standards; by giving St. David's the right to fire the chief executive officer; by giving St. David's the right to name the partnership board chairman; by giving St. David's the right to dissolve the partnership agreement and end the management services contract with HCA. In reversing the trial court judgment, the appellate court said

> If more than an insubstantial amount of the partnership's activities further noncharitable interests, then St. David's can no longer be deemed to operate exclusively for charitable purposes. Therefore, even if St. David's performs important charitable functions, St. David's cannot qualify for tax-exempt status . . . if its activities substantially further the private, profit-seeking interests of HCA.
>
> The appellate court has sent the case back to district court for trial (Taylor, 2003b).

In February of 2004, Illinois authorities revoked the tax-exempt status of a prominent Catholic hospital, Provena Covenant Medical Center, a 270-bed hospital in Urbana. The hospital was ordered to pay $1 million in property taxes, but the hospital plans to appeal. The decision by the Illinois Department of Revenue came after the Champaign County Board of Review had questioned the tax-exempt status of both major not-for-profit hospitals in the area over the last two years. The Board of Review had documented that the hospitals had used aggressive debt-collection tactics, including lawsuits, in order to collect bills from patients. The Board of Review had also documented the fact that Provena had contracted with several for-profit entities to fulfill key hospital functions. The American Hospital Association said that the decision, if extended to other not-for-profit hospitals "could turn the hospital industry upside down. A third of the nation's hospitals are operating in the red [Provena reported a $700,000 loss in 2003]. Suppose that all of a sudden local governments started taxing their [property and] buildings." (Lagnado 2004a).[5]

IRS Challenges to Tax-Exempt Status

In 1987, and in response to public pressure to reduce federal budget deficits, the IRS began auditing tax-exempt organizations, including healthcare organizations. By the end of 1992, the IRS had audited 233 tax-exempt healthcare organizations. Most frequently reported irregularities included inappropriate physician recruiting arrangements and taxable unrelated business income. In 1994, the IRS took action against Herman Hospital in Houston for violating the private inurement provisions that occurred during 1991. To protect the hospital's tax-exempt status, Herman Hospital agreed to pay nearly

$1 million in federal income taxes and penalties in response to IRS allegations that the hospital had offered lucrative physician recruitment and retention incentives including signing bonuses, income guarantees, free office space, malpractice insurance, equipment loans, and loan guarantees (Wang and Wambsganns 1997).

In 1991, the IRS initiated a new audit program for tax-exempt healthcare systems called the coordinated examination program (CEP). Using an interdisciplinary audit team of specialists in corporate restructuring, pensions, payroll taxes, income taxes, and tax-exempt bond financing, CEP audits focus on the system activities as well as each corporation of the system. In 1992, the IRS distributed a new audit guide for tax-exempt hospitals that called for an examination of the following (HFMA 1992):

- *Community benefit standard*: auditors check composition of the governing board, amount of charity care provided, and complaints of patient dumping (i.e., denying or transferring the patients based on inability to pay).
- *Unreasonable compensation and private inurement*: auditors check physician relationships to identify prohibited instances of private benefit, unreasonable compensation, improper disclosure, and inappropriate physician recruiting practices.
- *Financial analysis*: auditors check all affiliated entities to detect presence of prohibited proprietary purposes, inurement, serving of private interests, unrelated business income (i.e., income from business activities that is unrelated to the organization's tax-exempt purposes and therefore must be reported as taxable income), or lobbying activities.
- *Joint ventures*: auditors check joint ventures (a relationship established between two business entities for a specific purpose and point of time, for example, a hospital and radiologist purchasing and operating a computed tomography [CT] scanner together) between the hospital and a physician to determine if the ventures violate prohibitions on private benefit, inurement, or kickbacks (hospitals had until September, 1992, to rescind these relationships without penalty).
- *Independent contractors*: auditors check hospital contracts to determine whether contractors should be treated as contractors or employees for tax purposes.

As of June 30, 2000, the IRS had identified 875 candidates for CEP audits. Of these candidates, the IRS selected 787 based on a 20-point formula that is used to determine when exempt organizations should be audited. The formula includes both objective criteria like the size of the system as measured by gross revenues and total assets as well as subjective criteria like national significance or impact. Multihospital systems accumulate points quickly and therefore are subject to audits early in the audit schedule. The remaining 88 candidates for CEP audits did not meet the selection criteria of the 20-point formula, but were chosen by the IRS due to media coverage, reorganizations, or irregularities with forms filed with the IRS. According to the former director of exempt organizations in the national office of the IRS, the first 63 CEP audits closed resulted in average assessments or settlements of $2.5 million and an average audit length of three years (Kutak Rock 2001). The actions ranged from classifying and taxing unrelated business income to a $100 million tax bill for one unnamed system (Burda 1995). CEP audits resulted in the retroactive revocation of tax-exempt status of LAC facilities in Miami for private inurement to physicians and executives and a $10 million fine against Cape Coral Hospital in Florida for misspending proceeds from tax-exempt bonds (the CFO allegedly used the proceeds to pay off the mortgage on his home) (Greene 1995).

The IRS has intensified its review of tax-exempt organizations and has recently added side deals to its audit guide. To monitor side deals, auditors check the financial transactions, which are often made outside the purview of the organization and are designed to influence the sale of tax-exempt organizations to for-profit organizations (Wang and Wambsganns 1997). In its 1998, 389-page continuing education manual for healthcare organizations, the IRS provides guidance to not-for-profit hospitals. Amplifying their concern about side deals, the IRS published an entire chapter on whole-hospital joint ventures and included 24 questions that IRS agents ask during their examinations. For example, they ask, "Does participation in the joint venture by the exempt entity further its charitable purpose?" (Hallam 1998).

Legislative Challenges to Tax-Exempt Status

At the federal level, significant activity has been related to the tax privileges of tax-exempt organizations, but very little actual legislation has been effected. Representative Charles B. Rangel (D-NY), chairman of the House Ways and Means Committee's panel on select revenue measures, has held hearings on tax-exempt status and has voiced concerns that existing law regarding tax-exempt status is too lenient and too difficult to enforce. Representative Brian Donnelly (D-MA) has led legislative efforts to require tax-exempt hospitals to provide specific levels of charity care. In President Clinton's health reform bill, tax-exempt healthcare organizations were required to assess the health needs of the community on an annual basis and develop plans to meet those needs. But to date, the ideas proposed by Rangel, Donnelly, Clinton, and others have not been passed into law by Congress (Blankenau 1994).

The Taxpayer Bill of Rights II, which indirectly addresses tax-exempt issues, was signed into law on July 30, 1996. The act provides the IRS with intermediate sanctions prior to revoking an organization's tax-exempt status. The act also (Wang and Wambsganns 1997)

- Requires tax-exempt organizations to disclose excess benefit transactions (i.e., unreasonable compensation or any other transaction in which payment or benefit exceeds the value of the transaction) and excise taxes paid for such transactions on Form 990, which requires all not-for-profit organizations to substantiate their tax-exempt status;
- Expands public access to Form 990; and
- Subjects executives responsible for an excess benefit transaction, rather than the organization, to a 10-percent tax on the amount of excess benefit if corrected and reported, and a 200-percent tax on the amount of excess benefit if executives fail to correct a transaction in which they personally benefited (liability for uncorrected excess benefit transactions that include personal benefit may also extend to members of the governing board).

The IRS is considering obtaining additional information on Form 990 including information on

- Fund-raising expenses;
- Corporate responsibility practices; and
- Grants to foreign organizations. (IRS 2003).

At the state level, there has also been significant activity related to the tax privileges of tax-exempt organizations, and nine states have passed legislation that challenges, or at least defines more narrowly, tax-exempt status (Thompson Powers 1999).[6] As discussed earlier, the governor-appointed Texas Health Policy Task Force made policy recommendations regarding tax-exempt hospitals to the Texas Legislature in 1993. Later that same year, the legislature passed Texas Senate Bill 427. The purpose of the law was to establish the legal duty of not-for-profit hospitals to provide a certain amount for community benefits to retain their tax-exempt status. Community benefits included only charity care (i.e., unreimbursed costs of providing healthcare to the financially or medically indigent) and government-sponsored indigent care (i.e., unreimbursed costs of providing healthcare to patients whose eligibility was based on financial need—typically Medicaid patients). Under the law, not-for-profit hospital governing boards must develop a mission statement and community benefits plan for serving the community's healthcare needs. The plan must be based on a community-wide needs assessment and contain mechanisms for measuring the plan's effectiveness, including measurable objectives and a budget. The budget must include an amount for community benefits at least equal to one of the following:

- 4 percent of the hospital's net revenue;
- 100 percent of the hospital's state and local tax exemptions; or
- An amount that is reasonable in relation to community needs, available resources, and the hospital's state and local tax-exemptions.

The Texas Hospital Association (THA) provided member hospitals with an economic analysis of the bill before the bill was passed in 1993. In the aggregate, the analysis indicated that Texas not-for-profit hospitals were providing community benefits, as defined in the law, in excess of the required levels. For instance, in 1991 Texas not-for-profit hospitals provided community benefits valued at $367.6 million, after adjusting for charity care patients that had been classified as bad debt, while 4 percent of the hospitals' net patient service revenue requirement was $251.7 million and 100 percent of the hospitals' state and local tax-exemption requirement was $316.8 million. Although in the aggregate Texas not-for-profit hospitals appeared to be meeting the community benefit requirements of the new law, the THA warned member hospitals that individual hospitals might vary significantly and encouraged member hospitals to evaluate the options in relation to their own situation (Bailey 1993).

Individual organizations throughout the country would also do well to keep abreast of new developments as the tax status of healthcare organizations continues to be discussed at the state and federal levels.

Notes

1. For an informative history of the for-profit healthcare industry, see Columbia/HCA: *Healthcare on Overdrive*, by Lutz and Gee (1998).
2. Research exists that disputes the findings in the Herzlinger and Krasker study "Who Profits from the Nonprofits?" published in the Harvard Business Review in 1987. Arrington and Haddock published "Who Really Profits from Not-For-Profits" in *Health Services Research* in 1990. Using discriminant analysis on a larger data set over the same time period as the Herzlinger and Krasker study, Arrington and Haddock found that not-for-profit hospitals "appear more likely to be accessible to the uninsured and medically indigent than are the for-profits" and that "for-profit hospitals do not offer a scope of services—particularly community-oriented services—equivalent to that provided by not-for-profits" (p. 303).
3. Other court cases involve the appropriateness of tax-exempt status: *Fairview Haven v. Illinois Department of Revenue*, 506 N.E.2d 341 (1987), *Highland Park Hospital v. Illinois Department of Revenue*, 506 N.E.2d 1331 (Ill.App.Ct.1987), *Lutheran Home at Topton v. Board of Assessment*, 515 A.2d 59 (Pa. Commw.Ct.1986), and *School District v. Hamot Medical Center*, 602 A.2d 407 (1992).
4. PILOTs are common among universities and hospitals, both of which tend to be the largest owners of tax-exempt property in most jurisdictions. PILOTs are made to partially compensate the taxing authority for the loss of revenue on tax-exempt property. PILOTs may have started in 1929 when Harvard University agreed to pay the city of Cambridge. Harvard

continues to pay Cambridge about $1.1 million on $71 million worth of tax-exempt property.

5. In a related issue, in early 2004 HHS criticized the hospital industry for providing inadequate care to uninsured patients. The criticism was in response to a letter sent to HHS by the American Hospital Association that complained that federal policy prohibited hospitals from reducing prices to the uninsured and that federal rules required "aggressive efforts to collect from all patients" which would include the uninsured. HHS argued that hospitals had mischaracterized government policy and hospitals were simply "not correct" in arguing that complex federal rules left them no choice but to bill the uninsured full price, which is far more than most payers pay, including Medicare (Lagnado 2004b).

6. Of the nine states passing legislation, six states have passed mandatory community-benefit legislation: California, Georgia, Indiana, New York, Pennsylvania, and Texas; three states have passed voluntary community-benefit legislation: Massachusetts, Missouri, and Oregon.

References

Arrington, B., and C. C. Haddock. 1990. "Who Really Profits from Nonprofits?" *Health Services Research* 25 (2): 291–304.

Bailey, C. W. 1993. Texas Hospital Association Correspondence to Member Hospitals, August 19.

Bellandi, D. 2001. "IHC Must Show It's Tax-Exempt." *Modern Healthcare* 31 (20): 16.

Berman, H. J., S. F. Kukla, and L. E. Weeks. 1994. *The Financial Management of Hospitals, 8th ed.* Chicago: Health Administration Press.

Blankenau, R. 1994. "Measuring Up: Congress Reconsiders Tax-Exemption Standards Under Reform." *Hospitals & Health Networks* 68 (1): 14.

Bromberg, M. 1983. "The Medical-Industrial Complex: Our National Defense." *New England Journal of Medicine* 309: 1314–16.

Burda, D. 1995. "Justice Department Seeks IRS Referral Link." *Modern Healthcare* 25 (18): 16.

Government Accounting Office. 1992. "GAO Report on Non-Profit Hospitals." Washington, DC: Government Printing Office.

Gray, B. H. 1986. *For-Profit Enterprise in Health Care.* Washington, DC: National Academy Press.

Greene, J. 1995. "IRS Fines Cape Coral $10 Million." *Modern Healthcare* 25 (35): 3.

Hallam, K. 1998. "The IRS's List of No-Nos." *Modern Healthcare* 28 (33): 15.

Healthcare Financial Management Association. 1992. "UPDATA." *Healthcare Financial Management* 46 (6): 6.

Herzlinger, R., and W. Krasker. 1987. "Who Profits from Nonprofits?" *Harvard Business Review* 65 (1): 93–105.

Internal Revenue Service. 2003. [Online retrieval, 12/26/03]. http://www.irs.gov/ind_info/bullet.html.

Kuchler, J. A. 1992. "Tax-Exempt Yardstick: Defining the Measurements." *Healthcare Financial Management* 46 (2): 21–31.

Kutak Rock LLP. 2001. "IRS Coordinated Examination Program Update." [Online retrieval, 02/22/01]. http://www.kutakrock.com/Index/Memorand/body_irs_coordinated_examination_pr.html.

Lagnado, L. 2004a. "Hospital Found 'Not Charitable' Loses Its Status as Tax Exempt." *Wall Street Journal*, February 10, B1 and B7.

———. 2004b. "HHS Chief Scolds Hospitals for Their Treatment of Uninsured." *Wall Street Journal*, February 20, A1–2.

Lutz, S., and E. P. Gee. 1998. *Columbia/HCA: Healthcare on Overdrive*. New York: McGraw-Hill.

Morrisey, M. A., G. J. Wedig, and M. Hassan. 1996. "Do Nonprofit Hospitals Pay Their Way?" *Health Affairs* 15 (4): 132–144.

Piotrowski, J. 2003. "Yale–New Haven Sued." *Modern Healthcare* 33 (8): 16.

Relman, A. S. 1980. "The New Medical-Industrial Complex." *New England Journal of Medicine* 303: 963–70.

Sloan, F. A., J. Valvona, and R. Mullner. 1986. "Identifying the Issues: A Statistical Profile." In *Uncompensated Hospital Care: Rights and Responsibilities*, edited by Sloan, Blumstein, and Perrin. Baltimore, MD: Johns Hopkins University Press.

Board of Equalization of Utah County v. Intermountain Health Care. 1985. 709 P.2d 265.

Taylor, M. 2003a. "Exemption Denied." *Modern Healthcare* 33 (50): 16.

———. 2003b. "Partnerships Get Scrutiny." *Modern Healthcare* 33 (46): 8–9.

———. 2001a. "A Taxing Debate: City's Bid to Force Hospital to Pay Up Resurrects Exemption Issue." *Modern Healthcare* 31 (7): 41.

———. 2001b. "End to Legal Odyssey." Modern Healthcare 31 (20): 16.

Thompson Powers LLC. 1999. *The Politics of Exemption: Tax Revenue vs. Community Benefit—Not-for-Profit Hospitals Under Pressure*. Irving, TX: VHA Inc.

U.S. News and World Report. 1995. "Tax Exempt!" *U.S. News and World Report* October 2, 37–38.

Utah State Tax Commission. 1990. *Non-Profit Hospital and Nursing Home Charitable Property Tax Exemption Standard*. Salt Lake City: Utah State Tax Commission.

Wang, T., and J. R. Wambsganns. 1997. "Is Your Organization's Tax-Exempt Status at Risk?" *1997 HFM Resource Guide*. Chicago: Healthcare Financial Management Association.

Witek, J. E., D. L. Milligan, and J. B. Ryan. 1993. "Managing Charitable Purpose: Issues and Answers." Presented at the American College of Healthcare Executives Annual Administrative Congress on Healthcare Management, Chicago, 4 March.

Recommended Readings — Part I

Brigham, E. F. 1992. "Analysis of Financial Statements." *Fundamentals of Financial Management, 6th ed.* New York: Dryden Press.

Cleverly, W. O. 1997. *Essentials of Health Care Finance, 4th ed.* Gaithersburg, MD: Aspen Publishers.

Eastaugh, S. R. 2004. *Health Care Finance and Economics.* Sudbury, MA: Jones and Bartlett Publishers.

Gapenski, L. C. 2003. *Understanding Healthcare Financial Management, 4th ed.* Chicago: Health Administration Press.

Gray, B. H. (ed.) 1983. *The New Health Care for Profit: Doctors and Hospitals in a Competitive Environment.* Washington, DC: National Academy Press.

Griffith, J. R. 1993. *The Moral Challenges of Health Care Management.* Chicago: Health Administration Press.

Hankins, R. W., and J. J. Baker. 2004. *Management Accounting for Healthcare Organizations.* Sudbury, MA: Jones and Bartlett Publishers.

Herzlinger, R. E., and D. Nitterhouse. 1994. *Financial Accounting and Managerial Control for Nonprofit Organizations.* Cincinnati, OH: South-Western Publishing.

Lutz, S., and E. P. Gee. 1998. *Columbia/HCA: Healthcare on Overdrive.* New York: McGraw-Hill.

McLean, R. A. 2003. *Financial Management in Health Care Organizations, 2nd ed..* New York: Thomson Delmar Learning.

Person, M. M. 1997. *The Zero-Base Hospital: Survival and Success in America's Healthcare System.* Chicago: Health Administration Press.

Prince, T. R. 1992. *Financial Reporting and Cost Control for Health Care Entities.* Chicago: Health Administration Press.

Purtilo, R. 1993. *Ethical Dimensions in the Health Professions, 2nd ed.* Philadelphia: W. B. Saunders.

Southby, R. M. F., and W. Greenberg. 1984. *The For-Profit Hospital: Access, Quality, Teaching, Research.* Columbus, OH: Batelle Press.

Starr, P. 1982. The Social Transformation of American Medicine. New York: Basic Books.

Stevens, R. 1989. *In Sickness and in Wealth: American Hospitals in the Twentieth Century.* New York: Basic Books.

Suver, J. D., B. R. Neumann, and K. E. Boles. 1992. *Management Accounting for Healthcare Organizations, 3rd ed.* Chicago: Pluribus Press/HFMA.

Thompson Powers LLC. 1999. *The Politics of Exemption: Tax Revenue vs. Community Benefit—Not-for-profit Hospitals Under Pressure.* Irving, TX: VHA, Inc.

Zelman, W. A. 1996. *The Changing Health Care Marketplace: Private Ventures, Public Interests.* San Francisco: Jossey-Bass Publishers.

Zelman, W. N., M. J. McCue, and A. R. Millikan. 1998. "Health Care Financial Statements." *Financial Management of Health Care Organizations.* Malden, MA: Blackwell Publishers.

OPERATING REVENUE

4

THIRD-PARTY PAYMENT

Third-party payers are agents of patients who contract with providers (the second party) to pay all or a part of the bill to the patient (the first party), and have had an important affect on healthcare organizations over the last 70 years. As mentioned in Chapter 1 and illustrated in Figure 4.1, third-party payment, including payments from the federal government, private insurance, and state and local government, represented 81.3 percent of total personal healthcare expenditures in 2002.

History of Third-Party Payment

Third-party payment started in the 1920s, but not without significant opposition. Although labor unions supported compulsory health insurance for their members as early as 1915, their efforts failed as a result of opposition by the American Medical Association (AMA) and the antisocialist mood of the country during and after World War I. Physicians were wary of approving a payment system that would change the second-party payment system already in place (see Figure 4.2).

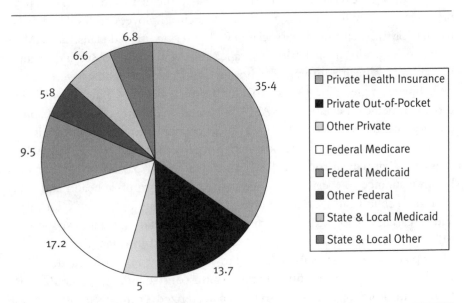

FIGURE 4.1
Percentage of Total Personal Healthcare Expenditures in the United States by Source of Funds, 2002

Legend:
- Private Health Insurance
- Private Out-of-Pocket
- Other Private
- Federal Medicare
- Federal Medicaid
- Other Federal
- State & Local Medicaid
- State & Local Other

Values: 6.8, 6.6, 5.8, 9.5, 17.2, 5, 13.7, 35.4

Source: Levit, K., C. Smith, C. Cowan, A. Sensenig, and A. Catlin. 2004. "Health Spending Rebound Continues in 2002." *Health Affairs* 23 (1): 147–159.

FIGURE 4.2
Second-Party
Payment

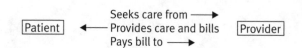

The second-party payment system was economically efficient in that patients sought only the amount and quality of care they could afford. However, the second-party payment system created ethical concerns because some patients who needed care could not afford care, and it prompted some employers to begin paying providers directly for the care received by their employees. The second-party system also created bad debt concerns because some patients sought emergency care and could not afford to pay the bill after the care was provided. This concern prompted Baylor University Hospital in Dallas to offer school teachers prepaid hospital care for $6 per year. Prior to this arrangement, teachers would deliver their babies in the emergency room and would be unable to pay the resulting hospital bills. In the next few years, several other hospitals offered similar arrangements to remain competitive with the Baylor plan, which later became the first Blue Cross plan. In 1933, Dr. Sidney Garfield began providing prepaid medical care to employees who worked on the California aqueduct system, and in 1938 he provided prepaid medical care to workers on the Grand Coulee Dam. Garfield's plan was later called the Kaiser-Permanente health plan (Henry J. Kaiser was the employer who contracted with Dr. Garfield) (Starr 1982).

The Depression in the 1930s made it difficult for employers to pay providers directly for the care received by their employees and for hospitals like Baylor to accept the risk associated with offering prepaid plans. The AMA softened its position on health insurance during the mid-1930s by accepting voluntary health insurance if hospital and medical benefits were separate. For example, Blue Cross provided hospital benefits, Blue Shield later provided medical benefits. The AMA remained adamantly opposed to compulsory health insurance and helped defeat proposals to include compulsory health insurance in President Roosevelt's Social Security Act in 1935. In 1945, President Truman introduced his health plan that if passed would provide health insurance to every citizen; increase funding for public health and maternal and child health services; initiate federal funding for medical education and research; and provide significant funding to build new, and expand existing, hospitals. In 1946, President Truman signed into law the only part of his plan that Congress passed: the Hospital Survey and Construction Act, which provided significant funding for hospital construction. The Republicans took control of Congress in 1946 and characterized Truman's health plan as socialized medicine, or publicly funded health benefits. Even with President Truman's surprising reelection in 1948, antisocialist sentiment and strong lobbying by the AMA prevented President Truman's plan from becoming reality (Starr 1982; Hepner and Hepner 1973).

Direct Service Plans

The defeat of compulsory health insurance in 1935 under President Roosevelt and again in the late 1940s under President Truman meant that health insurance in America would be largely voluntary and private. The early plans by Baylor University Hospital and Henry J. Kaiser were called direct service plans (employers prepaid specific hospitals and physicians to provide care to their employees) and were characteristic of most health insurance plans through the 1940s. Direct service plans were really an extension of second-party payment in that the employer prepaid the provider on behalf of the employee (see Figure 4.3).

In the mid-1940s plans called "commercial indemnity plans" allowed employers and/or employees to prepay to an insurance company that would reimburse a hospital or physician of the employee's choosing. These plans initiated the concept of the third party in that the insurance company was relatively independent from both the employer/employee and the provider (see Figure 4.4).

Between 1945 and 1949, group commercial indemnity plans increased from 7.8 million subscribers to 17.7 million subscribers, and individual commercial indemnity plans increased to 14.7 million subscribers. By 1953, commercial insurance plans, which were for-profit, provided coverage to 29 percent of Americans. Blue Cross, which was a not-for-profit plan, provided coverage to 27 percent of Americans. Through the 1950s, use of commercial indemnity plans grew steadily, often at the expense of the less aggressive Blue Cross plans.

Blue Cross typically set premiums using community rating (i.e., groups paid essentially the same premium, resulting in low-risk groups subsidizing

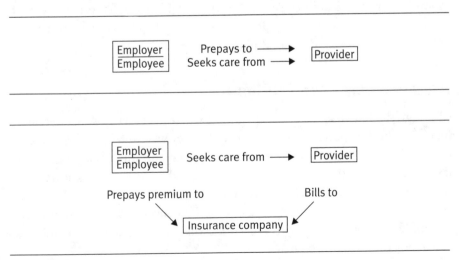

FIGURE 4.3
Direct Service Plans

FIGURE 4.4
Commercial Indemnity Plans

high-risk groups). Commercial insurance companies like Prudential and Metropolitan, which had had significant histories in life insurance, set premiums using experience rating (i.e., groups paid different premiums based on their risk). Commercial insurance companies often solicited low-risk Blue Cross groups by offering lower premiums.

By the late 1950s, 66 percent of Americans had some form of health insurance that was usually provided by the employer (Starr 1982). Part of this increase is attributable to the federal government's tax policies that allowed employers to deduct the cost of health benefits to employees. Medicare and Medicaid were introduced in 1966 (Medicare and Medicaid are discussed in more detail in Chapter 5); the percentage of covered Americans subsequently increased to 87 percent by 1968 (Harris 1975). Changes in federal Employee Retirement Income Security Act (ERISA) laws during the early 1980s allowed large employers to self-insure and gain the full benefit of any reductions in costs. Some of these reductions in costs were actually a transfer of costs to employees.[1] With the Deficit Reduction Act of 1984, the federal government began limiting the amounts employers could deduct for health benefits. As a result, the out-of-pocket costs to the patient grew, and the percentage of Americans covered by some form of health insurance dropped to its 2002 level of 85 percent.

While 85 percent of the total population has been insured with at least some health insurance coverage since 1995, there has been a significant decrease in the percent of nonelderly insured, offset by a significant increase in the percent of elderly insured as the country ages and more people become eligible for Medicare. The number of nonelderly people with health insurance decreased by 1.4 million in 2001 and 2.4 million in 2002—the largest single decrease in ten years. All of the decrease occurred among adults; children with health insurance actually increased slightly during 2002. The reason for the decrease among adults is attributed to decreases in the number of adults covered by employer-sponsored insurance. Decreases in the rates of employer-sponsored insurance are believed to be attributable to shifts in employment from large firms to small firms or self-employment and to the rising cost of healthcare (Holahan and Wang 2004).

Managed Care Organizations

Although the Baylor and Kaiser experiences with direct service plans were limited in the healthcare services they delivered, they were the first managed care organizations. Managed care organizations are organizations that manage the cost of healthcare, the quality of healthcare, and the access to healthcare. One way to classify managed care organizations is with Wagner's continuum (see Figure 4.5) (Wagner 1996). At one end of the continuum is the commercial indemnity plan, which requires precertification of elective admissions and case management of catastrophic illnesses.

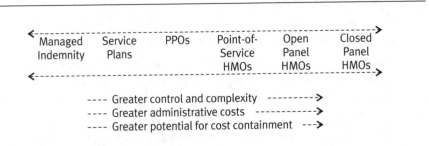

FIGURE 4.5
Managed Care
Continuum

Source: Adapted from Wagner, E. R. 1996. "Types of Managed Care Organizations." In *The Managed Health Care Handbook 3rd. ed.*, edited by P. R. Kongstvedt, p 33–45. Gaithersburg, MD: Aspen Publishers.

Service plans, like the typical Blue Cross plans, add contractual relationships with providers that often include maximum fee schedules and prohibitions on balance billing (i.e., providers cannot bill the patient for amounts over the fee schedules agreed to with the service plan). Preferred provider organizations (PPOs), are organizations that provide discounted provider services to insurance carriers and employers.

Providers usually agree to discount their prices in exchange for large volumes of patients. Health maintenance organizations (HMOs) are organizations that integrate the financing and delivery of healthcare into one organization (see Figure 4.6). Financial risk, and opportunity, shifts from the employer/employee under the commercial indemnity plans (i.e., the employer/employee pays for inappropriate use through increased premiums) to the HMOs (i.e., under prepayment, the HMO assumes the financial risk, and opportunity, for inappropriate use).

While most would agree that managed care reduced the rate of increase of healthcare costs, management care is not without its critics. Aggressive utilization review, including the requirement of pretreatment authorization practiced by most managed care organizations, is often criticized. In response to the criticisms, UnitedHealth Group, which insured 14.5 million people in 1999, found that medical reviews of physicians' treatments resulted in higher costs for the insurer. In December 1999, UnitedHealth decided to let their physicians have the final authority on medical treatments for their patients, even in cases where UnitedHealth might consider the medical treatments unnecessary. UnitedHealth found that they were spending over $100 million per year reviewing the physicians' orders and expected the new policy to save them over $25 million per year. While UnitedHealth physicians still must

FIGURE 4.6
Health
Maintenance
Organizations

notify UnitedHealth if they admit their patients, order home healthcare, or order expensive equipment, the final decision on medical necessity still rests with the patient's physician (HFMA 1998). Apparently this radical departure from convention has had little impact on UnitedHealth's bottom line. At the end of 2002, UnitedHealth reported 18 straight quarters of double-digit profit increases. UnitedHealth projected a 19 percent profit increase for 2003 (Rauber 2003a).

In response to a growing anti–managed care sentiment and in the face of possible legislation designed to hold managed care companies legally accountable for directly managing care through preadmission authorizations and utilization review, managed care companies like UnitedHealth are pursuing new methods to finance/deliver improved healthcare while holding down costs. One method is evidence-based case management where managed care companies partner with providers to determine the best, and thereby the most efficient, way to manage a case based on current evidence. For instance, Anthem Blue Cross and Blue Shield's Midwest Hospital Quality Program has been in effect for 11 years at more than 330 hospitals in Indiana, Ohio, and Kentucky. After Anthem collaborated with physicians and hospitals, the collaboration resulted in several targets being established: one was to increase the use of ACE inhibitors for health plan members diagnosed with congestive heart failure to 60 percent. In Indiana hospitals from 1998 to 2001, the use of ACE inhibitors increased from 52 percent to 60 percent. Hospitals and physicians who met the targets were reimbursed more than hospitals and physicians who do not meet the targets (Nowicki 2003).

Another method designed to give health plan members choices in coverage that also seems to save money is the move towards consumer-driven plans. As the cost of healthcare continues to rise, employers are passing more of the cost to their employees or not providing healthcare at all (about 37 percent of all employers and about 50 percent of small employers no longer offer health coverage). This economic phenomenon occurs at the same time as a demographic phenomenon—a large portion of the population, the baby boomers, are in their 50s and beginning to need and demand more healthcare. Baby boomers are used to getting what they want and should have large amounts of discretionary income to pay for what they want. Consumer-driven health plans allow the consumer to select the coverage they need or want, much like selecting the options on a car, and then the health plan costs out the coverage and converts the cost to a premium (Millenson 2003).

Humana, one of the nation's largest health plans, may have been the first to try a consumer-driven plan with its own employees. Humana's CEO Michael McCallister said "I'm a big believer that the most powerful player in understanding and managing costs is going to be the individual consumer. When people are spending their own money, given good and actionable information, they're going to do much better at controlling costs than the current model" (Rauber 2003b). From July, 2001, when Humana replaced its traditional coverage with consumer-driven coverage for its Louisville-area employees and their dependents, through June, 2002, Humana saved more than $2 million from its anticipated health benefits' costs. That included $1.4 million in savings attributable to changes in consumer behavior (switching to generic drugs or scheduling fewer doctor's visits); $400,000 attributable to a direct cost shift to employees through higher premiums, deductibles, and copays; and $200,000 attributable to the elimination of duplicated coverage between spouses. Originally, only about six percent of the employees selected the most "hard core" consumer-driven plan which included high deductibles and co-pays in exchange for much lower premiums. More recently, 18 percent of the employees selected the "hard core" plan, leading Humana officials to believe that the "hard core" plan is becoming more popular (Rauber 2003b).

HMOs

To manage increased risk, HMOs contain costs with aggressive methods of controlling use that include carefully selecting subscribers and providers, providing physician incentives, and providing subscriber/employer incentives. Eastaugh (1992) reported that HMOs used 37 percent fewer hospital days (341 days per 1,000 enrolled) for their nonelderly enrolled populations than commercial indemnity plans, which used 542 days per 1,000 enrolled. By 1995, some HMOs in California, a state that has had significant HMO market penetration for several years, reported 170 hospital-days per 1,000 enrolled (Robinson and Casalino 1995). Shortell and Hull (1996) reported that significant evidence exists that HMOs reduce the use of specialists and high-cost tests and procedures.

Because of their ability to control costs, HMOs have been attractive to employers that provide insurance coverage for their employees. As a result, HMOs have experienced growth since the passage of the HMO Act of 1973, which provided grant money to develop HMOs and required employers with 25 or more employees who already offered commercial indemnity insurance to also offer HMO coverage if an HMO plan was available. Rapid growth for HMOs occurred during the late 1980s and early 1990s as employers sought ways to reduce the healthcare costs for their employees. Group Health Association of America reported that 56 million people were enrolled in HMOs in 1995, compared to less than five million people that were enrolled in an HMO in 1973.

Historically HMOs have been classified based on the degree of control they have over their physician providers. Point-of-service plans (POSs) are HMOs that exert minimum to no control over their physician providers because they allow enrollees to seek care from providers not on contract with the HMO (i.e., out-of-network). Although the HMO reimburses the provider's fees, the HMO usually requires the enrollee to pay out-of-network providers larger deductibles and coinsurance, as well as higher premiums to the HMO, for the privilege of going out-of-network.

Enrollees have criticized HMOs for lack of choice, or lack of freedom of choice, in choosing physician providers, therefore, POSs have been a popular option for HMOs. Gabel (1994) reported that HMOs offering a POS option grew from less than 20 percent of HMO plans in 1990 to almost 60 percent in 1993. Zelman (1996) reported that by mid-1995, POS plans had approximately 20 million enrollees. Although growth of POS plans has been substantial, future growth is questionable as enrollees find that their needs are met by network physicians and reduce their reliance on out-of-network physicians. Gabel found that only about 16 percent of enrollees in the POS plans used the out-of-network option.

Open Panel HMOs   Open panel HMOs are HMOs that exert moderate control over physician providers; they contract with physicians to provide care for enrollees in the physicians' offices. Open panel HMOs include the direct contract model and the independent practice association (IPA) model. Direct contract HMOs contract with individual physicians to provide care, and IPAs contract with associations of physicians. Member physicians are not employees of the association. IPAs may be previously existing associations of physicians that contract with multiple HMOs, or the HMO may organize the association to provide physician services. In either model, as well as in the direct contract model, physicians see their own patients and HMO patients. The open panel HMO reimburses the physicians either on a fee-for-service basis, often with a discount, or by capitation (Wagner 1996).

Closed Panel HMOs   Closed panel HMOs are HMOs that exert maximum control over physician providers because the HMO contracts with or employs physicians to provide care for enrollees on an exclusive basis. Closed panel HMOs include the group model and the staff model. Group model HMOs contract with a multispecialty group of physicians to provide all physician care to enrollees, typically on capitation. In the group model HMO, physicians are employed by the group, not the HMO. Staff model HMOs employ individual physicians to provide all physician care to enrollees; primary care physicians are always employed, and some specialty and subspecialty physicians may actually be on contract. Closed panel HMOs provide incentive payments to physician providers based on performance (Wagner 1996).

Network HMOs   Network HMOs exert moderate to maximum control over physician providers because they contract with physician groups to provide care for enrollees. Network HMOs may be either open panel or closed panel. Typically, the network HMO relies on groups of primary care physicians and reimburses the groups on capitation. The primary care groups are often responsible for referring and reimbursing referrals to specialty physicians (Wagner 1996).

Post-Managed Care

When the managed care industry had a tough few years in the late 1990s with declining enrollments, poor public relations, and threatened anti–managed care legislation, many were predicting managed care's demise (Clarke 2000). The managed care industry adjusted with a "softer image" and more popular methods of controlling costs. Managed care continues to be a reliable method for payers including employers and the government to control healthcare costs. Managed care is also a cornerstone of President Bush's attempt to reform the Medicare program. However, employers and the government will continue to seek new ways to control costs like defined contribution plans and direct contracting.

Defined-Contribution Plans

Employers, faced with the reality that employees who face no personal economic consequences regarding healthcare spending will want, not necessarily need, more healthcare and higher quality healthcare, are turning from defined-benefit plans to defined-contribution plans. Under defined-benefit plans, the employee receives a defined benefit package and the employer/employee pays the premium which is adjusted each year based on experience. Employers have absorbed large, unpredictable premium increases for several years under these plans. Under defined-contribution plans, employees typically choose from a variety of healthcare options, with a specified amount of the premium paid for by the employer. Any healthcare costs above this amount are paid for by the employee. Defined-contribution plans shift more of the financial responsibility to the employee who will become more utilization and price conscious as a result. Employees will request more information about providers to evaluate more closely the benefit and risk associated with different treatment options before the employees agree to be treated. Defined-contribution plans put more pressure on providers of health services to be more price- and quality-competitive while at the same time more receptive to the idea of providing patients with information about treatment risks and options (Emery 2001).

Direct Contracting

As employers continue to seek strategies to reduce healthcare costs and as providers continue to consolidate resources in reaction to market forces, the answer may well be direct contracting, or large employers contracting directly with integrated delivery systems,[2] or systems of healthcare providers capable of accepting a financial risk and delivering a full range of healthcare services. Realizing that by transferring financial risk to HMOs, they have also transferred financial opportunity, many large employers or coalitions of smaller employers have decided to resume the financial risk and opportunity by self-insuring and then contracting directly with an integrated delivery system. Because the federal Employee Retirement Income Security Act of 1974 (ERISA) regulates direct contracting arrangements by large, self-insured employers, the employers are exempt from state insurance regulation and therefore avoid the associated costs that HMOs incur. Direct contracting also stimulates competition between integrated delivery systems and encourages local control and innovation. It also reduces administrative costs, which in turn reduces employer health plan costs (Burrows and Moravec 1997).

In 1996, Motorola hired an outside company to create a network of providers that included over 118,000 physicians by the end of 2000. Since Motorola, rather than the insurer, was in charge of credentialing, it set higher standards for physician participation than the standards set by previous health plans that had contracted with Motorola. Motorola estimated that every dollar it spent on its network saved $3 to $9 on medical care. Motorola's healthcare costs rose less than 5 percent per year since 1996 and Motorola projected no increase in healthcare costs for 2001. More than 70 percent of Motorola's 70,000 employees chose the company's plan over other options with an overall satisfaction rating of above 95 percent. In 1999, General Motors hired a pharmacist to track prescription drugs taken most by employees. The pharmacist used the information to negotiate discounts from drugmakers. In 1994, Safeway, Chevron, Bechtel, and other large San Francisco area companies used Pacific Business Group on Health to negotiate directly with providers for discounts to their 400,000 employees (Cohn, Eliopoulos, and Weintraub 2000).

Many healthcare organizations are positioning themselves for life after managed care. According to Zelman (1996), healthcare organizations are pursuing two major goals: access to and control over premium dollars, especially capitated premium dollars; and reorganizing to function as, or be a part of, an integrated delivery system. Zelman identifies the following strategies healthcare organizations are developing to accomplish these goals:

- Increase market power by making an organization and its affiliates more indispensable and influential;
- Expand the capacity of the organization to enable it to do what it could not do before, including expanding products and services and geographic markets;
- Increase capacity to accept capitated contracts;
- Improve administrative performance;
- Increase organizational efficiency;
- Generate economies of scale;
- Reduce duplicative costs;
- Improve information systems necessary to coordinate and integrate new, larger, and more complex systems, and to assist in integration;
- Secure access to capital; and
- Improve clinical performance and ability to compete on quality of care.

According to Zelman, functioning as or being a part of an integrated delivery system requires the following core elements:

- A certain level of clinical, not just administrative or financial, coordination among providers in a full continuum of care;
- A focus on the performance of the system as a whole, especially by the primary care physicians;
- Achievement of some level of physician integration or commitment of the physicians to the system, especially by the primary care physicians;
- System emphasis on prevention and primary care;
- Achievement of geographic and service breadth;
- Development of a sophisticated information system; and
- Capacity to identify, improve, and compete on quality.

The level of clinical coordination among physicians explains the rapid growth of physician-hospital organizations (PHOs), or joint ventures between hospitals and groups of physicians. In 1995, the Physician Payment Review Commission reported that 85 percent of all hospitals either had established a PHO or were in the process of establishing a PHO.

Methods of Payment

Third parties and patients use a variety of methods to pay providers for healthcare services. Methods of payment to healthcare organizations and other providers can be classified according to the amount of financial risk assumed by the healthcare organization.

Charges

Every healthcare organization has a list of charges (also called prices or rates) for care provided to patients. The organization may set charges based on the care provided; several other methods of setting charges are discussed in Chapter 7. If the healthcare organization sets charges correctly, and if the third party or patient pays the charges, the organization assumes no financial risk by accepting this method of payment. When patients responsible for their own bill do not pay and become a financial risk as a bad debt, it is assumed that the bad debt would result regardless of the method of payment. From the perspective of the third-party payer or patient, using set charges as the method of payment provides no financial incentive for the healthcare organization to provide only what is medically appropriate.

Charges Minus a Discount

Healthcare organizations offer discounted charges to third parties for several reasons, including as a return for large volumes of patients from a provider or to remain competitive with other organizations. If the healthcare organization does not discount its charges below its costs, the organization assumes very little financial risk accepting this method of payment. From the third-party payer's or patient's perspective, charges minus a discount as a method of payment provides no financial incentive for the healthcare organization to provide only what is medically appropriate.

Cost Plus a Percentage for Growth

Healthcare organizations receive the cost for care provided to the patients of third-party payers, plus a small percentage that allows the organization to develop new services and products. Typically, the healthcare organization bills charges to the third party, which reimburses the organization the projected cost, often expressed as a percentage of the charges. At the end of the year, the third party audits the healthcare organization to determine actual cost, and adjusts accordingly what it has reimbursed to the organization. Because the third party determines the final reimbursement after the organization delivers the care to the patient, this method of reimbursement is retrospective and therefore inflationary, because no incentive exists for the healthcare organization to contain costs. If the third party recognizes and approves the costs of the organization, the organization assumes very little financial risk accepting this method of payment.

Cost

Healthcare organizations receive the cost for care provided to the patients of third-party payers. Typically, the healthcare organization bills charges to the third party which reimburses the organization the projected cost, often expressed as a percentage of the charge. At the end of the year, the third party audits the healthcare organization to determine actual cost, and adjusts accordingly what it has reimbursed to the organization. The third party determines the final reimbursement after the organization delivers the care to the patient. This method of reimbursement is retrospective and therefore inflationary because little incentive exists for the healthcare organization to contain costs. If the third party recognizes and approves the costs of the organization, the organization assumes very little financial risk by accepting this method of payment. However, many third-party payers do not recognize the full costs incurred by healthcare organizations. As a result, the organization assumes financial risk for the patient and must pass on losses to other third parties and patients who pay more than cost (usually those paying charges and discounts from charges).

Per Diem

Healthcare organizations receive a per day reimbursement for care provided to the patients of third-party payers. Because the third-party payer sets the per diem rate prospectively, or prior to the provision of care, per diem as a method of payment provides both financial risks and financial incentives to the healthcare organization. In the event that the organization provides care for a cost greater than the per diem rate, the organization incurs a loss. In the event that the organization provides care for a cost less than the per diem rate, the organization realizes a profit. However, if the third-party payer does not monitor length of stays, the healthcare organization can extend length of stays to recover excessive per diem costs. Because per diem rates are generally the same for each day of a length of stay, this method of reimbursement assumes that costs are the same for each day of a length of stay. This assumption is true for many extended care organizations, but not for acute care organizations in which the patient incurs a greater proportion of the costs during the early days of the admission because of diagnostic testing.

Per Diagnosis

Healthcare organizations receive a per diagnosis reimbursement for care provided to the patients of third-party payers. Also prospective in nature, per diagnosis provides financial risks and financial incentives for the healthcare organization to control costs in a manner similar to per diem as a method of payment. However, organizations cannot extend length of stays to recover excessive per day costs. As a method of payment, per diagnosis adjusts for variable per day costs by reimbursing the diagnosis instead of the day.

Capitation

Healthcare organizations receive a fixed amount per person as compensation for providing care to a defined population in the future (AICPA 1996). Capitation as a payment method provides the most financial risk and opportunity to the healthcare organization because the fixed amount is based on the cost of care projected to be used by the covered population, rather than the cost of care actually used. Previously mentioned payment methods provide financial incentives to healthcare organizations to contain costs after the patient seeks care primarily by controlling use, but capitation also provides financial incentives to healthcare organizations to contain costs before the patient seeks care, primarily by encouraging prevention. Third-party payers and healthcare organizations negotiate capitated payments, often called premiums, based on their perceptions of the actuarial experience of the covered population. Whether the healthcare organization realizes a profit or incurs a loss depends on its ability to project demand for care by the covered population, and then to contain costs when a member of the enrolled population—a subscriber—seeks care.

Bad Debt and Charity Care

Although they are not actually methods of third-party payment, bad debt and charity care are important concepts to discuss in this context because the amounts are substantial in healthcare organizations.

Bad Debt   Healthcare organizations that use accrual accounting assume bad debt expense when the organization bills and expects payment from a patient or a third party, the organization receives no or partial payment, and the organization writes off all or part of the account. The *AICPA Audit and Accounting Guide for Health Care Organizations* (1996) requires that healthcare organizations report bad debt expense as an operating expense based on charges, not costs. While reporting charges overstates the value of bad debt, AICPA requires the reporting of charges because hospitals can uniformly report charges for bad debt whereas hospitals would have some difficulty reporting costs for bad debt due to the variety of ways to determine cost.

Charity Care   Healthcare organizations assume charity care expense when the organization provides care to a patient who the organization knows is unable to pay at the time of service. The *AICPA Audit and Accounting Guide for Health Care Organizations* (1996) requires that healthcare organizations do not report charity care as revenue, a deduction from revenue, or an operating expense. However, it requires that healthcare organizations do report the level of charity care (either charges, costs, or units) in a note to the statement of operations along with the organization's policy for providing charity care.

Uncompensated Care

According to American Hospital Association data for 2001 (see Table 4.1), hospital spending for uncompensated care, which is the total of bad debt and charity, dropped to its lowest level since 1983. Uncompensated hospital care as a percent of total expenses was 5.6 percent in 2001. A relatively strong economy before September 11 and the relative success of public programs like the State Children's Health Insurance Program (SCHIPS) were likely reasons for the decrease in 2001. Rising numbers of uninsured will likely cause the uncompensated hospital care cost to go up in 2002 and 2003 (Reilly 2003).

The Kaiser Commission study found that hospitals provided $23.6 billion of the total $35 in uncompensated care in 2001 (Tieman 2003). To

TABLE 4.1
Uncompensated
Hospital Care

Year	Uncompensate Care (in billions)	% of Total Expenses
1997	$18.5	6.0
1998	$19.0	6.0
1999	$20.7	6.2
2000	$21.6	6.0
2001	$21.5	5.6

Source: American Hospital Association. 2002. *American Hospital Association Health Forum Survey*. Chicago: AHA.

the extent they could, hospitals shifted these costs to paying patients through increased charges.

Cost Shifting

Cost shifting is the practice of shifting costs to some payers to offset losses from other payers. It occurs in every industry, usually to offset losses from bad debt and charity care. Evidence of cost shifting in healthcare is based on the fact that different payers pay different effective prices (charges minus a negotiated discount) for similar services. For instance, in 1990, Medicaid paid an average of 79.7 percent of the hospital's costs for caring for Medicaid's patients; Medicare paid an average of 89.2 percent of the hospital's costs for caring for Medicare's patients; and private payers paid an average of 126.8 percent of the hospital's costs for caring for private pay patients. Employers believe that cost shifting is unfair and the elimination of cost shifting is the primary reason that large employers favor an "all payer" system where each payer pays the same price for similar services. Cost shifting should not be confused with price discrimination which is the practice of setting prices based on what the market will bear (Feldstein 2003). However, according to a study by Lewin-ICF, a healthcare policy think tank, released by the HFMA in 1992 (Dobson and Roney 1992), most of the losses shifted in hospitals relate to losses attributed to Medicare and Medicaid. As shown in Table 4.2, the losses were large and grew from $20.1 billion, or 11 percent of hospital costs in 1989, to $34.6 billion, or 14 percent of hospital costs in 1992. The losses were passed to private payers, which increased their bills by 25 percent in 1989 and 38 percent in 1992 (Dobson and Clarke 1992).[3] The American Hospital Association (AHA) reported that uncompensated care, or the total of charity care and bad debt, was 20.7 billion for hospitals in 1999 and represented 6.2 percent of hospital total expenses (AHA 2001).

Recent evidence provided in Table 4.3 shows that cost shifting is on the decline as healthcare organizations lower their costs in response to Medicare

TABLE 4.2 Hospital Losses by Payer (in billions of dollars)

	1989	1992
Medicare	6.9	14.4
Medicaid	4.2	8.1
Other government	0.1	0.2
Total public	11.2	22.7
Charity/bad debt	8.9	11.9
Total losses	20.1	34.6
Percent of total hospital cost	11.1	14.0
Percent of private payer burden	25.0	38.0

Source: Adapted from Dobson, A., and J. Roney. 1992. *Cost-Shifting: A Self Limiting Process*. Washington, DC: Lewin-ICF.

TABLE 4.3
Hospital Payment-to-Cost Ratios by Source of Revenue

Payer	1990	1995	2000
Medicare	89.2	99.3	100.2
Medicaid	79.7	93.8	96.1
Private Payers	126.8	123.9	112.5

Source: MedPAC. 2003. *Report to Congress: Medicare Payment Policy*. [Online retrieval, 01/29/04]. http://www.medpac.gov/publications/congressional_reports/Mar02_AppB.pdf.

and Medicaid prospective payment rates and as competition lowers prices to private payers, thus making it more difficult for a healthcare organization to shift large losses to private payers. In the event that hospitals cannot shift the costs of uncompensated care and government program losses to private payers because the private payers either refuse to pay increased charges through competition or because the private payers refuse to pay for costs unrelated to their patients, the hospital must cut costs. Problem 4.1 demonstrates cost shifting first and then cost cutting. Chapter 5 will take a closer look at the history of Medicare and Medicaid and at governmental attempts at controlling the expenditures.

PROBLEM 4.1
Cost-Shifting/Cost-Cutting Problem

Cost Shifting
Next year, ABC healthcare organization will serve 100 patients analyzed in the following manner:

    30 Medicare patients who pay $850 per diagnosis
    20 Medicaid patients who pay $900 per diagnosis
    15 managed care patients who pay charges minus a 20 percent
        discount
    15 managed care patients who pay $700 per subscriber
    5 private insurance patients who pay charges
    5 self-pay patients who pay charges
    5 bad debt patients who pay nothing
    5 indigent patients who pay nothing

Next year, ABC's costs will be $1,000 per patient.

Calculate the charge necessary to recover ABC's cost (called cost-led pricing).

Step 1: Calculate the total projected loss by assuming the charge per patient equals the cost per patient.

Financial Class	No.	Costs	Charges	Collections	Profit
Medicare	30	30,000	30,000	25,500	−4,500
Medicaid	20	20,000	20,000	18,000	−2,000
MC #1	15	15,000	15,000	12,000	−3,000
MC #2	15	15,000	15,000	10,500	−4,500
Private	5	5,000	5,000	5,000	0
Self-pay	5	5,000	5,000	5,000	0
Bad Debt	5	5,000	5,000	0	−5,000
Indigent	5	5,000	5,000	0	−5,000
Total	100	100,000	100,000	76,000	−24,000

Step 2: Calculate the charge necessary to recover ABC's cost by dividing the loss by the number of patients who will pay an increased charge, or portion thereof, and then add the cost per patient to the answer.

$$\frac{24,000}{15(.80) + 5 + 5} + 1,000 = \$2,091$$

Step 3: Check the answer by calculating the loss using the new charge.

Financial Class	No.	Costs	Charges	Collections	Profit
Medicare	30	30,000	62,730	25,500	−4,500
Medicaid	20	20,000	41,820	18,000	−2,000
MC #1	15	15,000	31,365	25,092	10,092
MC #2	15	15,000	31,365	10,500	−4,500
Private	51	5,000	10,455	10,455	5,455
Self-pay	5	5,000	10,455	10,455	5,455
Bad debt	5	5,000	10,455	0	−5,000
Indigent	5	5,000	10,455	0	−5,000
Total	100	100,000	209,100	100,002	2

Note: The table produced in Step 3 can also be used to calculate contractual allowances (charges minus collections) for Medicare, Medicaid, and managed care. The total profit should be zero; "2" is due to a rounding error.

Cost Cutting

For the previously referenced cost-shifting problem, assume that those payers that pay charges, or charges minus a discount, limit ABC's charges to $1,070 per patient. Calculate the amount of costs that ABC will need to cut, or cover with additional revenues, to break even (realize no profit or loss).

Step 1: Calculate the total costs to be cut by using the new charge per patient to determine profit/loss.

Financial Class	No.	Costs	Charges	Collections	Profit
Medicare	30	30,000	32,100	25,500	−4,500
Medicaid	20	20,000	21,400	18,000	−2,000
MC #1	15	15,000	16,050	12,840	−2,160
MC #2	15	15,000	16,050	10,500	−4,500
Private	5	5,000	5,350	5,350	350
Self-pay	5	5,000	5,350	5,350	350
Bad debt	5	5,000	5,350	0	−5,000
Indigent	5	5,000	5,350	0	−5,000
Total	100	100,000	107,000	77,540	−22,460

Step 2: Check the answer by calculating the profit/loss using the new cost per patient, or $775.40. Remember, cost per patient day becomes $775.40, or $77,540/100, after reducing total costs by $22,460.

Financial Class	No.	Costs	Charges	Collections	Profit
Medicare	30	23,262	32,100	25,500	2,238
Medicaid	20	15,508	21,400	18,000	2,492
MC #1	15	11,631	16,050	12,840	1,209
MC #2	15	11,631	16,050	10,500	−1,131
Private	5	3,877	5,350	5,350	1,473
Self-pay	5	3,877	5,350	5,350	1,473
Bad debt	5	3,877	5,350	0	−3,877
Indigent	5	3,877	5,350	0	−3,877
Total	100	77,540	107,000	77,540	0

Notes

1. According to Eastaugh (1992), the proportion of healthcare costs paid by the patient were a record-low 12.9 percent in 1987. Since 1987, however, the proportion of healthcare costs paid by the patient has been climbing steadily to 13.7 percent in 2002 Although this increase in cost sharing (i.e., the transfer of costs to patients in the forms of increasing the employee share of premiums, and the existence of deductibles, and coinsurance) reduces unnecessary demand for services by the patient, Eastaugh (1987) warns of Feldstein's moral hazard (1981)—that the goal of cost sharing is to inhibit the worried well, but not the truly sick, from seeking care.
2. For a comprehensive discussion of integrated delivery systems including horizontal integration, or the expansion of a product or service line at the same point in the production process (e.g., nursing homes integrating with other nursing homes); and vertical integration, or the expansion of a product or service line at more than one point in the production process (e.g., hospitals integrating with nursing homes), see Zelman's *The Changing Health Care Marketplace: Private Ventures, Public Interests*, 1996.
3. To avoid antitrust claims of price discrimination, or the practice of charging different payers what the market will bear for the same service, healthcare organizations have typically charged different payers the same price for the same service and then discounted the price per agreement to some payers based on quantity. The healthcare organization records the difference between the price and the discounted price, or the amount collected per agreement, as a contractual allowance.

References

American Hospital Association. 2002. *American Hospital Association Health Forum Survey*. Chicago: AHA.

American Hospital Association. 2001. [Online retrieval, 02/08/01]. http://ww.aha.org/membersonly/factsheettbl.asp.

American Institute of Certified Public Accountants. 1996. *AICPA Audit and Accounting Guide: Health Care Organizations*. New York: AICPA.

Burrows, S. N., and R. C. Moravec. 1997. "Direct Contracting: A Minnesota Case Study." *Healthcare Financial Management* 51 (8): 50–55.

Clarke, R. 2000. "Beyond Managed Care" *Healthcare Financial Management* 54 (7): 16.

Cohn, L., P. Eliopoulos, and A. Weintraub. 2000. "What Comes After Managed Care?" *Business Week* October 23, 149–56.

Dobson, A., and R. L. Clarke. 1992. "Shifting No Solution to Problem of Increasing Costs." *Healthcare Financial Management* 46 (7): 25–32.

Dobson, A., and J. Roney. 1992. *Cost Shifting: A Self Limiting Process.* Washington, DC: Lewin-ICF.

Eastaugh, S. R. 1992. *Health Care Finance: Economic Incentives and Productivity Enhancement.* Westport, CT: Auburn House.

Eastaugh, S. R. 1987. *Financing Health Care: Economic Efficiency and Equity.* Dover, MA: Auburn House.

Emery, J. D. 2001. "The Defined-Contribution Plan: The Next Generation of Healthcare Financing." *Healthcare Financial Management* 55 (1): 37–39.

Feldstein, M. 1981. *Hospital Costs and Health Insurance.* Cambridge, MA: Harvard University Press.

Feldstein, P. 2003. *Health Policy Issues: An Economic Perspective, 3rd ed.* Chicago: Health Administration Press.

Gabel, J. R. 1994. *HMO Industry Profile.* Washington, DC: Group Health Association as cited in Zelman, W. A. 1996. *The Changing Healthcare Marketplace: Private Ventures, Public Interests.* San Francisco: Jossey-Bass Publishers.

Group Health Association of America. 1995. *Patterns in HMO Enrollment.* Washington, DC: GHAA.

Harris, S. E. 1975. *The Economics of Health Care: Finance and Delivery.* Berkeley, CA: McCutchan Publishing Corporation.

Healthcare Financial Management Association. 1998. *Healthcare Financial Management* 53 (12): 20–21.

Hepner, J. O., and D. M. Hepner. 1973. *The Health Strategy Game: A Challenge for Reorganization and Management.* St. Louis, MO: C. V. Mosby.

Holahan, J., and M. Wang. 2004. "Trends: Changes in Health Insurance Coverage During the Economic Downturn: 2000–2002." *Health Affairs*—Web Exclusive. [Online retrieval, 03/16/04]. http://content.healthaffairs.org/webexclusives/index.dt/?year=2004.

Levit, K., C. Smith, C. Cowan, A. Sensenig, and A. Catlin. 2004. "Health Spending Rebound Continues in 2002." *Health Affairs* 23 (1): 147–159.

MedPAC. 2003. *Report to Congress: Medicare Payment Policy.* [Online retrieval, 01/29/04]. http://www.medpac.gov/publications/congressional_reports/Mar02_AppB.pdf.

Millenson, M. (moderator). 2003. "Healthcare's Challenge: Rising Consumer Expectations." *HealthLeaders* 6 (1): RT1-RT15.

Nowicki, M. (moderator). 2003. "Care Management: Balancing Costs and Quality." *HealthLeaders* 6 (9): RT1–RT9.

Physician Payment Review Commission. 1995. *Annual Report to Congress, 1995.* Washington, DC: PPRC.

Rauber, C. 2003a. "Quiet Giant: What Hospitals and Other Health Plans Can Learn from UnitedHealth." *HealthLeaders* 6 (4): 38–46.

———. 2003b. "The New Face of Health Plans." *HealthLeaders* 6 (1): 37–43.

Reilly, P. 2003. "Charitable Dropoff: Uncompensated Care Drops to Lowest Level in Years." *Modern Healthcare* 22 (7): 4.

Robinson, J. C., and L. P. Casalino. 1995. "The Growth of Medical Groups Paid Through Capitation in California." *New England Journal of Medicine* 333 (25): 1684–1687.

Shortell, S. M., and K. E. Hull. 1996. "The New Organization of the Health Care Delivery Systems." In *Strategic Choices for a Changing Health Care System*, edited by S. H. Altman and U. E. Reinhardt, 101–148. Chicago: Health Administration Press.

Starr, P. 1982. *The Social Transformation of American Medicine.* New York: Basic Books.

Tieman, J. 2003. "Hope for the Uninsured." *Modern Healthcare* 22 (7): 6–7, 16.

Wagner, E. R. 1996. "Types of Managed Care Organizations." In *The Managed Health Care Handbook, 3rd. ed.*, edited by P. R. Kongstvedt, 33–45. Gaithersburg, MD: Aspen Publishers.

Zelman, W. A. 1996. *The Changing Health Care Marketplace: Private Ventures, Public Interests.* San Francisco: Jossey-Bass Publishers.

MEDICARE AND MEDICAID

President Johnson and the 89th Congress changed the philosophy of healthcare in the United States from an individual responsibility to a social responsibility, and changed access to healthcare from a privilege to a right. However, historians credit President Kennedy with reopening the debate on compulsory health insurance. President Kennedy strongly supported compulsory health insurance for the elderly during his campaign and called for legislation in his State of the Union address in 1963. President Johnson made compulsory health insurance a central issue in the 1964 presidential campaign and, once elected, called for legislation in his State of the Union address in 1964. The country's empathy after the assassination of President Kennedy and President Johnson's adroit legislative skills facilitated the passing of 12 major pieces of health legislation by Congress as part of President Johnson's Great Society[1] (Hepner and Hepner 1973). President Johnson signed Medicare and Medicaid into law as part of the Social Security Amendments of 1965 (P.L. 89-97) at the Truman Library, with former President Truman in attendance.

Many believe that President Johnson's Great Society was built on the backs of future generations. When President Johnson assumed office in 1963, the economy was projected to soar to extraordinary levels by the end of the century. This projected growth in the economy would pay later for the guns and butter agenda of the president. This agenda included escalating the conflict in Viet Nam while initiating significant social programs in the United States—a costly agenda funded without significant tax increases. President Johnson thought that tax increases would have forced Congress to choose between fighting the Communists in Southeast Asia and fighting poverty in the United States (Peterson 1996).

Medicare

Medicare Eligibility

Medicare, Title XVIII of the Social Security Amendments of 1965, is a federally funded program that provides health insurance to Americans at age 65. Significant expansion in eligibility for Medicare occurred only in 1972. At that time, the disabled under age 65 who qualified for Social Security disability benefits and those with end-stage renal disease were included. Within the context of balancing the federal budget, considerable discussion has taken place regarding increasing the eligibility age of Medicare in a fashion similar to Social Security.[2] However, Democratic party leadership has proposed using future budget surpluses to reduce the eligibility age for Medicare to age 62.

Medicare Benefits

In 1966, Medicare covered seven basic services. Covered under Part A of the program known as hospital insurance (HI) were inpatient hospital services; outpatient diagnostic services; and home health agency services following hospitalization. In 1967, extended care facilities services following hospitalization were added. Covered under Part B of the program known as supplemental medical insurance (SMI) were physician and other medical services; outpatient therapeutic services; and home health agency services (Harris 1975). Since 1966, certain preventive services have been added including pneumococcal, influenza, and hepatitis B vaccines; mammography screening; and Pap smears. In 1982, hospice coverage was added for Medicare beneficiaries who were certified as terminally ill. The most significant expansion of services occurred in 1988 with the passage of the Medicare Catastrophic Coverage Act, which included a cap on the Medicare beneficiaries' liability for catastrophic illness, outpatient prescription coverage, and additional skilled nursing facility (SNF) coverage. The Medicare Catastrophic Coverage Act, which was intended to be funded solely by Medicare beneficiaries, was repealed in 1989 as a result of opposition to additional taxes to fund the program (Gornick et al. 1996).

Benefits for Part A of Medicare include 90 days of inpatient coverage per benefit period, which begins the first day of hospitalization and ends 60 days after the last discharge from a hospital or SNF. Beneficiaries may have an unlimited number of benefit periods during their lifetime. In addition, beneficiaries have one lifetime reserve of 60 days that the beneficiary can use if the 90 days are exhausted in any given benefit period. Part A also covers up to 100 posthospital days in a SNF and unlimited visits by a home health agency. Medicare beneficiaries must pay an inpatient hospital deductible set at the cost of one hospital day ($776 in 2000) each benefit period in which they are hospitalized. Medicare beneficiaries must pay hospital coinsurance set at 25 percent of the hospital deductible for days 61 through 90. Medicare beneficiaries must pay hospital coinsurance set at 50 percent of the hospital deductible for each lifetime reserve day. For SNF care, Medicare beneficiaries must pay a coinsurance set at 12.5 percent of the hospital deductible for days 21 through 100 (Hoffman, Klees, and Curtis 2000).

Benefits for Part B include physician and other professional services and certain supplies. Medicare beneficiaries must pay a $100 annual deductible. Hospitals must accept assignment, or accept what Medicare pays as full payment, but physicians can accept or reject assignment. If the physician accepts assignment, Medicare pays 80 percent and beneficiaries pay 20 percent. Prior to 1989, if the physician rejected assignment, he or she could charge any amount and balance bill beneficiaries the amount not paid by Medicare.

The Omnibus Budget Reconciliation Act of 1989 (OBRA 1989) established a physician fee schedule and limited the amount physicians' charges could exceed the fee schedule. In so doing, OBRA of 1989 also limited the amount physicians who rejected assignment could balance bill Medicare beneficiaries (Gornick et al. 1996).

Medicare+Choice (Part C) is an expanded set of options for the delivery of healthcare under Medicare. While all Medicare beneficiaries can receive benefits through the original fee-for-service program, most beneficiaries enrolled in HI and SMI can now choose to participate in a Medicare+Choice plan instead. Organizations that contract as Medicare+Choice plans must meet specific organizational, financial, and other requirements. Primary types of Medicare+Choice plans include:

- Coordinated care plans that include HMOs, PSOs, and PPOs, as well as other coordinated care plans certified by Medicare;
- Private, unrestricted fee-for-service plans that allow beneficiaries to select certain private providers; and
- Medical savings account (MSA) plans that provide benefits after a single, high deductible is met.

Except for MSA plans, all Medicare+Choice plans are required to provide the current Medicare benefit package, excluding hospice services. To remain competitive, Medicare+Choice plans frequently offer additional benefits (Hoffman, Klees, and Curtis 2000). About 15 percent of Medicare beneficiaries were enrolled in Medicare+Choice plans in 2000 (DeLew 2000).

On December 8, 2003, President Bush signed into law the Medicare Prescription Drug, Improvement, and Modernization Act (MMA) of 2003, which provides Medicare beneficiaries (seniors and the qualified disabled) with the most significant improvement in Medicare benefits (Part D) since the beginning of Medicare in 1965. In addition to giving all Medicare beneficiaries access to prescription drug coverage, the Act also provides enhanced coverage to low-income seniors, access to an immediate drug discount card, increased coverage for certain preventive services, and savings for many state governments (HHS 2003).

Medicare Financing

Medicare was initially (1966) financed by assessments on employers for Part A (0.35 percent of payroll up to $6,500), by a coinsurance of $3 per month paid by beneficiaries for Part B, and by general revenue allocations to Part B (Harris 1975). Initial Medicare expenditures had been grossly under-projected, however. President Johnson reportedly believed that Medicare spending would run about $500 million a year (Peterson 1996). Medicare expenditures were $4.2 billion in 1967, the first full year of the program (Helbing 1993). Medicare expenditures growth was also grossly under-projected. Critics of the program exaggerated an end-of-the-century annual expenditure of $10 billion (Frum 1994). 2002 Medicare spending was $267.1 billion with growth projected at an additional $13 billion per year through the year 2013 (Heffler et al. 2004). The program has remained solvent by:

- Increasing assessments to employers and employees (2.9 percent of payroll with no limit in 2000);
- Increasing cost sharing (i.e., deductibles, coinsurance, and balance billing) by beneficiaries to 16.5 percent of all program expenditures;
- Increasing the allocation from general revenues (general revenues represented 58.4 percent of Part B funding in 1967 and 73.4 percent of Part B funding in 1991 (Petrie 1993); and
- Enacting legislation designed to slow the rate of growth, which averaged 10 percent per year between 1970 and 1998 (DeLew 2000).

Medicare Reimbursement to Providers

Funded by the federal government, Part A of Medicare reimbursed hospital services based on retroactive, reasonable cost, or cost-based reimbursement. Recognizing that hospitals charged more than cost, Medicare reimbursed hospitals a percentage of the charge at the time of service, and then made adjustments based on cost reports that Medicare required hospitals to file. To ensure quality, Medicare required hospitals to either pass a Joint Commission accreditation visit, called deemed status, or undergo a Medicare certification visit. This certification visit was thought by most to be more difficult by design; Medicare did not want to be in the inspection business and preferred that hospitals seek deemed status provided by the Joint Commission. Part B of Medicare reimbursed physician and outpatient services based on reasonable and customary charges, which allowed physicians to realize a profit by providing services to Medicare patients.

President Reagan introduced the first significant reimbursement reform in his Tax Equity and Fiscal Responsibility Act of 1982 (TEFRA). While the act reduced taxes in response to President Reagan's campaign promise, it also contained significant reimbursement reform for Medicare. Specifically, the act introduced cost limits per case and cost limits per year (known as TEFRA limits). The act directed the Department of Health and Human Services (HHS) to develop a prospective payment system (PPS) for hospitals. It also introduced the option of managed care plans to beneficiaries and made Medicare the secondary payer when beneficiaries had additional insurance.

President Reagan signed into law the Social Security Amendments of 1983, which included provisions for prospective payment. Prospective payment applied to Part A reimbursement only, with the exception of capital costs, which were still reimbursed on cost, and was intended to replace cost-based reimbursement. The amendments established prospective payment rates for diagnostic-related grouping (DRG), or similar cases that should require similar resource consumption.[3] Hospitals that provided care for less cost than the established rate for a DRG realized a profit. Hospitals that provided care for more cost than the established rate realized a loss. Because hospitals were thus given a financial incentive to under-use the system and realize a profit, the federal government relied on peer review organizations (PROs), established under the TEFRA legislation, to ensure that Medicare beneficiaries were receiving appropriate care.[4] Medicare implemented the PPS over a three-year period to give hospitals time to adjust their costs. During that three-year period, Medicare used hospital-specific data to establish the DRG rates. At the end of the three-year period, hospitals were subject to a national rate with an adjustment for labor costs, which varied between regions. Currently, three different national rates exist: a teaching hospital rate; an urban hospital rate; and a rural hospital rate.[5] Medicare used the DRG rate schedule to provide incentives and penalties for certain physician ordering patterns. For instance, hospitals that performed open-heart surgery before trying angioplasty were punished with a low rate of reimbursement, whereas hospitals that performed successful angioplasty without open-heart surgery were rewarded with high reimbursement.

The Omnibus Budget Reconciliation Act of 1990 folded capital costs into the DRG rate over a ten-year period. Prior to 1990, Medicare had reimbursed capital costs based on reasonable cost, meaning that Medicare reimbursed its share of capital costs regardless of use. By folding capital costs into the DRG rate, hospitals risked losing substantial reimbursement if their buildings and equipment were not properly used. Hospitals that had overextended their capital were forced to consolidate their assets through a sale or a joint venture (joint ventures with proprietary organizations were popular because the proprietaries had access to additional sources of capital).

The HCFA Resource-Based Relative Value System (RBRVS) of 1992 changed the way Medicare reimbursed physicians. Prior to 1992, Medicare had reimbursed physicians based on reasonable and customary charges. By reimbursing physicians on a RBRVS, Medicare established a prospective, flat fee per visit similar to PPS for hospitals. Physicians who provided care for less cost than the established rate realized a profit; physicians who provided care for more cost than the established rate realized a loss. Furthermore, Medicare used the RBRVS rate schedule to provide incentives and penalties for certain medical specialties. Visits to primary care physicians resulted in favorable reimbursement, but visits to specialists resulted in unfavorable reimbursement.

The Balanced Budget Act of 1997 (BBA of 1997) reduced Medicare reimbursements to providers by $115 billion over five years according to the following schedule (Ernst & Young 1997):

- $43.8 billion from hospitals: PPS rates frozen and capital payments reduced 2.1 percent;

- $25.7 billion from post-acute care: PPS implemented in SNFs in 1998, in home health agencies in 2000, and in rehabilitation hospitals in 2004;
- $21.8 billion from managed care: Provider-sponsored organizations (PSOs) were allowed to enter the market and bid on Medicare business, which was to be capitated;
- $11.7 billion from physicians: RBRVS declared budget neutral, but substantially increased primary care reimbursement and substantially decreased specialist reimbursement; updates to RBRVS payment schedule will be tied to a composite index; physician extenders, like physician assistants and nurse practitioners, paid directly and allowed to practice without direct physician supervision; and
- $12.1 billion from other sources.

The Balanced Budget Refinement Act of 1999 (BBRA of 1999) provided approximately $16 billion in Medicare relief over five years after the government discovered that BBA of 1997 had cut two to three times more than the $115 billion originally intended. Major reimbursement provisions of BBRA of 1999 included the following (VHA 1999):

- $7.9 billion to hospitals including $6.1 billion to hospital outpatient, $0.8 billion to rural hospitals, $0.6 billion to teaching hospitals, $0.3 billion to PPS-exempt hospitals, $0.1 billion to disproportionate share hospitals;
- $4.0 billion to Medicare+Choice;
- $2.7 billion to skilled nursing facilities; and
- $1.3 billion to home health care.

The Medicare, Medicaid, and SCHIP Benefits Improvement and Protection Act of 2000 (BIPA of 2000) provided $35 billion in reimbursement relief over five years by increasing certain Medicare and Medicaid provider payments; adding preventive benefits and reducing beneficiary cost sharing under Medicare; and improving insurance options for low-income children, low-income families, and low-income seniors. Major reimbursement provisions of BIPA of 2000 included the following (HFMA 2000a):

- $12 billion to hospitals;
- $11 billion to managed care;
- $5 billion to Medicare and Medicaid beneficiaries;
- $3 billion to other providers;
- $2 billion to skilled nursing facilities and therapy services; and
- $2 billion to home health care.

The Medicare Prescription Drug, Improvement, and Modernization Act of 2003 (MMA of 2003) provided more than drug coverage for seniors.

Regarding reimbursement, the Act provided an estimated $25 billion in payment improvements to providers over ten years (HFMA 2004; Scott 2004a):

- Hospitals
  - Payment increases of full market basket to hospitals that submit quality data from 2005 through 2007; hospitals that do not submit quality data will receive market basket minus 0.4 percent.[6]
  - Indirect medical education payment increases of 6.0 percent for the last half of 2004; 5.8 percent for 2005; 5.55 percent for 2006; and 5.35 percent for 2007.
  - Changes to the labor share of the wage index, from 71 percent to 62 percent for low-wage areas, with all other areas held harmless.
  - An increase to 12 percent (up from the current 5.7 percent) in the cap for Medicare disproportionate share (DSH) payments for small rural and urban hospitals.
  - A 16 percent Medicaid DSH increase in 2004; low-DSH states will get 16 percent annually for five years.
  - Increased payments to critical access hospitals (CAHs) to costs plus one percent (hospitals that might otherwise qualify to become a CAH except for their having a psychiatric or rehabilitation unit may still qualify if the units are not more than 10 beds—hospitals will also be allowed to use 25 beds for acute [the previous limit for acute care was 15 beds]).
  - Continuation of the outpatient PPS hold harmless provisions for two years for rural hospitals with fewer than 100 beds and sole community providers (SCHs).
- Physicians (and others paid under the Medicare physician fee schedule)
  - Payment increase of 1.5 percent in 2004 and provisions for another 1.5 percent increase in 2005 (instead of the planned reduction of 4.5 percent).
  - Future changes to the physician payment formula will be based on a 10-year rolling average of the gross domestic product instead of the current single year measure.
  - Areas of the country with geographic payment adjustments below 1.0 will be increased to 1.0 in 2004 through 2006.
  - Bonus payments of 5.0 percent for three years to all physicians delivering care in underserved areas of the country.
  - A temporary moratorium on therapy caps for 2004 while Congress and Centers for Medicare and Medicaid Services (CMS) research an alternative to the caps.
- Home Health
  - Elimination of the proposed co-payment provision.
  - Payment increases of market basket minus 0.8 percent in 2004 through 2006.
  - Bonus payments to rural providers, amounting to 5 percent for 2004.

- Ambulances
    - Payments will be based on regional floors, with adjustments for low-population rural areas.
    - Across-the-board adjustments of 1.0 percent for urban areas and 2.0 percent for rural areas in 2004 through 2006.
- Durable medical equipment
    - Payment rates frozen from 2004 through 2006 with rates for the top five services adjusted to reflect rates paid in the Federal Employees Health Benefit Program.
    - Competitive bidding for the largest metropolitan statistical areas (MSAs) to begin in 2007, expanding to 80 MSAs in 2009.

Medicare Expenditures

The cost of the Medicare program has been a problem for Congress from the very beginning (see Figure 5.1). Use was under-projected and revenue sources, particularly projected economic growth, were overly optimistic. Attempts have been made to control costs through federal legislation (which is discussed in the next section), increased assessments to employers and employees, increased cost sharing to beneficiaries, and increased program allocation from general revenues. Even with these attempts, the HHS—which has the overall responsibility for the administration of the Medicare program—projects that the Medicare Trust Fund will go bankrupt in 2019.

The very low average growth rate in Medicare expenditures during 1996 projected to 2005 stands in stark contrast to previous years, which averaged more than 10 percent growth. The 1996 to 2000 rate can be attributed to the implementation of the BBA of 1997, the intense efforts to identify and

FIGURE 5.1
Average Annual Percentage Increase in Total Medicare Expenditures

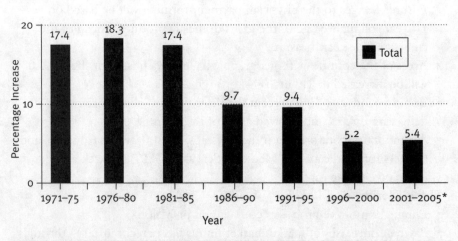

*2001–2005 is projected
Source: HCFA. 2000a. *Healthcare Financing Review: Medicare and Medicaid Statistical Supplement 2000*, p. 89.

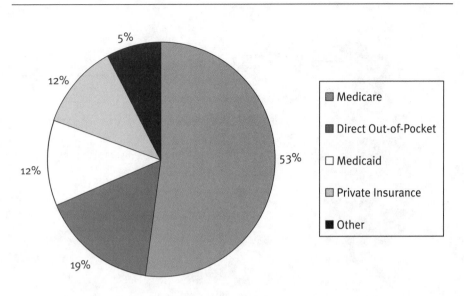

FIGURE 5.2
Sources of
Payment for
Medicare
Beneficiaries,
1999

Source: CMS Web-Based Chart Series. 2004. "Program Information on Medicare, Medicaid, SCHIP, and Other Programs." [Online retrieval, 02/04/04]. http://www.cms.gov.

correct fraud and abuse in the Medicare program, and the very low rate of general and Medicare inflation (Foster 2000).

It is important to note that Medicare pays only a little more than half of a Medicare beneficiary's healthcare expenditures. For instance, in 1999, the per capita Medicare beneficiary spent $9,573 on healthcare of which Medicare paid 53 percent (see Figure 5.2) Direct out-of-pocket expenditures, which does not include beneficiary payments for Medicare Part B premium or private health insurance premiums, is comprised of Medicare cost sharing (27 percent of out-of-pocket expenditures) and expenditures that are outside the Medicare Benefit package (see Figure 5.3). In 1999, the per capita Medicare beneficiary spent $1,825 on direct out-of-pocket expenditures, of which 53 percent was attributable to Medicare cost sharing.

Total healthcare expenditures (from all sources) for Medicare beneficiaries for 1999 were $385.2 billion. Hospitals received 40 percent of those expenditures while medical providers received 22 percent (see Figure 5.4).

Slowing the growth of Medicare spending is particularly important in relation to the "graying of America"—the increasing proportion of the population that is aged 65 years and older.

This demographic phenomenon is caused by the very large baby-boom population (those born between 1946 and 1964) that makes up approximately one-third of the existing U.S. population. This age segment will begin to turn 65 starting in the year 2011 (see Table 5.1). The phenomenon is also caused by the longer life expectancy of those over 65 years (see Table 5.2).

FIGURE 5.3
Direct
Out-of-Pocket
Spending by
Medicare
Beneficiaries,
1999

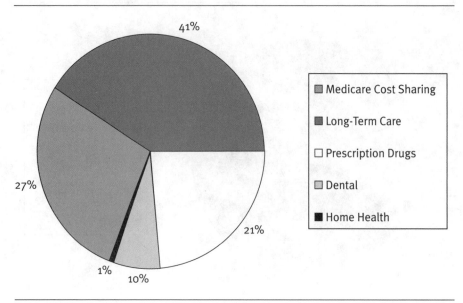

Source: CMS Web-Based Chart Series. 2004. "Program Information on Medicare, Medicaid, SCHIP, and Other Programs." [Online retrieval, 02/04/04]. http://www.cms.gov.

The "graying of America" has special significance to healthcare organizations, because the 65 years and older population uses healthcare services at a much higher rate than the under-65 population. As a result, healthcare expenditures are disproportionately high for the 65 years and older population. Although 12.6 percent of the total population was 65 years and older

FIGURE 5.4
Total Health
Care
Expenditures
for Medicare
Beneficiaries,
1999

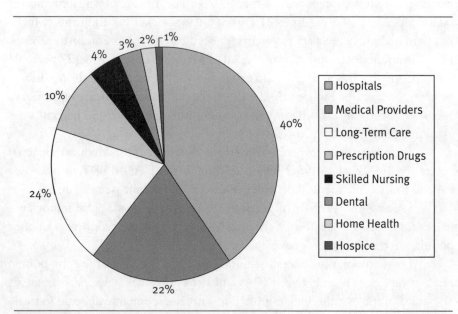

Source: CMS Web-Based Chart Series. 2004. "Program Information on Medicare, Medicaid, SCHIP, and Other Programs." [Online retrieval, 02/04/04]. http://www.cms.gov.

Year	Percent
1930	5.4
1940	6.8
1950	8.1
1960	9.3
1970	9.8
1980	11.3
1990	12.5
2000	12.8
2010	13.3
2020	16.4
2030	20.1
2040	20.7
2050	20.4

TABLE 5.1
Percentage of U.S. Population 65 and Older

Source: U.S. Bureau of the Census. *Current Population Reports Series P-23*, No. 128 and *P-25*, No. 1018. In Rice, D. P. 1996. "Beneficiary Profile: Yesterday, Today, and Tomorrow." *Health Care Financing Review*, 18 (2): 23–97.

Year	Life Expectancy	
	Male	Female
1950	12.8	15.0
1960	12.8	15.8
1970	13.1	17.0
1980	14.1	18.3
1990	15.1	18.9
2000	16.4	20.0
2010	17.2	20.8
2020	18.0	21.5
2030	18.9	22.3
2040	19.8	23.2
2050	20.8	24.0

TABLE 5.2
U.S. Life Expectancy at 65

Source: U.S. Bureau of the Census. *Current Population Reports Series P-23*, No. 128 and *P-25*, No. 1018. In Rice, D. P. 1996. "Beneficiary Profile: Yesterday, Today, and Tomorrow." *Health Care Financing Review*, 18 (2): 23–97.

in 1994, they represented 89.2 percent of nursing home residents; 74.5 percent of home health visits; 40.1 percent of hospital days; and 22.2 percent of physician visits (Rice 1996). The 65 years and older population accounted for 36 percent of all healthcare expenditures (Waldo et al. 1989).

Medicaid

Medicaid Eligibility

Medicaid, Title XIX of the Social Security Amendments of 1965, is a jointly funded program that provides health insurance to the medically indigent (i.e., individuals who may be able to pay for normal living expenses, but cannot afford healthcare expenses).[7] Historically, eligibility for Medicaid has been linked to eligibility for two federal cash assistance programs: Aid to Families with Dependent Children (AFDC) and Supplemental Security Income (SSI). The Omnibus Budget Reconciliation Act of 1986 (OBRA of 1986) expanded eligibility for low-income pregnant women, children, and infants, regardless of their eligibility for a state's AFDC program. The Medicare Catastrophic Coverage Act of 1988 required states to pay Medicare premiums, coinsurance, and deductibles for the elderly who earned less than the state's poverty limit (Tudor 1995).

The Balanced Budget Act of 1997 provided $23.4 billion over five years to Kids Care, a program to expand health coverage for children whose parents' income was too high to qualify for Medicaid, but too low to afford private insurance (Ernst & Young 1997).

Medicaid Benefits

Although the federal government finances 50 to 83 percent of Medicaid costs in any given state, each state has significant authority in administrating its Medicaid program. Each state is allowed considerable discretion in: establishing its own income and resource criteria for program eligibility; determining the amount, duration, and scope of optional services beyond the mandatory services required by the federal government; and determining provider reimbursement methodologies. Mandatory services required by the federal government include the following:

- Inpatient hospital;
- Outpatient hospital;
- Rural health clinic;
- Lab and x-ray services;
- Nurse practitioner services;
- Nursing facility services (limited to age 21 years and older);
- Home health services (limited to age 21 years and older);
- Early and periodic screening, diagnosis, and treatment services (EPSDTS) (limited to under age 21 years);
- Family planning services and supplies;
- Physician services;
- Nurse-midwife services;
- Dental services (medical/surgical); and
- Transportation services.

Optional services vary by state (HCFA 1996).

In 1997, the State Children's Health Insurance Program (SCHIP) was enacted as part of BBA of 1997 in response to increasing numbers of uninsured children in families with incomes too high to qualify for Medicaid and declining Medicaid enrollment because of the delinking of welfare and Medicaid in the Personal Responsibility and Work Opportunity Reconciliation Act of 1996. SCHIP allows states to implement three options to expand coverage for children in families with incomes up to 200 percent of the poverty level: (1) expanded Medicaid coverage, (2) separate coverage, or (3) a combination of coverages. The goal of SCHIP is to provide health insurance coverage to 50 percent of the nation's 10 million uninsured children. In 1997, SCHIP was appropriated $24 billion over 5 years and $40 billion over 10 years to help states reach that goal (Hakim, Boben, and Bonney 2000; Hoffman, Klees, and Curtis 2000).

Medicaid Financing

The Medicaid program has two categories of costs: costs for provider services, which are determined by formula (see note 6); and costs for administrative services, which are shared equally by the federal and state government. The federal portion of costs is financed from general revenues. The state portion of costs for provider services may be financed from state and local revenues; however, the state's portion must be at least 40 percent. The state portion of costs for administrative services is financed by state revenues (HCFA 1996).

Medicaid Reimbursement to Providers

The Medicaid program operates as a vendor payment program—providers are reimbursed directly by the state. Reimbursement is subject to federal conditions that all states must satisfy. First, reimbursement must be such to recruit a sufficient number of providers. Second, participating providers must accept the Medicaid reimbursement as payment in full. Third, reimbursement to providers must be conditional on appropriate efficiency, economy, and quality standards. Each state has significant authority over reimbursement methods and rates with the following exceptions (HCFA 1996):

- Reimbursements to institutions cannot exceed amounts that would be paid for similar services under the Medicare program.
- Disproportionate share hospitals are exempt from the Medicare limit.
- For hospice services, Medicaid reimbursements cannot be lower than Medicare reimbursements.

Regarding the first exception that reimbursements to institutions cannot exceed amounts that would be paid for similar services under the Medicare program, HCFA uses an upper payment limit (UPL) for Medicaid reimbursement to the states. The UPL is not based on the Medicare payment for individual procedures, but rather is based on an aggregate amount of payments made to states on behalf of three classes of providers—all outpatient providers, state-owned inpatient providers and non-state-owned providers. This allows states to redirect federal Medicaid reimbursements within classes. For instance, in the non-state-owned class, a state could increase the reimbursement to county-owned hospitals at the expense of private-owned hospitals. HHS has identified 28 states that currently have or are proposing UPL arrangements that increase Medicaid reimbursements to public providers. HCFA believes that this loophole could cost the federal government $20 billion over five years in inappropriate federal reimbursements to the states. In response to media coverage of such Medicaid system abuse by states, HHS published a final rule in December, 2000 to restrict a state's ability to use the UPL option to enhance public hospital Medicaid reimbursement. In essence, the proposed rule creates a fourth and separate class of providers—local government-owned providers. If the rule is finalized, public hospitals in states that use the UPL option will see reduced Medicaid reimbursements. Private hospitals could also be affected by reduced Medicaid reimbursements to cover the state losses or by increased expectations to provide uncompensated care (Ferman 2001).

From the beginning, most states used reimbursement methodologies either identical to or similar to the reimbursement methodologies used by Medicare. For reimbursement to institutional providers, this meant that most Medicaid programs used cost-based reimbursement as their basis for reimbursement.

As use and costs grew, most Medicaid programs implemented the same reimbursement controls as Medicare. During the late 1970s, many Medicaid programs were more aggressive than Medicare in recognizing reasonable costs. As Medicare moved into prospective reimbursement methodologies in the early 1980s, most Medicaid programs adopted methodologies based on case mix, or DRGs, similar to Medicare methodologies. However, some Medicaid programs set payment levels based on the historic costs of each institution. This practice had the effect of rewarding providers whose costs had historically been high and penalizing providers who had been cost-conscious in the past (Berman, Kukla, and Weeks 1994). Some Medicaid programs also deviated from Medicare's case-mix methodology, using other prospective methodologies like rate-of-increase and negotiated budget methodologies. For reimbursement to physician providers, Medicaid programs used either fee schedules or reasonable charges methodologies. Medicaid programs using fee schedules set a flat maximum reimbursement for each service. Medicaid programs using reasonable charges limit reimbursement to the lowest of the physician's actual charge, the physician's customary charge for similar services, or the prevailing physicians' charges in the area. A few Medicaid programs have requested permission, via Section 1115 research and demonstration waivers, to develop managed care programs for their Medicaid beneficiaries (HCFA 1996).

The Balanced Budget Act of 1997 effectively eliminated this waiver requirement by giving states the option to require Medicaid beneficiaries to enroll in managed care plans. The act permits provider-sponsored organizations (PSOs) to bid on Medicaid business, which will be capitated (Ernst & Young 1997).

Medicaid Costs

In the early 1990s, the Medicaid program experienced average annual expenditure increases of 19.4 percent (see Figure 5.5). This was extraordinary growth compared to growth in Medicare (10.8 percent for Part A and 7.2 percent for Part B), and in private insurance (6.0 percent). State governments were concerned with the rate of Medicaid cost growth and with the disproportionate revenue growth, which averaged only 7 percent annually over the same time period (Tudor 1995).

Wade and Berg (1995) studied the causes for the rapid growth in the Medicaid program during the early 1990s and reported that growth in Medicaid enrollment, federal Medicaid policy, and state Medicaid policy are all significantly related to Medicaid expenditure growth. Growth in Medicaid enrollment was defined using the following variables: adult Medicaid enrollment; child Medicaid enrollment; blind and disabled Medicaid enrollment; aged Medicaid enrollment; and AIDS Medicaid enrollment. These variables were significantly related to growth in Medicaid expenditures at the 0.01 level, except AIDS enrollment, which was significant at the 0.05 level.

Federal Medicaid policy was defined using the Boren amendment and the Budget Reconciliation Act of 1987. The Boren amendment required states to set "reasonable" payment rates for nursing facilities and hospitals. The amendment resulted in providers suing state Medicaid programs in more than 30 states. In most cases, providers prevailed and states were required to raise Medicaid payment rates; in some cases, states were required to retroactively raise Medicaid payment rates.[8] OBRA of 1987 established a single category of skilled nursing care facilities (SNFs). In effect, the legislation required intermediate care facilities (ICFs) to meet the higher standards of SNFs, and required the states to recognize the increased costs associated with compliance

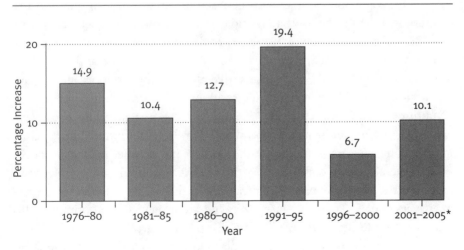

FIGURE 5.5

Average Annual Percentage Increase in Medicaid Expenditures

*2001–2005 is projected

Source: HCFA. 2000a. *Healthcare Financing Review: Medicare and Medicaid Statistical Supplement 2000*, p. 89.

in their payment rates. Wade and Berg (1995) identify, but did not include in their definition, other federal policies that might have caused an increase in Medicaid expenditures: the Medicare Catastrophic Coverage Act of 1988, which required states to cover low-income Medicare beneficiaries; and the Zebley decision, which retroactively expanded Medicaid coverage for disabled children. The Boren amendment and OBRA of 1987 were significantly related to growth in Medicaid expenditures at the 0.01 level.

State Medicaid policy was defined by Wade and Berg using the following variables as crude measures of the state's political ideology: tax price, tax capacity, and the governor's political party affiliation. Tax price is an estimate of the median voter's share of the unit cost of providing an additional unit of service to a Medicaid enrollee and was expected to be negatively related to growth in Medicaid expenditures. Tax capacity is the median household income and was expected to be positively related to growth in Medicaid expenditures.

According to Wade and Berg, the effect of state policy variables on the growth of Medicaid expenditures is more evident by category of expenditures than expenditures as a total. However, tax price was usually a negative indicator—(sometimes a significant one); as tax price decreases, Medicaid expenditures increase. Tax capacity was usually a positive indicator (sometimes significant); as tax capacity (i.e., state income) increases, Medicaid expenditures increase.

The governor's political party affiliation suggests that Republican governorship is associated with significantly greater growth in Medicaid expenditures than Democratic governorships, but was statistically significant only in the expenditure models for the aged Medicaid enrollees. Statistical significance was reported by Kronebusch (1993) for aged, blind, disabled, and child Medicaid enrollees, but not for adult Medicaid enrollees.

The Wade and Berg and Kronebusch research calls into question the commonly accepted belief that Democrats spend more on social programs than Republicans. Kronebusch offers two plausible explanations for the positive relationship between conservative ideology of the state and growth in Medicaid expenditures. First, conservative ideology may support higher payment rates to providers, which would result in higher growth in Medicaid expenditures. Second, conservative ideology may support spending a relatively generous amount on groups that conservatives have determined deserve, or merit, public support—groups like the aged, blind, disabled, and children.

Several factors contribute to the relatively slow growth in Medicaid expenditures in recent years (Medicaid expenditures have increased an annual average of 8.4 percent since 1996 and are projected to continue at this rate through 2005): a strong economy that slowed enrollment growth, lower healthcare provider prices, increased managed care penetration into Medicaid populations, and restrictions on disproportionate share hospital (DSH) payments (Provost and Hughes 2000).

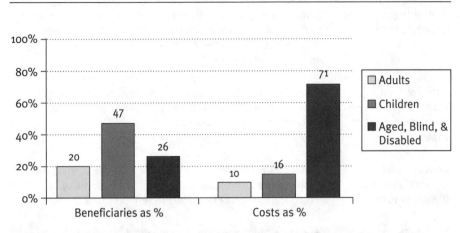

FIGURE 5.6
Medicaid
Beneficiaries
by Eligibility
Category
and Cost

Source: CMS Web-Based Chart Series. "Program Information on Medicare, Medicaid, SCHIP, and Other Programs." [Online retrieval, 02/04/04]. http://www.cms.gov.

In relation to Medicaid costs, it is important to point out who is served by the Medicaid program. In 1998, 41.4 million people were enrolled in the Medicaid program and 40.6 million people actually accessed services costing $175 billion with per capita cost of $4,310. However, an analysis of the Medicaid beneficiary cost by eligibility grouping indicates that a relatively small proportion of Medicare beneficiaries are responsible for the majority of Medicaid costs (see Figure 5.6). For instance, while the aged, the blind, and the disabled represent 26 percent of all Medicaid beneficiaries, they account for 71 percent of all Medicaid costs.

Legislative Attempts to Control Costs of Medicare and Medicaid

The federal government discovered early that Medicare and Medicaid use and resulting costs had been under-projected, and that retroactive, cost-based reimbursement to hospitals and charge-based reimbursement to physicians was inflationary. As early as 1971, the federal government attempted to control healthcare costs through legislation and regulation. Table 5.3 lists the attempts to control costs.

Wage and Price Controls of 1971	Imposed wage and price controls in an attempt to deal with inflation throughout the economy. In the healthcare industry, price increases were limited according to federal price guidelines through 1974.
Social Security Amendments of 1972	Authorized price controls in the healthcare industry and directed the Department of Health, Education, and Welfare (DHEW) to develop a prospective payment method of reimbursement.

TABLE 5.3
Legislation and
Regulation to
Control
Healthcare
Costs

continued on next page

TABLE 5.3 (*Continued*)	**Professional Standards Review Organizations (PSROs) of 1972**	Established a peer-review program to determine appropriateness and quality of care delivered in hospitals to beneficiaries of federal programs. Inappropriate admissions, length of stays, or surgeries resulted in reductions in reimbursements.
	National Health Planning and Resource Development Act of 1974	Established certificate-of-need regulations, which required hospitals to obtain approval for capital expenditures and improvements that cost over $100,000.
	Omnibus Budget Reconciliation Act (OBRA) of 1980	Eliminated the "prior hospitalization" requirement for home health services reimbursement, and eliminated the limitation on the total number of home health services visits.
	Tax Equity and Fiscal Responsibility Act (TEFRA) of 1982	Placed rate-of-increase limits on inpatient hospital services; replaced Professional Standards Review Organizations (PSROs) with Peer Review Organizations (PROs); extended Medicare coverage to hospice care for those certified as terminally ill; made Medicare the secondary payer for working beneficiaries covered by their employers.
	Social Security Amendments of 1983	Introduced hospital prospective payment based on DRGs to replace retroactive, cost-based payment; required federal workers to pay Medicare hospital insurance payroll tax (federal workers had been exempt from the tax prior to 1983).
	Deficit Reduction Act (DEFRA) of 1984	Froze physician fees and established the Participating Physician and Supplies Program (PAR), which allowed physicians to accept assignment (i.e., physicians would accept the Medicare-approved charge as full payment and would not balance bill the Medicare beneficiaries). In return, Medicare would list physicians in a directory available to beneficiaries, and expedite billing.
	Consolidated Omnibus Budget Reconciliation Act (COBRA) of 1985	Made Medicare coverage mandatory for state and local government employees hired after 1985; directed HHS to develop a prospective payment system for physicians. As part of COBRA, Section 9121, or the Emergency Medical Treatment and Active Labor Act (EMTALA), also known as the anti-dumping law, requires that hospitals with emergency rooms 1) must provide a medical screening examination to anyone requesting such examination in order to determine whether the individual is in an emergency medical condition; 2) in the event that the hospital determines that the individual is in an emergency condition, the hospital must provide medical treatment to stabilize the condition; and 3) must not transfer individuals in emergency medical conditions unless a) the patient requests the transfer after knowing the hospital is obligated to continue treatment or b) the transfer is medically appropriate. Hospitals and emergency room physicians that violate EMTALA can be fined up to $50,000 each per violation (see http//www4.law.cornell.edu/uscode/42/1395dd.html).[9]

Omnibus Budget Reconciliation Act (OBRA) of 1986	Placed maximum allowable actual charge (MAAC) limits on the amounts physicians could bill Medicare beneficiaries above the Medicare-approved charge.
Medicare Catastrophic Coverage Act of 1988	Expanded Medicare benefits to include outpatient prescriptions, placed a cap on patient costs for catastrophic medical expenses, and expanded SNF coverage. Funded by increases in the Part B premium and a new supplemental income premium.
Medicare Catastrophic Coverage Act Repeal of 1989	Restored benefits to previous levels and canceled new premium; directed HHS to develop a prospective payment system for physicians.
Omnibus Budget Reconciliation Act (OBRA) of 1989	Introduced new fee schedule for physician services and limited the amount above the fee schedule that physicians could bill beneficiaries; tied increases in fee schedule to volume performance standards. Prohibited physician referrals under Medicare for clinical lab services when the referring physician has a financial relationship (known as self-referrals) with the lab unless the terms of certain statutory or regulatory exceptions are met (known as Stark I regulations, named after the bill's sponsor, Congressman Pete Stark D-CA).
Omnibus Budget Reconciliation Act (OBRA) of 1990	Increased Part B deductible to $100; moved the reimbursement for inpatient hospital capital costs from cost-based reimbursement to prospective reimbursement based on DRGs.
HCFA Resource-Based Relative Value System (RBRVS) of 1992	Introduced a prospective payment system for physicians over a three-year implementation period.
Omnibus Budget Reconciliation Act (OBRA) of 1993	Removed cap on wages subject to Medicare Part A payroll tax; introduced new tax on Social Security benefits above certain incomes. Expanded Stark I prohibitions on physician self-referrals to include additional designated health services: physical therapy, occupational therapy, radiology including MRI, CT, and ultrasound, radiation therapy, durable medical equipment and supplies, parental and enteral nutrients, prosthetics, orthotics and prosthetic devices, home health services, outpatient prescription drugs, and inpatient and outpatient hospital services (known as Stark II). Final rules published in January, 2001, "generally permit" self-referrals as long as compensation paid to the physician with an ownership interest is not more than would be paid to a physician who did not have an ownership interest.
Personal Responsibility and Work Opportunity Reconciliation Act of 1996	Made restrictive changes to welfare eligibility that in turn restricted eligibility to Medicaid.

continued on next page

TABLE 5.3 (*Continued*)	**Health Insurance Portability and Accountability Act (HIPAA) of 1996**	Protected currently insured people from losing coverage because of job change or family illness; required insurers who offer small group coverage to make policies available to all small groups; allowed for a pilot study of medical savings accounts (MSAs) or insurance accounts for the self-employed and small-employers which would allow the beneficiaries substantial rebates if use is low; mandated standardized, electronic billing by 2000; allowed the self-employed to increase their tax deduction for health insurance costs from 30 percent to 80 percent of the cost by 2006; and tightened fraud and abuse rules.
	Balanced Budget Act (BBA) of 1997	Cut Medicare program expenditures by $115 billion over five years; froze disproportionate share hospital payments in 32 states and cut payments in 18 states; gave states the option to require Medicaid beneficiaries to enroll in managed care; allowed provider-sponsored organizations (PSOs) to bid on Medicare and Medicaid business; and introduced SCHIP, which provided funding over five years to expand health coverage for children.
	Balanced Budget Refinement Act (BBRA) of 1999	Recognized as BBA relief, BBRA restored Medicare program expenditures by $16 billion over five years.
	Medicare, Medicaid, and SCHIP Benefits Improvement and Protection Act (BIPA) of 2000	Recognized in part as BBA relief, BIPA restored Medicare program expenditures to hospitals by $35 billion over five years. The $109 billion appropriations bill includes increased funding for the National Institutes of Health's medical research; increased funding for the Centers for Disease Control; increased funding for Ryan White CARE Act; and increased funding for independent children's hospitals to train pediatricians.
	Medicare Prescription Drug, Improvement, and Modernization Act (MMA) of 2003	Recognized as the most extensive Medicare reform in its history, MMA introduced prescription drug benefits; provided $25 billion in payment improvements for providers with incentives for hospitals to report quality data to the government and bonuses to underserved areas; imposed an 18-month moratorium on the development of specialty hospitals; replaced Medicare+Choice with Medicare Advantage; allowed people with high-deductible health insurance policies to shelter some income from taxes in Health Savings Accounts (HSAs); and allowed drug importation from Canada after the drugs are certified as safe.

Health Insurance Portability and Accountability Act (HIPAA) of 1996

The Health Insurance Portability and Accountability Act (HIPAA) of 1996, which was jointly sponsored by Sen. Edward Kennedy (D-Mass.) and Sen.

Nancy Kassebaum (R-Kan.), approved virtually unanimously by both the House and Senate and signed into law by President Clinton on August 21, 1996, was designed to improve the availability of health insurance to working families and their children. HIPAA includes important new protections for an estimated 25 million Americans who move from one job to another, who are self-employed, or who have pre-existing medical conditions.

For details on the most important provisions of HIPAA, see Appendix 5.1.

HIPAA Administrative Simplification Standards

As mandated by HIPAA, HHS has published final rules on five standards that make up the administrative simplification program, a program to streamline the processing of healthcare claims, to reduce the volume of paperwork, and to save the healthcare system billions of dollars while providing better service for providers, insurers, and patients (see Table 5.4 for timetable). By promoting the greater use of electronic transactions and the elimination of inefficient paper forms, HHS estimates that administrative simplification standards will provide a net savings of $29.9 billion to the healthcare industry over the next ten years (HHS 2000a).

HHS published final rules on transactions and code sets in August, 2000. By law, health plans, healthcare clearinghouses, and healthcare providers that choose to transmit their financial transactions in electronic format must comply with these rules by October, 2002. Small health plans (i.e., less than

Standard	Final Rule Published	Compliance Required	
			TABLE 5.4
Transactions & Code Sets	08/17/00	10/16/02 (2003 < $5 million)	Timetable for Adoption of Administrative
National Provider Identifier	01/23/04	10/23/07 (2007 < $5 million)	Simplification Standards
National Employer Identifier	05/31/02	07/30/04 (2005 < $5 million)	
Privacy	08/14/02	04/13/03 (2004 < $5 million)	
Security	02/20/03	04/20/05 (2006 < $5 million)	

Source: CMS. 2004. "HIPAA Administrative Simplification." [Online retrieval, 02/05/04]. http://www.cms.gov/hipaa/default.asp.

$5 million in receipts) must comply by October, 2003. Provisions of the final rules include the following:

- Health plans will be able to pay providers, authorize services, certify referrals, and coordinate benefits using a standard electronic format for each transaction. Providers will be able to use a standard format to determine eligibility for insurance coverage, determine the status of a claim, request authorizations for services or specialist referrals, and receive electronic remittance to post receivables.
- Rules also include new standards for other common transactions and coding standards for reporting diagnoses and procedures in the transactions.
- Employers who provide health insurance to their workers and their dependents also will be able to use a standard electronic format to enroll or disenroll employees and to submit premium payments to any health plans with whom the employer contracts.
- The rules outline a process for maintaining the format and content of the standard transactions system. National healthcare standard organizations and data content committees will accept and review requests for changes to the standards.

HHS cautioned that these transactions and code sets final rules were being released under the assumption that national identifiers for employers and providers and final health information privacy rules would take effect at approximately the same time (HHS 2000a).

While HIPAA administrative simplification is intended to save health plans, healthcare clearinghouses, and healthcare providers over the long term, initial expenditures required to implement the requirements of the final rules on transactions and codes sets will be significant. Most of these initial costs will be in the form of consulting and legal fees, additional operations personnel, and information systems development (DeMuro and Gantt 2001). HHS originally projected that administrative simplification would cost hospitals about $3.8 billion over five years, but later revised that projection to $17.6 billion. The American Hospital Association believes the cost will be closer to $22.5 billion and that the implementing regulations go far beyond what Congress intended with the original legislation (Tieman 2000).

HHS published final rules on national employer identifiers in May of 2002. In the past, a single employer would use multiple identification numbers, which slows activities such as health plan enrollments and premium payments. Under the final rule on national employer identifiers, employers must use only their already existing Employer Identification Number (EIN), which is issued and maintained by the Internal Revenue Service. Potential savings are accounted for in the $1.5 billion already referenced under transactions and code sets and national provider identifiers (HHS 2001). Compliance is set for July of 2004 for larger organizations and July of 2005 for smaller organizations.

HHS published final rules on national provider identifiers in January of 2004 with compliance expected in May of 2007 for larger organizations and May of 2008 for smaller organizations. In the past, healthcare providers were assigned different identification numbers by private health plans, hospitals, nursing homes, and public programs like Medicare and Medicaid. Under the final rule, every healthcare provider must apply for an eight-digit identifier that they would use whenever processing claims electronically.

HHS published proposed rules on privacy of electronically transmitted personal health information in November, 1999. The proposed rules generated over 52,000 comments to HHS. Comments represented a wide variety of concerns; the primary concern expressed by providers was the cost of implementation.

HHS published final rules on health information privacy in December, 2000. By law, health plans, healthcare clearinghouses, and healthcare providers that choose to transmit their financial and administrative transactions in electronic format had to comply with these rules by April, 2003 and February, 2004 for smaller organizations. The final rules covered all medical records and other individually identifiable health information held or disclosed by a health plan, healthcare clearinghouse, and healthcare providers in any form, whether communicated electronically, on paper, or orally. The Office of Civil Rights is responsible for enforcing the rules (OCR 2001).

The final rules strengthen the security of medical records and extend coverage to include paper records, oral communications, and electronic information. The new rules apply to all consumers whether they are privately insured, publicly insured through Medicare or Medicaid, or uninsured. Both public and private sector organizations are covered by the rules and are prohibited from using or disclosing protected health information except as stipulated in the final rules (HHS 2000b).

HHS intends the privacy rules to accomplish three broad objectives: (1) define the circumstances in which protected health information may be used and disclosed; (2) establish certain patient rights regarding protected health information; and (3) require that organizations adopt administrative safeguards to ensure the privacy of protected health information. Penalties for noncompliance include civil fines up to $25,000 per calendar year for each violation and criminal penalties up to $250,000 or a 10-year prison term, or both. For criminal liability, HHS must prove that the organization intended to disclose protected information or that the organization somehow profited from the disclosure (DeMuro and Gantt 2001).

Provisions of the final rules on health information privacy include the three following (HHS 2000b).

1. Circumstances in which protected health information may be used and disclosed. An individual's health information can be used for health purposes only.
   - Health plans, clearinghouses, and providers can use patient health information only for the purposes of treatment, payment, or operations. Patient health information cannot be used for non-health purposes—such as by employers making personnel decisions or financial organizations making financial decisions—without the expressed authorization of the patient.
   - Health plans, clearinghouses, and providers should provide only the minimum health information necessary for purposes of the disclosure. This provision does not apply to the transfer of medical records for treatment purposes.
   - Health plans, clearinghouses, and providers must ensure informed and voluntary patient authorization for all nonroutine disclosures of health information.
   - Health plans, clearinghouses, and providers may disclose patient health information without patient authorization for the following reasons which the government deems in the public's best interest:
     - Oversight of the healthcare system, including quality assurance activities;
     - Public health concerns;
     - Research limited to a waiver of authorization by a privacy board or Institutional Review Board;
     - Judicial and administrative proceedings;
     - Limited law enforcement activities;
     - Emergency circumstances;
     - Identification of the deceased, or cause of death;
     - Facility patient directories; and
     - Activities related to national defense and security.
2. Patient rights regarding protected health information. Patients have significant new rights to understand and control how health plans, clearinghouses, and providers should use patient health information.
   - Health plans and providers must give patients a clear written explanation of how health plans and providers will use, keep, and disclose the patient's health information.
   - Health plans and providers must give patients access to their medical records. Patients must be able to see and obtain copies of their records, amendments to their records, and a history of disclosures.
   - Health plans and providers must receive patient authorization before information is disclosed to others. Patient authorization must meet specific requirements. Providers are required to obtain patient authorization before sharing information for treatment, payment, and operational purposes. Patients must authorize disclosure for all

nonroutine and non-treatment purposes such as releasing information to financial institutions that might be determining mortgage or loan qualification or life insurance premiums. Patients have the right to request restrictions on the uses and disclosures of their protected health information.

- Health plans and providers generally cannot condition treatment based on a patient's agreement to disclose health information for non-routine uses.
- Patients have the right to complain to the health plan or provider, or HHS, concerning perceived violations of patient rights regarding protected health information.

3. Administrative safeguards to ensure the privacy of protected health information. Final rules establish administrative safeguard standards that health plans and providers must adopt, but the final rules leave implementing policies and procedures to the discretion of the health plans and providers to account for their business, size, and available resources. However, at a minimum health plans and providers must provide the following:

- Written privacy procedures including who has access to protected information, how protected information will be used, and under what conditions protected information would be disclosed to business associates. Health plans and providers must report privacy breaches of business associates (any outside organization that handles confidential health information).
- Employee training on privacy protection procedures and the designation of a privacy officer.
- Grievance procedures to provide patients with a mechanism to make inquiries and complaints regarding the privacy of their records.

In August of 2002, HHS released final amendments to the privacy rule (many healthcare providers had hoped that the privacy standard would either be abandoned in its entirety by the Bush administration or struck down in court). As anticipated, the amended final privacy rule permits, but does not require, covered entities to obtain written patient consents before the entity uses protected health information (PHI). Covered healthcare providers that have a direct treatment relationship with patients must make a "good faith effort" to obtain from the patient a signed acknowledgment of receipt of the provider's notice of privacy practices the first time treatment is rendered. HHS also adopted most of the proposed changes regarding the permissable use of PHI for marketing without a patient's specific authorization. Likewise, HHS adopted many of the proposed changes regarding de-identification and generally permits uses and disclosures of limited data sets of PHI for the purposes or research, public health activities, and healthcare operations provided that the data set does not include directly identifiable information (HFMA 2002).

Unlike the costs associated with the final rules for transactions and code sets (the majority of which are initial costs associated with implementation), health information privacy costs will include not only implementation costs, but significant ongoing costs associated with ongoing maintenance of compliance systems and processes that may not be offset by future savings. HIPAA health information privacy rules may also impede the flow of health information to healthcare providers trying to coordinate patient care.[10] Another difficulty for health plans and providers will be ensuring HIPAA compliance with business associates like vendors, attorneys, and consultants. Monitoring and influencing how business associates use protected health information will be difficult for health plans and providers. In most cases, health plans and providers will need to negotiate new contracts that address privacy issues. Probably the most difficult compliance issue for health plans and providers will be the privacy rule to provide patients with an accounting of all disclosures of protected information while also giving patients the opportunity to amend or correct the information (DeMuro and Gantt 2000).

On February of 2003, HHS published its final rules for security with compliance set for April of 2005 for larger organizations and April of 2006 for smaller organizations. The final rules provide a series of implementation specifications for the security of protected health information in electronic form. Broadly, covered entities must (HFMA 2003):

• Ensure the confidentiality, integrity, and availability of all electronic protected health information that the covered entity creates, receives, maintains, or transmits;
• Protect against any reasonably anticipated threats or hazards to the security and integrity of such information;
• Protect against any reasonably anticipated uses or disclosures of such information that are not otherwise permitted or required; and
• Ensure compliance by its workforce.

All organizations that transmit health information electronically will be required to develop a security plan, to provide training for employees, and to secure the electronic and physical access. The rule also includes provisions for electronic signatures (HHS 2001b). The final rule did clarify that because paper-to-paper faxes, person-to-person telephone calls, video teleconferencing, or messages left on voice mail were not in electronic form before the transmission, those activities are not covered by the rule (HFMA 2003).

Pawola et al. (2000) have identified ten critical success factors designed to ensure a compliance with the security rule:

1. Establish an overall information security plan for all systems.
2. Secure user authorization by implementing identifiers, passwords, and other devices (e.g., biometric systems).
3. Access new control mechanisms that will restrict the ability to view, update, and print patient data according to who the users are and why they need access to the record.
4. Develop audit trails to monitor and identify who accesses secured data.
5. Implement physical security and disaster recovery protocols to ensure that essential data can be restored quickly during a disaster situation.
6. Protect remote access points and external electronic communications to ensure security at the point of entry and during transmission.
7. Monitor data integrity to ensure that systems have built-in non-repudiation functionality.
8. Train users on organizational practices for communication and awareness of security and confidentiality practices.
9. Integrate risk management with all systems to analyze the strengths and weaknesses in regard to security and confidentiality.
10. Maintain complete documentation on compliance as a record for Federal Security Audits as well as other audits.

HIPAA Civil Monetary Penalty (CMP) Authority

HIPAA of 1996 provided the legislative authority to HHS Office of Inspector General (OIG) to implement changes to the agency's civil monetary penalty (CMP) authority. OIG issued the final rule on April 26, 2000 to become effective on its publication date (see http://dhhs.gov/progorg/oig/oigreg/cmpfinal.pdf). Changes in the agency's CMP authority include the following:

• Expands the OIG's authority to impose CMPs to all federal healthcare programs;
• Increases the maximum monetary penalty for violations occurring after January 1, 1997, from $2,000 to $10,000; and
• Creates additional CMPs for individuals retaining control or ownership interest in a facility to which they refer Medicare patients, upcoding and claims for medically unnecessary services, providing medically unnecessary services, inducing beneficiaries to choose a particular provider or supplier, and making false certification of patient eligibility to home health agencies.

The Balanced Budget Act of 1997 gave OIG the authority to grant safe harbors, that is, technical violations that would warrant a CMP, but would not result in federal prosecution. While OIG has 23 published safe harbors under the anti-kickback law, which is a criminal statute, OIG proposed its first CMP safe harbor on May 2, 2000. The CMP safe harbor applies, under certain conditions, to independent dialysis facilities that pay Medicare Part

B and Medigap premiums for financially needy Medicare beneficiaries with end-stage renal disease. The OIG noted its concern that by offering financial assistance to needy Medicare beneficiaries as part of an advertisement or solicitation, providers might influence a beneficiary's choice of provider; therefore, providers are prohibited from advertising that they would pay premiums as one of the conditions under this safe harbor (HFMA 2000b).

Balanced Budget Act (BBA) of 1997

The Balanced Budget Act (BBA) of 1997 represents the most significant Medicare reform since the advent of prospective payment in 1983. The BBA promised to balance the federal budget by 2002, but the projected bankruptcy of the Medicare Trust Fund in 2029 fuels continued debate over entitlement programs. Ernst & Young warned clients that the BBA was not the end of a budget-cutting process, but rather just the beginning (Ernst & Young 1997). BBA includes incremental steps toward reforming Medicare and makes a move toward universal healthcare coverage through SCHIP. BBA charges a federal commission with proposing structural changes to Medicare while introducing Medicare+Choice, a new program intended to give Medicare beneficiaries new choices of private health plans. For details on the most important provisions of BBA of 1997, see Appendix 5.2.

Balanced Budget Refined Act (BBRA) of 1999

After significant evidence that BBA was cutting more than the projected $115 billion from the federal budget (some estimated that BBA was cutting two to three times more than the $115 billion originally intended)[11], Congress passed and the president signed the Balanced Budget Refinement Act (BBRA) in November of 1999. The plan provided an estimated $16 billion in Medicare relief over five years. For details on the most important provisions of BBRA, see Appendix 5.3.

Medicare, Medicaid, and SCHIP Benefits Improvement and Protection (BIPA) Act of 2000

In December of 2000, Congress passed and the president signed the Medicare, Medicaid, and SCHIP Benefits Improvement and Protection (BIPA) of 2000. BIPA provided about $35 billion over five years and increased Medicare and Medicaid provider payments; added preventive benefits and reduced beneficiary cost sharing under Medicare; and improved insurance options for low-income children, low-income families, and low-income seniors. For details of the most important provisions of BIPA, see Appendix 5.4.

Medicare Prescription Drug, Improvement, and Modernization Act (MMA) of 2003

In late November 2003, Congress passed the Medicare Prescription Drug, Improvement, and Modernization Act (MMA) of 2003 which President Bush then signed in early December. Heralded as the most significant expansion of the Medicare program since its inception, the Act was a compromise between Republicans who wanted to privatize Medicare and Democrats who wanted to expand Medicare benefits. In addition to the increased payments to health-care providers referenced earlier in the chapter, MMA provides the following (HHS 2003) as discussed below.

Medicare beneficiaries without drug coverage will be eligible for the Medicare-endorsed Prescription Drug Card, available in 2004 and effective until the full drug benefit is available in 2006. The card is estimated to save beneficiaries between 10 and 25 percent on most prescription drugs. Low-income seniors (incomes below 135 percent of poverty) will be given immediate financial assistance of $600 per year annually in addition to the card.

Medicare-Endorsed Prescription Drug Discount Care

Beginning in 2006, Medicare beneficiaries will have access to at least the standard drug benefit described below:

Medicare Drug Benefit

- Monthly premium of about $35 (which may be means tested along with Part B premiums).
  - Annual deductible of $250.
  - Coinsurance of 25 percent up to an initial coverage limit of $2,250.
  - No coverage for prescription drug costs between $2,250 and $3,600.
- Protection against high out-of-pocket prescription drug costs, with copays of $2 for generics and $5 for all other drugs, once an enrollee's out-of-pocket prescription drug costs reach $3,600.

Low-income seniors will not be required to pay the monthly premium or the annual deductible, will have no coverage gap, and will not be required to pay copays.

Private companies will administer the drug benefit on a regional basis. Beginning in 2010, traditional Medicare will face competition from private plans in six metropolitan areas in which at least two private plans enroll a minimum of 25 percent of the existing Medicare beneficiaries. For those who remain in traditional Medicare, premium increases will be capped at five percent per year and waived for low-income seniors. The competition will serve as a demonstration project and will last for six years.

MMA will speed generic drugs to the market by limiting the ability of pharmaceutical companies to block cheaper equivalents.

Generic Drugs

MMA generally maintains the ban on drug importation, but permits Canadian imports if deemed safe by HHS.

Drug Importation

Savings for State Governments and Employers

In addition to helping Medicare beneficiaries, MMA helps states by paying an increasing percentage of current state costs for prescription drugs (states paid $7 billion for prescription drugs for dual eligibles in 2002). The percentage starts at 10 percent initially and increases to 25 percent over the next ten years.

For employers who offer (or continue to offer) their Medicare-eligible retirees prescription coverage, MMA provides a 28 percent subsidy for each enrollee's annual prescription drug cost between $250 and $5,000.

New Preventive Benefits

Beginning in 2005, all newly enrolled Medicare beneficiaries will be covered for an initial physical exam, and all beneficiaries will be covered for cardiovascular screening blood tests, and those beneficiaries at risk will be covered for a diabetes screen.

Modernizing Drug Delivery Systems

MMA also calls for the use of electronic prescribing in the delivery systems in order to reduce transcribing errors and help prevent costly adverse drug interactions.

Specialty Hospitals

MMA imposes an 18-month moratorium on the development of new specialty hospitals and the expansion of existing specialty hospitals in order to research the effects of specialty hospitals on overall costs.

Health-Related Savings Accounts

MMA allows people with high-deductible health insurance policies (at least $1,000 deductible for singles and $2,000 deductible for couples) to shelter income from taxes equal to the amount of the deductible.

Medicare Advantage

MMA establishes Medicare Advantage to replace Medicare+Choice as Medicare's managed care product. Medicare Advantage should have higher payments to healthcare providers and less cost and more choices of providers available to the enrollee.

Early criticism of MMA has focused on its cost (the White House projected a ten-year cost of $534 billion in its 2004/05 budget) which will be addressed in Chapter 16 and its popularity with Medicare beneficiaries, many of whom already have prescription drug coverage provided by employers after the beneficiaries retired or through Medigap policies. A well-respected study indicated that 73 percent of Medicare beneficiaries had some drug coverage in 1998 (Poisal and Murray 2001). MMA prohibits Medicare beneficiaries from having insurance coverage that would cover the beneficiary's share of drug costs under the new benefit. Congress cited two reasons for this controversial provision: to prevent duplication of coverage and to ensure that beneficiaries would bear some of the cost out-of-pocket to help reduce overutilization (Pear 2003).

TABLE 5.5
What Does
MMA Really
Give Seniors?

Senior's Yearly Rx Cost	Senior Pays	Medicare Pays	Percentage of Rx Cost Paid by Senior*
$ 250	$ 250	$ 0	268%
500	313	188	147
1,000	438	562	86
1,500	563	937	66
2,000	688	1,313	55
2,500	1,000	1,500	57
3,000	1,500	1,500	64
4,000	2,500	1,500	73
5,000	3,500	1,500	78
7,500	3,720	3,780	55
10,000	3,845	6,155	43
15,000	4,095	10,905	30

*Percentages assume the estimated $420 in yearly premiums paid by the seniors. Including premiums, the senior break-even point would be around $825 a year in drug spending.
Note: In 1998, the average senior without drug coverage spent $550 per year on prescription drugs and the average senior with drug coverage spent $1,003 per year on prescription drugs (Poisal and Murray, 2001).
Source: Scott, J. S. 2004b. "Tackle Your Healthcare Problems." Presentation at the Winter meeting of the HFMA South Texas/ACHE San Antonio Chapters, San Antonio, 30 January.

Scott (2004b) developed a chart (Table 5.5) that provides Medicare beneficiaries an idea of what the drug benefit provides them.

Medicare/Medicaid Fraud and Abuse

One of the most significant initiatives by the federal government to control healthcare costs has been the recent emphasis on enforcing fraud and abuse statutes. Fraud is an intentional misrepresentation of fact designed to induce reliance by another. Abuse is an unintentional misrepresentation of fact. The Coalition Against Insurance Fraud estimated that public and private health insurance fraud cost the industry $53 billion in 1994. According to the coalition, categories of fraud and their incidence of occurrence include (Ernst & Young 1996):

- Services billed but not rendered (49 percent);
- Forgiveness (i.e., kickbacks) of deductibles and coinsurance (12 percent);
- Fraudulent coding (i.e., upcoding) (7 percent);
- Billing two parties for the same service (4 percent);
- Billing for brand-name drugs when generics were dispensed (3 percent);
- Billing for unlicensed practitioners (2 percent); and
- Other (2 percent).

Fraudulent or abusive practices can result in criminal and civil liability and administrative sanctions. Criminal liability under the Fraud and False Statements Act can result in fines and imprisonment. Civil liability under the False Claims Act can result in fines of $10,000 for each false claim plus three times the total amount of the loss by the government. Civil liability under the False Claim Act extends to those who submit the fraudulent claim and to those who have knowledge that the claim is fraudulent. Knowledge is defined as either actual knowledge or reckless disregard for the claim's validity. Therefore, the government does not have to prove that false claims were submitted with the intent to defraud (i.e., the healthcare organization knew), but that the false claims were submitted in an environment that was likely to produce false claims (i.e., the healthcare organization should have known). Furthermore, the government must prove its case by a preponderance of evidence in civil cases; the burden of proof in criminal cases is beyond a reasonable doubt (Russo 1997).

The Anti-Kickback Act, which is a criminal statute, can result in criminal fines up to $25,000 and civil fines up to $50,000 as well as five years in prison. Administrative sanctions can result in possible exclusion from federal programs as specified in the Balanced Budget Act of 1997. The Anti-Kickback Act was passed in 1972 and prohibits anyone from knowingly or willfully soliciting or accepting any type of remuneration to induce referrals for health services that are reimbursed by the federal government.

The Stark law is similar to the Anti-Kickback Act, and as a result is often confused with the Anti-Kickback Act. The Stark law is a federal civil statute passed in 1989 (Stark I) with amendments passed in 1993 (Stark II). The Stark law prohibits physicians from referring patients to an entity with which the ordering physician has an ownership interest or compensation arrangement if patient payments come from either the Medicare or Medicaid programs (Watnik 2000). Final rules on Stark II were released in January, 2001, after years of vigorous debate between the American Medical Association and the federal government. While prohibiting physician self-referral to most organizations that they own in whole or in part, the final rules "generally permit" self-referrals as long as compensation paid to the physician with an ownership interest is not more than would be paid to a physician who did not have an ownership interest (Romano 2001a). Current federal government initiatives regarding fraud and abuse are listed in Table 5.6.

Federal Safe Harbors

The 1972 purpose of the federal anti-kickback law is to protect the federal healthcare programs and their patients from fraud and abuse by limiting the influence of money on healthcare decisions. The law states that anyone who knowingly and willfully receives or pays anything of value to influence the referral of federal healthcare program business, including Medicare and Medicaid, is committing a felony punishable by up to five years in prison, criminal fines up to $25,000, civil fines up to $50,000, and possible exclusion from participating in federal programs. Most healthcare providers argued that the law was overly broad and punishment was severe for commercial arrangements

Health Insurance Portability and Accountability Act (HIPAA) of 1996	Appropriates a new trust fund to pay for expanded investigations and broadens the authority of the FBI in investigations.	**TABLE 5.6** Government Initiatives on Fraud and Abuse
Operation Restore Trust	A two-year pilot program initiated in 1995 to detect and punish fraud and abuse in the home health agencies, nursing homes, and durable medical equipment (DME) companies in five states (Texas, California, Florida, New York, and Illinois), which represent over 50 percent of all Medicare business. On May 20, 1997, HHS announced that the program had recovered $188 million and extended the program to 13 additional states (HFMA 1997a).	
DRG Payment Window (72-Hour Rule)	Prohibits a hospital from billing for outpatient services provided by a controlling entity within 72 hours of an admission. This initiative has recovered $71.3 million from 2,672 hospitals through 2000.	
Billings for Teaching Physicians	Prohibits a hospital from billing for teaching physician services when the teaching physician is not actually present at the time of service. This initiative has recovered $75 million from six institutions through 2000.	
Qui Tam Provisions	Protects and rewards (15 to 25 percent of the total recovery) whistleblowers who identify instances of fraud and abuse to the federal government. Total recoveries from qui tam lawsuits exceed $2.915 billion in 2,981 cases filed since 1986. The Department of Justice (DOJ) filed 483 qui tam lawsuits in 1999 resulting in recoveries of $458 million. In cases either settled or won by DOJ, the average recovery was $5.8 million and the average whistleblower (relator) award was $1.0 million (HFMA 2000d). However, DOJ takes court action on one of about 20 whistleblower complaints filed (HFMA 1999).	
Voluntary Disclosure	Limits liability for healthcare organizations that discover, identify (to the federal government), and correct billing errors and other fraudulent or abusive practices.	
Federal Safe Harbors	Payment practices to physicians that are safe from federal prosecution under the Anti-Kickback Act (see following section).	
Medicare Integrity Program	Permits HHS to contract with private organizations to decrease fraud and abuse.	

continued on next page

TABLE 5.6 *continued*	Hospital Outpatient Lab Project	Prohibits a hospital from improper unbundling and double-billing of laboratory tests. This initiative has recovered $56 million from 249 hospitals.
	Prospective Payment System Patient-Transfer Project	Prohibits a hospital for billing for a discharge when the patient was in fact transferred and only eligible for a per diem of the DRG at discharge. This initiative has recovered $429 million. Hospitals typically receive more reimbursement for a discharge than for a transfer. Medicare has specific conditions for both discharge billing and transfer billing. A discharge occurs when a patient is formally released from the hospital, dies in a hospital, or is transferred to a non-PPS hospital or facility. A transfer occurs when a patient is moved from one PPS hospital or facility to another, moved to a non-PPS hospital that is under a statewide cost control project or demonstration project, or moved to a PPS hospital whose first PPS cost-reporting period has not yet begun.
	Pneumonia Upcoding Project	This initiative has recovered $19 million from 16 hospitals (see Gundling 1998).
	Corporate Integrity Agreements (CIA)	Agreements between the Office of the Inspector General and healthcare organizations that are usually required as part of a settlement in a civil fraud investigation. The agreement identifies how the organization will ensure that compliance occurs after the settlement.

that can be beneficial to federal programs and their patients. Agreeing with this argument, in 1987 Congress authorized the OIG to identify specific safe harbors for various commercial arrangements that, while prohibited by law, would not be prosecuted.

The following 1991 safe harbors address the types of business and payment practices to physicians that are safe from federal prosecution when certain conditions are met:

- *Investment Interests.* Protects payment to an investor that is a return on an investment interest if the investment is either a) in an entity with assets greater than $50 million, of which payments are based solely on the amount of the investment interest, or b) in a smaller entity where the activities of the investors are limited.
- *Space Rental.* Protects payment by a lessee to a lessor for the use of space if the payment is set in advance and not based upon referrals or business between the parties.

- *Equipment Rental.* Protects payment by a lessee of equipment to a lessor for the use of the equipment if the payment is set in advance and not based on referrals or business generated between the parties.
- *Personal Services and Management Contracts.* Protects payment by a principal provided by the agent if the compensation is set in advance and not based on referrals or other business generated between the parties.
- *Sale of Practice.* Protects payment to a practitioner by another practitioner for the sale of the former practitioner's practice.
- *Referral Services.* Protects payment for the cost of operating the referral service made to an entity serving as a referral service.
- *Warranties.* Protects payment or exchange of anything of value under a warranty provided by a manufacturer or supplier to a buyer.
- *Discounts.* Protects a discount or other price reduction on a good or service received by a buyer if the discount is related to the purchase of a specific good or service and the discount is reported on a claim for payment.
- *Employment Relationships.* Protects payments by an employer to an employee for employment in the furnishing of any item or service.
- *Group Purchasing Organizations.* Protects payments by a vendor of goods or services to a group purchasing organization as part of an agreement to furnish goods or services to an individual entity.
- *Waiver of Beneficiary Coinsurance and Deductible Amounts.* Protects the reduction or waiver of any coinsurance or deductible amount either by a hospital if the reduction is not related to the beneficiary's stay and is not made as part of a price reduction or to an individual if the patient qualifies for certain subsidized services.

The following 1992 safe harbors (published in final form in 1996) address the types of business or payment practices to physicians that are safe from federal prosecution in managed care settings when certain conditions are present:

- Increased coverage, reduced cost-sharing amounts, or reduced premium amounts offered by health plans to beneficiaries.
- Price reductions offered by health plans to beneficiaries.

The following 1999 safe harbors address the types of business and payment practices to physicians that are safe from federal prosecution when certain conditions are met (Glasser and Bloomquist 2000):

- *Investments in Ambulatory Surgical Centers.* Protects certain investment interests in four categories of freestanding Medicare-certified ASCs: surgeon-owned ASCs, single-specialty ASCs, multi-specialty ASCs, and hospital/surgeon-owned ASCs (hospital investors must not be in a position to influence referrals).

- *Joint Ventures in Underserved Areas.* Relaxes several of the conditions of the 1991 Investment Interest safe harbor if the joint venture is in an underserved area as defined by OIG regulations.
- *Practitioner Recruitment in Underserved Areas.* Protects recruitment payments made by entities to attract needed physicians and other healthcare professional to rural and urban health professional shortage areas (HPSAs). This safe harbor requires that at least 75 percent of the recruited practitioner's revenue be from patients who reside in the HPSA and this safe harbor limits the duration of payments to three years.
- *Obstetrical Malpractice Insurance Subsidies in Underserved Areas.* Protects a hospital or other entity that pays all or a portion of the malpractice insurance premiums for practitioners engaging in obstetrical practices in HPSAs. This safe harbor requires that at least 75 percent of the effected practitioner's patients must be from the HPSA.
- *Sale of Physician Practices to Hospitals in Underserved Areas.* Protects hospitals in HPSAs that buy and hold the practice of a retiring physician until a new physician can be recruited. This safe harbor requires that the sale must be completed within three years and that the hospital must engage in good faith efforts to recruit a new practitioner.
- *Investments in Group Practices.* Protects investments by physicians in their own group practices, if the group practice meets the physician self-referral (Stark) law definition of a group practice.
- *Referral Arrangements for Specialty Services.* Protects certain arrangements when an individual or entity agrees to refer a patient to another individual or entity for specialty services in return for the party receiving the referral to refer the patient back at a certain time and under certain conditions.
- *Cooperative Hospital Services Organization.* Protects cooperative hospital service organizations (CHSOs) that qualify under section 501(e) of the Internal Revenue Service Code. CHSOs are organizations formed by two or more not-for-profit hospitals, known as patron hospitals, to provide specifically enumerated services, such as purchasing, billing, or clinical services solely for the benefit of patron hospitals.

Violations of the fraud and abuse statutes appear to be both widespread and serious. Citing widespread violations in 1995, the OIG identified 4,660 hospitals (approximately 80 percent of all hospitals) that had violated the DRG payment window (OIG 1995). Representative of the more serious violations, the Clinical Practice of the University of Pennsylvania, an approved faculty practice plan of the University of Pennsylvania Health System, agreed to a $30 million federal False Claims Act settlement in 1995. The settlement resulted from a federal audit of 100 patient records to determine if the physician billing for the patient's procedure was actually present during the procedure. Using the audit's findings, the OIG extrapolated the amount of overpayment during a six-year period. The resulting $10 million was then tripled consistent with the provisions of the False Claims Act (Eiland 1996).

In 1998, the Daughters of Charity agreed to a $586,000 settlement involving four of its hospitals that had allegedly filed false Medicare cost reports. The hospitals were accused of "knowingly" failing to report discounts on radiology film purchased from Eastman Kodak. The alleged false Medicare cost reports were brought to the government's attention by a whistleblower. Daughters of Charity admitted to no wrongdoing in the settlement (Bellandi 1998).

In 1999, Olsten Corporation, which provides staffing services for home health care agencies worldwide, and its subsidiary, Kimberly Home Health Care, agreed to pay $61 million in civil and criminal fines and penalties to settle allegations that the companies paid illegal kickbacks to secure management agreements and submitted fraudulent claims to Medicare. The federal government charged the company with selling home health agencies to Columbia/HCA below market value in exchange for an agreement to later manage them. In addition, the government charged that Olsten filed fraudulent cost reports to Medicare seeking payment for nonreimbursable expenses. A whistleblower in the case, a former Olsten vice president, received $9.8 million from the qui tam lawsuit (HFMA 1999).

In 2000, Fresenius Medical Care North America agreed to the most comprehensive corporate integrity agreement ever imposed on a company doing business with the federal government. Terms of the agreement include paying $486 million to settle federal charges that one of the subsidiaries, National Medical Care, conspired to overbill Medicare and other federal programs. While corporate integrity agreements usually run for five years, the Fresenius agreement lasts for eight years. Indictments are pending against several former executives of National Medical Care (HFMA 2000c).

In 2001, HCA (formerly Columbia/HCA) entered into the largest healthcare fraud agreement ever reached with the Department of Justice (DOJ). Under the civil settlement, HCA will pay $745 million plus interest for its alleged false billing practices. HCA also agreed to pay $95 million in criminal fines. The $745 million civil settlement includes the following civil penalties: $95 million for outpatient lab billing practices; $403 million for upcoding; $50 million for claiming unreimbursable marketing and advertising costs HCA reported were community education costs; $90 million for charging Medicare for nonreimbursable costs incurred in the purchase of home health agencies; and $106 million for billing Medicare, Medicaid, and TRICARE for home health visits that either did not occur or occurred on patients without proper authorization. HCA also signed an eight-year corporate integrity agreement with HHS. The agreement, which covers only corporate liability for certain fraud, does not resolve the allegations that HCA filed false cost reports with the federal government and that HCA paid kickbacks to physicians for referrals, nor does the agreement resolve individual wrongdoing (HFMA 2001). Several private insurance companies considered claims against HCA for hundreds of millions of dollars the private insurance companies insist were paid to HCA for fraudulent claims (Taylor 2001a) (a motion for class action certification was denied in 2003 in *Smallwood v. HCA*).

In 2002, HCA entered into settlements with the Department of Justice for $898.5 million. The settlement ended the longest and costliest healthcare fraud case which started in 1993. In the settlement, HCA paid $631 million to the Justice Department to resolve eight whistleblower lawsuits that alleged HCA falsified Medicare cost reports, paid kickbacks to physicians for patient referrals and submitted false wound-care claims. In addition, HCA committed to pay $17.5 million to state Medicaid departments to resolve similar allegations. HCA proceeded to pay $250 million in non-fraud-related cost report overpayments to CMS. HCA also paid undisclosed amounts for plaintiffs' legal bills (Taylor 2002).

In 2003, the Department of Justice filed a $323 million lawsuit against Tenet and claimed that Tenet had violated a 1994 corporate integrity agreement (CIA) signed by its predecessor, National Medical Enterprises. The CIA was signed in conjunction with a $379 million settlement against the company's psychiatric hospital subsidiary. The $323 million civil action filed under the False Claims Act alleged that Tenet illegally submitted more than 19,300 false claims for $115 million in wrongfully upcoded Medicare bills in order to maximize revenue (Taylor 2003). In an unrelated case also in 2003, Tenet agreed to a $54 million settlement with the Department of Justice to settle civil claims that might result from an investigation of two physicians who practice at a Tenet hospital. The physicians allegedly performed medically unnecessary procedures and falsely billed Medicare (Galloro 2003).

The federal government has brought a series of civil actions against nursing homes for alleged violations of the False Claims Act. When a nursing home submits a claim to the federal government for care that was substandard, the government argues that the home submitted a false claim because the claim is an "implicit certification" of compliance with all statutes and regulations including those that govern quality of care. The government first advanced the implicit certification theory for nursing homes in the case known as Tucker House (1996). The nursing home agreed that the quality of care (nutrition and wound care) was substandard and that the submission of the claim constituted a certification that the services billed (quality services) were in fact the services provided. The nursing home settled the case with the government for $600,000. While some cases similar to Tucker have been settled in the government's favor, many cases that have gone to trial have been won by the nursing homes (see *United States ex rel. Mikes v. Straus* 1999). Nursing homes argue that quality of care problems are not a legitimate basis for claims under the False Claims Act and that an expressed certification that medically necessary care was provided via the provider agreement does not mean that an implied certification exists to meet all applicable statutes and regulations for billing purposes (Landsberg and Keville 2001).

In 2000, the DOJ announced that it had reached an agreement with Lafayette General Medical Center of Louisiana regarding allegations that the hospital had improperly billed Medicare for patients that had been transferred to other facilities. When a PPS hospital admits but later transfers a patient to another PPS hospital, the first hospital is entitled to payment based on a per diem of the DRG at discharge, not the full DRG payment. Lafayette General agreed to pay $365,000 in total damages and implement a corporate integrity program that will be administered by HHS (HFMA 2000d).

In 2001, the DOJ joined a civil whistleblower lawsuit against Catholic Healthcare West (CHW), one of the nation's most prominent Roman Catholic hospital systems. The suit alleged that the Sacramento regional office and three of its hospitals padded annual Medicare cost reports and kept reserve Medicare cost reports to document disallowed costs and set aside reserves in case Medicare reimbursement had to be returned (Bellandi 2001).

Violations of fraud and abuse statutes have not been limited to providers. Blue Cross/Blue Shield of Illinois, the Medicare fiscal intermediary for Illinois and Michigan, pled guilty to eight felony counts in 1998, and agreed to pay $144 million in penalties. Blue Cross/Blue Shield of Illinois admitted to manipulating work records, falsifying records to cover up poor performance as the Medicare fiscal intermediary, and obstructing a federal investigation. The wrongdoing was brought to the government's attention by a whistleblower, who will receive more than $20 million as a reward (HFMA 1998). In 2000, the DOJ joined a civil whistleblower lawsuit against the national healthcare accounting firm of KPMG. The lawsuit accuses KPMG of helping five Florida hospitals owned by HCA to falsify Medicare cost reports that they used to inflate their payments from Medicare. The government said KPMG prepared reserve Medicare cost reports for the hospitals to set aside funds to repay the government in the event unallowable costs were eventually determined by the government in the submitted cost reports. Both AHA and HFMA have filed amicus curiae briefs in the case defending the practice of maintaining reserve cost reports. Their contention is that reserve cost reports are a way of estimating the effects of potential adjustments to costs by the government and do not necessarily mean that the submitted cost reports were incorrect or fraudulent (Taylor 2000).

Regarding violations of the Anti-Kickback Act, in 1996, Bethany Medical Center paid $1.2 million to settle charges that the medical center paid kickbacks to a physician group in exchange for patient referrals from area nursing homes (Eiland 1996).

In 1997, OrNda Healthcorp paid $12.6 million to settle charges that several of its hospitals had paid physicians for Medicare patient referrals and had received referrals from other physicians with whom the hospitals had improper financial relationships (HHS 1997).

In November, 1999, the OIG announced a new safe harbor to protect certain ambulance restocking arrangements. Previously, OIG had issued several advisory opinions regarding their concerns that certain ambulance restocking arrangements by hospitals could induce ambulance operators to refer patients to particular hospitals. Under the safe harbor, hospitals can restock ambulances for supplies used during the transport of emergency patients to the hospital if the ambulance supplier pays the hospital the fair-market value for the supplies. In addition, OIG proposed that hospitals can restock ambulances for free or for reduced prices if the hospital meets certain conditions to ensure that inducements do not occur (HFMA 2000e).

Because fraud and abuse violations appear to be both widespread and serious, and because HHS Inspector General June Gibbs Brown declared in September 1997 a policy of "zero tolerance for fraud" (HFMA 1997), most healthcare executives are seeking ways to prevent and detect fraud in their organizations.

In 1991, the U.S. Sentencing Commission issued guidelines for federal judges to use in sentencing corporations that had been found guilty of criminal misconduct including fraud and abuse. The guidelines allow for lighter sentences for corporations that have corporate compliance programs in place:

> An effective program to prevent and detect violations means a program that has been reasonably designed, implemented, and enforced so that it generally will be effective in preventing and detecting criminal conduct. . . . The hallmark of an effective program to prevent and detect violations of the law is that the organization exercised due diligence in seeking to prevent and detect criminal conduct by its employees and other agents. (USSC 1991)

The guidelines provide seven requirements for an effective compliance program (Eiland 1996):

1. Establishes reasonable compliance standards and procedures that are organization-specific and that address the areas of greatest risk of liability, such as patient billing and medical record coding;
2. Appoints a high-level employee, typically called a corporate compliance officer, who is charged with overseeing compliance with established standards and procedures;
3. Exercises due care in delegating discretionary authority so that discretionary authority is not delegated to employees likely to engage in wrongdoing (e.g., fraudulent and abusive acts, or other illegal and unethical conduct);

4. Communicates compliance standards and procedures to employees through training programs on an initial and ongoing basis;
5. Designs, implements, and monitors auditing systems to detect wrongdoing by employees, and has a system for employees to report suspected wrongdoing;
6. Enforces compliance standards and procedures on a consistent basis through appropriate disciplinary mechanisms, including disciplining employees who fail to detect wrongdoing; and
7. Responds to wrongdoing in a consistent and timely manner, including disclosure of the wrongdoing to the appropriate government officials.

The OIG, in conjunction with a $325 million dollar settlement with SmithKline Beecham Laboratories, announced the pending release of model corporate compliance plans.[12] To date, HHS has published model corporate compliance plans for clinical laboratories, hospitals, home health agencies, third-party medical billing companies, DME suppliers, hospices, Medicare+Choice organizations, and nursing facilities. All model compliance plans are based on the following seven core elements (HHS 2000c):

1. Implementation of written policies, procedures, and standards of conduct;
2. Designation of a compliance officer;[13]
3. Development of training and educational programs;
4. Creation of a hotline or other measures for receiving complaints and procedures for protecting callers from retaliation;[14]
5. Performance of internal audits to monitor compliance;
6. Enforcement of standards through well-publicized disciplinary directives; and
7. Prompt corrective action in response to detected offenses.

Corporate compliance with the core recommendations will not only reduce the incidence of fraud and abuse, but it will also protect an organization from liability and administrative sanctions.

In certain cases, DOJ has filed civil and sometimes criminal charges against individuals in charge of organizations involved in fraud and abuse. In 1998 and one year after the federal raid on Columbia/HCA, four executives were indicted in connection with a scheme to overbill federal health agencies (Limbacher 1998). Also in 1998, seven Baptist Medical Center (Kansas City, MO) executives, including the CEO, were indicted for authorizing kickbacks. In 1997, Baptist Medical Center settled civil charges and agreed to pay $17.5 million for kickbacks to obtain nursing home referrals (Moore 1998). In 2001, a jury in federal bankruptcy court in Dallas found a former hospital chief executive officer of Tri-City Health Centre liable for breaching his fiduciary duty to his hospital by filing 141 false claims to Medicare in which he personally profited. The jury focused on two transactions by the former CEO: buying a CT scanner and then selling it to the hospital for a large profit (the cost of which was passed on to Medicare beneficiaries) and owning a construction company that completed a $5 million dollar renovation project for his hospital and then charged the hospital, and consequently Medicare, $12 million. The former CEO was ordered to pay $1 million to Medicare and $9.8 million to the trustee of the now-bankrupt hospital (Taylor 2001b). Also in 2001, a county grand jury in Kentucky returned indictments against the CEO, a former nurse, of a bankrupt 25-bed hospital. The CEO was indicted on seven counts of theft by deception for taking frequent trips to a condominium in Florida and charging the expenses to the hospital (Romano 2001b).

Notes

1. The purpose of President Johnson's legislative program was to eradicate poverty in the United States. While most health legislation in general— and Medicare in particular—was not aimed at those living in poverty, health legislation is often included in the "Great Society." President Johnson benefited from a robust economy set in motion by President Kennedy's economic policies, and by a liberal majority in Congress.

2. *Those born in*   *Can retire with full Social Security benefits at age*
   1937 and before   65
   1938–1942   add 2 months to 65 for every year after 1937
   1943–1954   66
   1955–1959   add 2 months to 66 for every year after 1954
   1960 and later   67

3. In *Who Will Tell the People*, Greider reports that the federal government used unaudited cost reports during the phase-in period, and as a result hospitals were grossly overpaid.

4. PROs replaced PSROs established by the Social Security Amendments of 1972. While PSROs were intended to protect the Medicare beneficiary from overuse rewarded under retroactive cost-based reimbursement, PROs were intended to protect the Medicare beneficiary from underuse rewarded under prospective DRG-based reimbursement.

5. Rural hospitals lost money under PPS for different reasons. First, the federal government set the rural hospital rate lower than the urban hospital rate, reflecting what the federal government believed to be lower healthcare costs in the rural community. Second, rural hospitals were reimbursed a per diem rate of the final DRG rate if they transferred the patient. Because the majority of hospital costs occur in the first few days of hospitalization, a per diem rate seldom fully reimbursed a rural hospital for the costs incurred during the first few days.

6. In order to qualify for the full market basket update to their PPS payments in 2005, hospitals must enroll with the Quality Improvement Organization's data warehouse by June 1, 2004 and transmit the required data by July 1, 2004. The required data includes 10 quality measures related to heart attack, heart failure and pneumonia for patient discharges during the hospital's most recent quarter.

7. Both the federal and state governments fund Medicaid. The state contribution ranges from 17 to 50 percent depending on the poverty status of the state (Gurny, Baugh, and Davis 1992) based on the formula (Tudor 1995):

$$\text{State share} = \frac{\text{state per capita personal income}}{\text{national per capita personal income}} \times .45$$

8. The Boren amendment was repealed in the Balanced Budget Act of 1997, giving back to the states the authority to establish payment rates.

9. Under EMTALA, Mercy Health Center in Oklahoma City settled a case for $18,250 in connection with the refusal to accept a patient transfer who later died. In an unrelated case, St. Anthony's Hospital in Oklahoma city lost an anti-dumping case and paid a $35,000 fine (Taylor 2000).

10. According to Scott (2000), the problem with the rules on health information privacy is that HHS based the rules on the wrong premise: that with very few exceptions, every use and disclosure of personal health information should be prohibited. Under this premise, innovative strategies for using and disclosing an individual's health information will be discouraged, and perhaps made illegal. Scott recommends that a better approach would be for HHS to identify what uses of health information are not allowed, and punish the violators.

11. The SNF industry is a good example of excessive BBA cuts. HFMA reported that the Congressional Budget Office budget figures indicate Medicare spending for SNF services from 1998 to 2002 would be $12.2 billion less than intended by the BBA and will reach $15.8 billion less than intended by 2004 (HFMA 2000f).

12. It was alleged that SmithKline Beecham had performed and received Medicare reimbursement for unnecessary lab tests, had billed Medicare for tests that had not been performed, and had engaged in code jamming (i.e., coding by nonphysician personnel for procedures that the ordering physician had omitted) (Watnik 1998).

13. OIG recommends that the chief compliance officer not be the chief financial officer or anyone else that might have a conflict of interest pertaining to the billing process. When pressed on this point, OIG has recommended the director of nursing or the director of medical records be the chief compliance officer.

14. Centralized billing operations present special problems for healthcare systems that must find a way to respond to patient complaints regarding billing problems at each institution.

Appendix 5.1
Health Insurance Portability and Accountability Act (HIPAA) of 1996

The most important provisions of HIPAA include the following.

- Guaranteed Access for Small Business—Small businesses with 50 or fewer employees are guaranteed access to health insurance because no insurer can exclude an employee or family member from coverage based on health status.
- Guaranteed Renewal of Insurance—Once an insurer sells a policy to any individual or group, the insurer is required to renew coverage regardless of the health status of the individual or any member of the group.
- Guaranteed Access for Individuals—People who lose their group coverage (through loss of employment or job transfer, for example) will be guaranteed access to coverage without regard to health status in individual markets or state-provided programs.
- Preexisting Conditions—Workers covered by group insurance policies cannot be excluded from coverage for more than 12 months due to a pre-existing medical condition. Such limits can only be placed on conditions treated or diagnosed within the six months prior to their enrollment in an insurance plan. Insurers cannot impose new pre-existing condition exclusions for workers with previous coverage.
- Enforcement—States have primary responsibility to enforce HIPAA. If states fail to enforce HIPAA, the Secretary of HHS can impose civil monetary penalties on insurers who violate HIPAA. The Secretary of Labor will enforce HIPAA through self-insured (ERISA) plans. The Secretary of Treasury will impose tax penalties on employers or insurance plans that fail to comply with HIPAA.
- Self-Employed Individuals—HIPAA gradually increases the tax deductions for health insurance for self-employed individuals from 30 percent in 1996 to 80 percent in 2006.
- Medical Savings Accounts—HIPAA allows businesses with 50 or fewer employees and self-employed individuals enrolled in a high-deductible health plan to establish tax-favored medical savings accounts (MSAs). Annual deductibles are $1,500 to $2,250 for individuals and $3,000 to $4,500 for families. Maximum out-of-pocket expenses are $3,000 for individuals and $5,500 for families. HIPAA limits the maximum number of MSAs established under this provision to 750,000 for the four-year demonstration project.

- Fraud and Abuse—HIPAA creates a new fraud and abuse program known as the Medicare Integrity Program to be coordinated by the HHS Office of the Inspector General and the Department of Justice with funding appropriated from the Medicare Hospital Insurance (HI) trust fund. HIPAA also provides the following related to fraud and abuse:
  - Requires exclusion from Medicare and Medicaid for felony convictions related to healthcare fraud or controlled substances;
  - Creates a program encouraging Medicare beneficiaries to report fraud and abuse and to offer suggestions to improve efficiency of the Medicare program, and provides incentive payments to beneficiaries in certain cases;
  - Requires issuance of advisory opinions, additional safe harbors, and fraud alerts regarding the anti-kickback statute;
  - Creates a new exception to the anti-kickback statute for certain risk-sharing organizations;
  - Expands conditions under which civil monetary penalties and intermediate sanctions can be imposed on HMOs participating in Medicare;
  - Establishes a database of final adverse actions taken against healthcare providers; and
  - Makes knowing and willful transfer of assets to gain Medicaid eligibility subject to criminal penalties.
- Long-Term Care Insurance—HIPAA establishes minimum federal consumer protection and marketing requirements for tax-qualified long-term care insurance policies, including a requirement that insurers start benefit payments when a policy holder cannot perform at least two "activities of daily living." HIPAA also provides that long-term care insurance premiums and unreimbursed long-term care services costs are tax deductible as a medical expense, and benefits received under long-term care insurance are excludable from taxable income. Employer-sponsored long-term care insurance receives the same tax treatment as health insurance.
- Medigap Insurance—HIPAA revises the notices requirement for health insurance policies that pay benefits without regard to Medicare coverage or other insurance coverage.
- Viatical Insurance Settlements—HIPAA allows a person who is within 24 months of death to have a portion of their death benefit prepaid tax free by the insurance company. HIPAA also allows a chronically ill person to sell their life insurance tax free if the proceeds of the sale are spent on long-term care.
- Administrative Simplification—HIPAA requires that all healthcare providers and health plans that engage in electronic administrative and financial transactions use a single set of national standards and identifiers. Electronic health information systems must meet security standards. If

Congress does not enact privacy legislation within three years, HIPAA will require healthcare providers, health plans, and healthcare clearinghouses to follow privacy regulations as promulgated by HHS for individually identifiable electronic health information (HHS 1996).

Appendix 5.2
Balanced Budget Act of 1997

1. Reduced reimbursements to providers by $115 billion over five years.
   - $43 billion from hospitals. PPS rates frozen, capital payments reduced, and PPS for hospital outpatient services by 1999 (see following section on Medicare Hospital Outpatient Prospective Payment System).
   - $25.7 billion from post-acute care. PPS in SNFs by 1998 (see following section), home health agencies by 2000 (see following section), and rehab hospitals by 2004.
   - $21.8 billion from managed care. PSOs allowed to enter markets and bid on Medicare business, which will be capitated.
   - $11.7 billion from physicians. While RBRVS is budget neutral, updates to RBRVS will be tied to the composite index; physician extenders can be paid directly and are allowed to practice without direct physician supervision.
   - $12.5 billion from other sources.
2. Froze disproportionate share payments in 32 states and cut payment in 18 states.
3. Gave states the option to require Medicaid beneficiaries to enroll in managed care.
4. Allowed PSOs to bid on Medicare and Medicaid business.
5. Introduced SCHIP, which provided $23.4 billion over five years to expand health coverage for children (HCFA 1997).
6. Introduced Medicare+Choice, which took effect in 1999. Medicare+Choice replaced the risk contracting program and permits participation by a wide variety of private insurance plans.

Medicare Skilled Nursing Facility (SNF) Prospective Payment System

Prior to July 1, 1998, HCFA paid for most Medicare services performed in SNFs on a reasonable cost basis. BBA of 1997 required HCFA to replace the cost-based system with a prospective payment system (PPS). The PPS for SNFs that went into effect on July 1, 1998 pays SNFs a per diem rate for all routine, ancillary, and capital costs related to the services furnished to Medicare beneficiaries. Per diem payments for each admission are case-mix adjusted using a resident classification system called Resource Utilization Groups III (RUG-III) based on data from resident assessments. The labor portion of the federal rates is adjusted for geographic variation in wages. The SNF PPS had a three-year transition that took into account both the facility-specific rate determined from cost reports as well as the national rate adjusted for geographic variation in wages (HCFA 1998).

Medicare Hospital Outpatient Prospective Payment System

Prior to August 1, 2000, HCFA paid for most Medicare services performed in the hospital outpatient setting based on cost. On average, Medicare beneficiary coinsurance accounted for about 50 percent of total Medicare payments to hospitals for outpatient services (beneficiary coinsurance was based on 20 percent of the hospital's billed charges for the outpatient services, while Medicare's payment for the same services is cost-based). BBA of 1997 required HCFA to replace the cost-based system with a prospective payment system (PPS), which pays hospitals' specific predetermined payments for outpatient services. BBA also changed the way beneficiary coinsurance is determined. Outpatient PPS will save beneficiaries billions of dollars of coinsurance while ensuring more accurate and equitable payments under Medicare. Proposed regulations were published September 9, 1998, and the final regulations were published on April 7, 2000, with a compliance date of August 1, 2000 (HCFA 2000b; Gambil 1999).

Medicare hospital outpatient PPS will cover all Medicare participating hospitals, except critical access and Indian Health Services hospitals and hospitals in Maryland. The new PPS will include most hospital outpatient services and Medicare Part B services furnished to hospital inpatients who have no Part A coverage. Services covered under the new PPS are surgical procedures, radiology, clinic visits, emergency department visits, diagnostic services and tests, surgical pathology, chemotherapy, surgical dressings, certain preventive services, splints and casts, antigens, certain vaccines, and partial hospitalization. Services not covered are ambulance services, occupational, physical, and speech therapy, laboratory services, home visits, durable medical equipment, prosthetics, and orthotics, and services requiring inpatient care (Rich and Kreitzer 1999). Under the new PPS, HCFA bases payments on the ambulatory payment classification (APC) system, which divides all outpatient services included in the new payment system into 451 groups. The services within each group are clinically similar and require comparable resources. HCFA assigns a relative payment weight to each APC based on the median cost of the services within the APC. The APC payment rates were initially determined on a national basis, then the wage component of the APC (60 percent) was adjusted based on a geographic area's wage level (HCFA 2000b).

Duncan (1999) suggests hospitals implement the following steps to reduce potential losses under the Medicare hospital outpatient PPS.

1. Form a planning team to analyze the effect of APCs on hospital operations.
2. Identify financial effect of APCs to determine the net profit or loss compared to the previous cost-based Medicare reimbursement.

3. Analyze billing processes to ensure that the hospital submits all codes related to the outpatient service to the fiscal intermediary for payment.
4. Review superbills (which list the commonly used CPT code for easy check-off in the outpatient setting) and charge masters (which assign current CPT codes to outpatient services) to ensure current information.
5. Improve coding quality through seminars, coding courses, and other educational courses for coders.
6. Appoint an APC coordinator to oversee the APC program.
7. Educate caregivers and ancillary staff members about making justifiable decisions regarding the best use of hospital resources and about the importance of good documentation regarding the decisions.
8. Modify technology accordingly to take advantage of new APC software.

The American Hospital Association (AHA) has expressed concern that, given the complexity of the new outpatient reimbursement system, coding and billing errors would almost certainly occur, at least in the implementation stages, thus putting hospitals at the mercy of federal prosecutors. In a June 23, 2000, letter to AHA (available online at http://www.hhs.gov/progorg/oig/testimony/aha.htm), the HHS Inspector General June Gibbs Brown reiterated her office's position that the OIG does not subject providers "to civil or criminal penalties for innocent errors, mistakes, or even negligence." Brown noted that should allegations of improper billing arise under the new outpatient reimbursement system, the OIG would consider a variety of factors before determining whether to prosecute (HFMA 2000e):

• The clarity of the relevant rule;
• The complexity and novelty of the billing system;
• The guidance issued by HCFA and its agents including fiscal intermediaries;
• The extent to which the provider has attempted to ascertain an understanding of the relevant rule;
• The quality of the efforts of the provider to train personnel on the billing system; and
• Whether the provider has an effective compliance program in place.

Medicare Home Health Prospective Payment System

BBA of 1997 required implementation of a prospective payment system for home health services by 2000. HCFA published final regulations on July 3, 2000 and on October 1, 2000 Medicare began paying providers of home health services a prospective rate for services and supplies bundled into 60-day episodes of care. No transition period was given, nor were PPS rates blended with previous Medicare reimbursements. Episodes of care begin with the first billable visit. Information taken from a patient-assessment instrument are recorded in the Outcome and Assessment Information Set (OASIS) and then used to classify patients into groups based on clinical characteristics (80 different home health resource groups [HHRGs]) that affect expected resource requirements. Payments would be made for each group and then adjusted for certain differences between cases (e.g., transfers and deaths) and home health agencies (wage differences based on facility location). Services covered include home health aide services, medical social services, occupational therapy, physical therapy, skilled nursing care, and speech language pathology. Medical supplies covered include routine and nonroutine medical supplies needed for the above services and approved in a plan of care. Durable medical equipment (DME) is not included and Medicare continues to reimburse DME on a fee schedule (Grimaldi 2000). The law originally mandated that payment rates be reduced by 15 percent in 2000. This reduction in payment was delayed until 2002 by BIPA of 2000.

Medicare Inpatient Rehabilitation Prospective Payment System

BBA of 1997 required implementation of a discharge-based PPS system by October 1, 2000. For a variety of reasons, final implementation has been delayed and implementation is now set for cost reporting periods that occur on or after April 1, 2001. Based on the proposed regulations for the new system, information taken from a patient-assessment instrument—the currently proposed instrument is the Minimum Data Set for Post Acute Care (MDS-PAC)—would be used to classify patients into groups based on clinical characteristics—97 different case-mix groups (CMG) are currently proposed—that affect expected resource requirements. Payments would be made for each group and then adjusted for certain differences between cases (e.g., transfers, short stays, interrupted stays) and facilities (e.g., wage differences based on facility location). The law originally mandated that payment rates be set at 2 percent less than reimbursement under the current system. This reduction in payment was removed by BIPA of 2000. The proposed regulations call for a two-year optional transition period (Gundling 2001).

Appendix 5.3
Balanced Budget Refinement Act (BBRA) of 1999

After significant evidence that BBA was cutting more than the projected $115 billion from the budget (some estimate that BBA was cutting two to three times more than the $115 billion originally intended), Congress passed and the president signed the Balanced Budget Refinement Act (BBRA) in November of 1999. The plan provides an estimated $16 billion in Medicare relief over five years. BBRA, also known as the Balanced Budget of 1997 Amendments, was passed as part of the Consolidated Appropriations Act.

Major provisions of BBRA of 1999 include the following (VHA 1999):

1. *$7.9 billion to hospitals*
   - $6.1 billion to hospital outpatient. Provides two to three years of payments in addition to outpatient PPS payments for certain devices, drugs, and biologicals; provides additional payments for certain high-cost cases; extends the 5.8 percent reduction in hospital operating costs and the 10 percent reduction for capital-related costs until outpatient PPS is fully implemented; provides payments in addition to PPS payments to hospitals during the first 3 years of PPS if a hospital's payments are less than the pre-PPS payments would have been in 1996; delays for two years the implementation of the volume expenditure cap; delays for two years the expansion of the list of DRGs to which the transfer provision applies; holds certain rural hospitals harmless from payment reductions under PPS; holds cancer hospitals harmless from payment reductions under PPS; requires BBA beneficiary copayment amounts to be unaffected by any BBRA provisions; limits the amount for which a Medicare beneficiary can be billed for an outpatient procedure to the Medicare deductible amount for an inpatient stay ($776 in 2000) and provides funds to compensate hospitals for the difference; and clarifies the budget-neutral implementation of PPS and eliminates the additional 5.7 percent on top of the formula-driven overpayment.
   - $0.8 billion to rural hospitals. Applies the 96-hour length of stay limitation on an average annual basis rather than on a per case basis; updates the criteria used to designate outlying rural counties as part of metropolitan statistical areas (MSAs); permits sole community hospitals that are now paid using the federal rate to transition over time to payment based on their hospital-specific FY1996 cost; extends the Medicare Dependent Hospital program through FY2006; updates the FY2000 target amount by market basket for discharges from sole community hospitals occurring in FY2001; permits rural hospitals to increase their resident limits by 30 percent for both direct medical education and indirect medical education payments; permits nonrural facilities that operate separately accredited rural training programs to increase their resident limits; permits rural hospitals with fewer than 50 beds to apply for grants not to exceed $50,000 for meeting the costs associated with implementing new PPS systems.
   - $0.6 billion to teaching hospitals. Changes direct graduate medical education (DGME) to incorporate a national average amount based on FY1977 hospital-specific per resident amounts; freezes indirect medical education (IME) adjustments at 6.5 percent through FY2000, reduces the adjustment to 6.25 percent in FY2001 and then to 5.5 percent in FY2002 and subsequent years; establishes a national average "per

resident" payment amount, adjusted for differences in area wages, starting on or after October 1, 2000.

- $0.3 billion to PPS-exempt hospitals. Adjusts the 75-percent cap to reflect differences in wage-related costs across geographic areas beginning for cost reporting periods on or after October 1, 1999; increases continuous bonus payments to eligible long-term care and psychiatric providers 1 to 1.5 percent for cost reporting periods beginning on or after October 1, 2000, and 2 percent for cost reporting periods beginning on or after October 1, 2001.

- $0.1 billion to disproportionate share hospitals. Freezes the reduction in the disproportionate share hospital (DSH) formula to 3 percent in FY2001, changes the reduction to 4 percent in FY2002; requires the secretary of HHS to collect hospital cost data on uncompensated inpatient and outpatient care, including non-Medicare bad debt and charity care as well as Medicaid and indigent care charges for cost reporting periods beginning on or after October 1, 2001.

2. *$4.0 billion to Medicare+Choice.* Changes the phase-in of the new risk adjustment method based on health status to a blend of 10 percent new health status method/90 percent old demographic method in 2000 and 2001; provides a new entry bonus of 5 percent on the monthly Medicare+Choice payment rate in the first 12 months and 3 percent in the subsequent 12 months to organizations that offer a plan in a payment area without a Medicare+Choice plan since 1997; sets aside graduate medical education funds to pay hospitals with nursing and allied health education programs that serve Medicare+Choice patients (total payment may not exceed $60 million); allows cost contracts with HMOs to be renewed through 2004; eases requirements that limit how plans design and market Medicare+Choice plans to beneficiaries; reduces exclusion period from five years to two years for organizations seeking to re-enter the program after withdrawing; provides for submission of adjusted community rates by July 1 instead of May 1; reduces national per capita Medicare+Choice growth percentage of 0.3 percent in 2002 instead of 0.5 percent as previously scheduled.

3. *$2.7 billion to skilled nursing facilities.* Increases temporarily the federal per diem payment by 20 percent for 15 categories of Medicare patients in skilled nursing facilities (SNFs) starting April 1, 2000; increases the federal rates for all categories by 4 percent in FY2001 and FY2002; increases payments paid from April 1, 2000, through September 30, 2000; includes the cost of Part B services in the computation of the facility-specific component of the SNF per diem payment, during the transition, to the federal per diem PPS for SNFs that had participated in the Nursing Home Case Mix and Quality Demonstration Project; permits SNFs to elect, on or after December 15, 1999, to receive Medicare payments based 100 percent on the federal per diem rate rather than partially on

a federal per diem rate and partially on a pre-PPS facility-specific rate; provides that from enactment to September 30, 2001, PPS payments to certain SNFs will be based 50 percent on the facility-specific rate and 50 percent on the federal per diem rate for SNFs in operation before July 1, 1992, and if at least 60 percent of the SNF's patients in cost reporting periods beginning in 1998 were immuno-compromised secondary to an infectious disease; requires the secretary of HHS to assess and report, within 18 months of enactment, on the variations in state licensure and certification standards regarding providers of respiratory therapy in SNFs and the need for Medicare to require examinations for, or certification of, workers providing respiratory therapy.

4. *$1.3 billion to home health care.* Delays the 15-percent reduction in payment rates until one year after implementation of PPS; provides $10 per beneficiary for administration of the OASIS questionnaire to new home health patients for services furnished during cost periods in FY2000; raises the "per beneficiary" limit by 2 percent for agencies subject to the per beneficiary limit in cost reporting periods starting in FY2000; establishes the lesser of $50,000 or 10 percent of a home health agency's Medicare payments in the previous year as the annual amount of an agency's surety bond requirement; requires the bond to be in effect for 4 years or longer if agency ownership changes; allows prior periods covered by a bond to be counted; excludes DME, including oxygen and oxygen supplies, from the home health consolidated billing program; clarifies that the increase in home health PPS in FY2002 and FY2003 will be the market basket minus 1.1 percent.

Appendix 5.4
Medicare, Medicaid, and SCHIP Benefits Improvement and Protection Act of 2000

Major provisions of BIPA of 2000 include the following (HFMA 2000a):

- *$12 billion to hospitals.* Increases inflation update for hospitals to full market basket in 2001 and market basket minus 0.55 percent in 2002 and 2003; adjusts teaching hospital payments for medical education by increasing the IME payment to 6.5 percent in both 2001 and 2002; provides greater hospital bad debt reimbursement by increasing the amount of a beneficiary's bad debt to a hospital that is reimbursable under Medicare to 70 percent beginning with the 2001 cost reports; raises hospital outpatient department prospective payments by increasing the annual adjustment in 2001 to full market basket; increases Medicaid payments to safety net hospitals by setting 2001 state-specific allotments at 2000 levels adjusted for inflation and by setting 2002 allotments at 2001 levels adjusted for inflation; improves rural hospital programs by making more equitable the treatment of rural hospitals under the Medicare disproportionate share hospital system by expanding program eligibility and by strengthening the Critical Access Hospital (CAH) program by exempting CAH swing beds from SNF prospective payments, by reimbursing physicians at 115 percent of the fee schedule, by paying emergency room physicians and ambulances at reasonable cost, and by allowing rural hospitals to choose among three cost reporting periods to determine eligibility for the Medicare Dependent Hospital (MDH) program; increases payments for PPS-exempt hospitals by increasing payments for rehabilitation hospitals in 2002 to 100 percent of pre-BBA levels; increasing bonuses for psychiatric hospitals to 3 percent; and raises the national cap on long-term care hospital reimbursement by 2 percent and increases the individual long-term care hospital target by 25 percent.

- *$11 billion to managed care.* Increases rates to $525 in urban areas and $475 in all other areas; enhances managed care plan accountability by increasing the civil penalties that the secretary of HHS might assess on plans that violate their contracts; codifies risk adjustment phase-in period for managed care plans to an explicit seven-year phase-in schedule; changes provider participation rules and quality standards including permitting premium reduction as a benefit, providing for elections to be effective when made, permitting uniform coverage policies for multistate plans, requiring HCFA to approve marketing materials on a timely basis, and allowing cost contractors to expand service areas and enroll more beneficiaries; and provides for interaction with fee-for-service policies by linking Medicare+Choice rates to growth in Medicare fee-for-service rates.

- *$5 billion to Medicare and Medicaid beneficiaries.* For Medicare beneficiaries, adds preventive benefits including nutrition therapy and glaucoma screening and improves preventive benefits including colon cancer screening and cervical cancer screening; increases coverage for immunosuppressive drugs; accelerates beneficiary hospital outpatient coinsurance phase-down; extends immediate coverage to beneficiaries with Lou Gehrig's Disease; expands homebound definition to include adult day care; for Medicaid beneficiaries, permits enrollment of uninsured children at school and other sites; continues healthcare coverage for those leaving welfare for work to 12 months after leaving welfare; and simplifies enrollment for low-income Medicare beneficiaries.

- *$3 billion to other providers.* Increases payments to hospices by adding 5 percent to the hospice payment base rate; raises payments for renal dialysis by 1.2 percent in addition to the 1.2 percent provided by BBRA; and adjusts updates for durable medical equipment, orthotics and prosthetics, and ambulances by providing a full CPI inflation update for DME suppliers in 2001, a full market basket update for suppliers of orthotics and prosthetics in 2001; and a full CPI update for ambulance providers in 2001.

- *$2 billion to skilled nursing facilities and therapy services.* Increases inflation update for SNFs to full market basket in 2001 and market basket minus 0.5 percent in 2002; allows for improved nursing staffing ratios by increasing the nursing component of the resource utilization groups (RUGs) by 16.66 percent in 2001 and requires SNFs to post staffing ratios to ensure that residents are informed; delays $1,500 annual payment caps per beneficiary for physical/speech therapy and occupational therapy until after 2002; provides increases in payment for high-cost rehabilitation therapy by increasing rehabilitation RUGs by 6.7 percent starting in 2002.
- *$2 billion to home health care.* Delays 15-percent reduction in payments until 2002; increases inflation update to full market basket in 2001; assists rural home health agencies by adding a 10-percent add-on payment to rural agencies in 2001 and 2002.

References

Bellandi, D. 2001. "CHW Faces Medicare Fraud Charges." *Modern Healthcare* 31 (8): 12.

———. 1998. "Daughters of Charity Agrees to Settlement." *Modern Healthcare* 28 (32): 8.

Berman, H. J., S. F. Kukla, and L. E. Weeks. 1994. *The Financial Management of Hospitals, 8th ed.* Chicago: Health Administration Press.

CMS. 2004. "HIPAA Administrative Simplification." [Online retrieval, 02/05/04]. http://www.cms.gov/hipaa/default.asp..

CMS Web-Based Chart Series. 2004. "Program Information on Medicare, Medicaid, SCHIP, and Other Programs." [Online retrieval, 02/04/04]. http://www.cms.gov.

DeLew, N. 2000. "Medicare: 35 Years of Service." *Health Care Financing Review* 22 (1): 75–86.

DeMuro, P. R., and A. H. Gantt. 2001. "HIPAA Privacy Standards Raise Complex Implementation Issues." *Healthcare Financial Management* 55 (1): 42–47.

Duncan, D. G. 1999. "Preparing for Medicare's APC System." *Healthcare Financial Management* 53 (7): 40–45.

Eiland, G. W. 1996. "The Scary New World of Health Care Fraud and Abuse: Recent Medicare Settlements." Presented to the South Texas Chapter of Healthcare Financial Management Association. Corpus Christi.

Ernst & Young. 1997. *Just Another Day in Healthcare.* Washington, DC: Ernst & Young.

———. 1996. *Corporate Compliance.* Washington, DC: Ernst & Young.

Ferman, J. H. 2001. "Medicaid's Upper Payment Limit Issue." *Healthcare Executive* 16 (1): 61–62.

Foster, R. S. 2000. "Trends in Medicare and Financial Status, 1996–2000." *Health Care Financing Review* 22 (1): 35–51.

Frum, D. 1994. *Dead Right.* New York: Basic Books.

Galloro, V. 2003. "Not Quite Over Yet." *Modern Healthcare* 33 (32): 10–11.

Gambil, M. A. 1999. "Ambulatory Payment Classifications: Impact on Hospital Operations." Paper presented at the annual meeting of the Oklahoma Chapter of Healthcare Financial Management Association, Oklahoma City, 27 May.

Glasser, D. L., and D. E. Bloomquist. 2000. "New and Clarified Safe Harbors May Ease Certain Provider Transactions." *Healthcare Financial Management* 54 (2): 42–47.

Gornick, M. E., J. L. Warren, P. W. Eggers, J. P. Lubitz, N. D. Lew, M. H. Davis, and B. S. Cooper. 1996. "Thirty Years of Medicare: Impact on the Covered Population." *Health Care Financing Review—Medicare: Advancing Towards the 21st Century 1966–1996* 18 (2): 179–234.

Grimaldi, P. L. 2000. "Medicare's New Home Health Prospective Payment System Explained." *Healthcare Financial Management* 54 (11): 46–54.

Gundling, R. L. 2001. "HCFA Proposes PPS for Inpatient Rehabilitation Services." *Healthcare Financial Management* 55 (2): 72–73.

———. 1998. "Hospital Transfers and Discharges Defined." *Hospital Financial Management* 52 (11): 72–73.

Gurny, P., D. K. Baugh, and F. A. Davis. 1992. "A Description of Medicaid Eligibility." *Health Care Financing Review: Medicare and Medicaid Statistical Supplement*: 207–26. Baltimore, MD: USDHHS.

Hakim, R., P. Boben, and J. Bonney. 2000. "Medicaid and the Health of Children." *Health Care Financing Review* 22 (1): 133–41.

Harris, S. E. 1975. *The Economics of Health Care: Finance and Delivery.* Berkeley, CA: McCutchan Publishing Corporation.

Health Care Financing Administration. 2000a. *Health Care Financing Review: Medicare and Medicaid Statistical Supplement 2000*: 89.

———. 2000b. "Factsheet of a Medicare Outpatient PPS." [Online retrieval, 01/25/01]. http://www.hcfa.gov/facts/fs0004b.htm.

———. 1998. "Skilled Nursing Facility PPS." [Online retrieval, 02/12/01]. http://www.hcfa.gov/medicare/snfpps.htm.

———. 1997. "BBA of 1997 Subtitle A—Medicare+Choice." [Online retrieval, 01/18/01]. http://www.hcfa.gov/regs/budget97.htm.

———. 1996. "Overview of the Medicaid Program." *Health Care Financing Review: Medicare and Medicaid Statistical Supplement 1996*: 144–187.

Healthcare Financial Management Association. 2004. "Highlights: Medicare Prescription Drug, Improvement, and Modernization Act." [Online retrieval, 02/03/04]. http://www.hfma.org/resource/focus_areas/medicare/400246.htm.

———. 2003. "HIPAA Final Security Rule Worksheets." [Online retrieval, 02/03/04]. http://www.hfma.org/resource/focus_areas/HIPAA.htm

———. 2002. "Highlights: The Final Modifications to the HIPAA Privacy Rule." [Online retrieval, 02/03/04]. http://www.hfma.org/resources/focus_areas/HIPPA.htm.

———. 2001. "Administrative Simplification Timetable." [Online retrieval, 02/14/01]. http://www.hfma.org/kn/Timetable.htm.

———. 2000a. "Happy-Holidays." [Online retrieval, 01/10/01]. http://www.hfma.org/kn/happy-holidays.htm

———. 2000b. "Updata." *Healthcare Financial Management* 54 (7): 10–11.

———. 2000c. "Industry Scan." *Healthcare Financial Management* 54 (3): 21.

———. 2000d. "Industry Scan." *Healthcare Financial Management* 55 (12): 22–23.

———. 2000e. "Industry Scan." *Healthcare Financial Management* 54 (10): 21.

———. 2000f. "Industry Scan." *Healthcare Financial Management* 54 (7): 20.

———. 1999. "Industry Scan." *Healthcare Financial Management* 53 (9): 18.

———. 1998. "Updata." *Healthcare Financial Management* 52 (9): 10.

———. 1997. "Updata." *Healthcare Financial Management* 51 (7): 9–10.

Heffler, S., S. Smith, S. Keehan, M. R. Clemens, M. Zezza, and C. Truffer. 2004. "Trends: Health Spending Projections Through 2013." *Health Affairs*—Web Exclusive. [Online retrieval, 03/16/04]. http://content.healthaffairs.org/webexclusives/index.dt/?year=2004.

Helbing, M. 1993. "Medicare Program Expenditures." *Health Care Financing Review: Medicare and Medicaid Statistical Supplement 1992*. Baltimore, MD: USDHHS.

Hepner, J. O., and D. M. Hepner. 1973. *The Health Strategy Game: A Challenge for Reorganization and Management*. St. Louis, MO: C.V. Mosby.

Hoffman, D., B. Klees, and C. Curtis. 2000. "Overview of the Medicare and Medicaid Programs." *Healthcare Financing Review* 22 (1): 175–93.

Kronebusch, K. 1993. "Medicaid Politics." Ph.D. diss., Harvard University.

Landsberg, B. S., and T. D. Keville. 2001. "Nursing Homes Face Quality-of-Care Scrutiny under the False Claims Act." *Healthcare Financial Management* 55 (1): 54–58.

Limbacher, P. B. 1998. "Columbia Case Grows." *Modern Healthcare* 28 (30): 12.

Moore, D. 1998. "Baptist Execs Indicted." *Modern Healthcare* 28 (29): 2, 14.

Office of the Inspector General. 1995. Medicare and Medicaid Guide, Report #A-03-94-00021. Washington, DC: OIG.

Office of Civil Rights. 2001. "HIPAA Penalties." [Online retrieval, 01/05/01]. http:www.hhs.gov/ocr/hipaa.html.

Pawola, L. M., S. Diwan, B. Patterson, and E. Rabinovitch. 2000. "Understanding the Implications of HIPAA." *Advance for Health Information Executives* 4 (2): 33–38.

Pear, R. 2003. "Medigap Insurance Barred." *New York Times*, December 7, F71.

Peterson, P. G. 1996. *Will America Grow Up Before It Grows Old?* New York: Random House.

Petrie, J. T. 1993. "Overview of the Medicare Program." *Health Care Financing Review: Medicare and Medicaid Statistical Supplement*, 1–12. Baltimore, MD: USDHHS.

Poisal, J.S., and L. Murray. 2001. "Growing Differences Between Medicare Beneficiaries With and Without Drug Coverage." *Health Affairs* 20 (2): 74–85.

Provost, C., and P. Hughes. 2000. "Medicaid: 35 Years of Service." *Health Care Financing Review* 22 (1): 141–75.

Rice, D. P. 1996. "Beneficiary Profile: Yesterday, Today, and Tomorrow." *Health Care Financing Review* 18 (2): 23–46.

Rich, D., and M. H. Kreitzer. 1999. "Ambulatory Patient Classification." Presented at a Quorum CFO/HIM/PFS networking meeting, San Antonio, TX, 9 July.

Romano, M. 2001a. "Less Stark, More Clarity." *Modern Healthcare* 31 (2): 2–3, 9.

———. 2001b. "Hospital's Ex-CEO Indicted." *Modern Healthcare* 31 (8): 20.

Russo, J. J. 1997. "Health Care Fraud/Abuse: Recent Developments." Presented to the Healthcare Financial Management Association Annual National Institute, Orlando, FL, 1 July.

Scott, J. S. 2004a. "Winners and Losers Under the New and Improved Medicare." *hfm* 58 (1): 28–29.

———. 2004b. "Tackle Your Healthcare Problems." Presentation at the Winter meeting of the HFMA South Texas/ACHE San Antonio Chapters, San Antonio, 30 January.

———. 2000. "On Privacy: What We Don't Share Can Hurt Us." *Healthcare Financial Management* 54 (3): 26–27.

Taylor, M. 2003. "A Question of Integrity." *Modern Healthcare* 33 (2): 6–7, 16.

———. 2002. "Some Fraud Fight Left." *Modern Healthcare* 32 (51): 6–7, 12.

———. 2001a. "Private Payers Pressure HCA." *Modern Healthcare* 31 (6): 16.

———. 2001b. "Ex-hospital CEO Guilty of Fraud." *Modern Healthcare* 31 (6): 6.

———. 2000. "Bean Counters Beware." *Modern Healthcare* 30 (51): 2, 12.

Tieman, J. 2000. "One Huge HIPAA." *Modern Healthcare* 30 (52): 8.

Tudor, C. G. 1995. "Medicaid Expenditures and State Responses." *Health Care Financing Review* 16 (3): 1–10.

U.S. Bureau of the Census. *Current Population Reports Series P-23*, No. 128 and *P-25*, No. 1018. In Rice, D. P. 1996. "Beneficiary Profile: Yesterday, Today, and Tomorrow." *Health Care Financing Review* 18 (2): 23–97.

U.S. Department of Health and Human Services. 2003. "Backgrounder: Prescription Drug Coverage for Medicare Beneficiaries." [Online retrieval, 02/02/04]. http://www.hhs.gov/news/press/2003.htm.

———. 2001a. "National Employer Identifiers." [Online retrieval, 02/15/01]. http://aspe.hhs.gov/adminsimp/nprm/press2.htm.

———. 2001b. [Online retrieval, 02/15/01]. http://aspe.hhs.gov/adminsimp/nprm/press3.htm.

———. 2000a. "Administrative Simplification." [Online retrieval, 08/11/00]. http://www.aspe.os.dhhs.gov/admnsimp/final/press1.htm.

———. 2000b. "Privacy." [Online retrieval, 12/20/00]. http://aspe.os.dhhs.gov/admnsimp/pvcfact1.htm.

———. 2000c. "SNF." [Online retrieval, 02/13/01]. http://oig.hhs.gov/medadv/snffinal.htm.

———. 1997. "OrNda." [Online retrieval, 02/13/01]. http://oig.hhs.gov/medadv/ornda.html.

———. 1996. "Summary of HIPAA of 1996." [Onlive retrieval, 08/28/96]. http://www.netreach.net/wmanning/hr3103.htm.

United States Sentencing Commission. 1991. *United States Sentencing Guidelines*, 8A1.2.

United States v. GMS Management-Tucker, Inc. et al., No. 96–1271 (E.D. Pa. 1996).

United States ex rel. Mikes v. Straus, 84 F. Supp. 2d 427 (S.D.N.Y. 1999).

Voluntary Hospitals of America (VHA). 1999. "BBA Relief." [Online retrieval, 01/10/01]. http:www.vha.com/publicpolicy/bbarelief.shtml.

Wade, M., and S. Berg. 1995. "Causes of Medicaid Expenditure Growth." *Health Care Financing Review* 16 (3): 11–25.

Waldo, D. R., S. T. Sonnenfeld, D. R. McKusick, and R. H. Arnett. 1989. "Health Expenditures by Age Group, 1977 and 1987." *Health Care Financing Review* 10 (4): 111–120.

Watnik, R. 2000. "Antikickback versus Stark: What's the Difference?" *Healthcare Financial Management* 54 (3): 66–67.

———. 1998. "Healthcare Compliance: National Perspective." Presented at a meeting of the South Texas Chapter of the Healthcare Financial Management Association, San Antonio, 30 January.

6

COST ACCOUNTING

Cost accounting is the analysis of costs including methods for classifying costs, allocating costs, assembling costs, and determining product costs. The purpose of cost accounting is to provide management with cost information for a variety of reasons including cost management, setting charges, and profitability analysis.

Cost accounting in healthcare has increased in importance and degree of sophistication with the advent of prospective payment in 1983 and the rapid growth of managed care in the mid-1980s, both of which required cost information by product (Eastaugh 1987). With a fixed charge set by the government for diagnosis-related groups (DRGs) and managed care organizations for contracts, healthcare organizations should know the cost of providing the service to determine profitability. Prior to 1983, cost accounting was driven by the Medicare cost report, which required aggregate data; most insurance companies paid the full charge regardless of cost.

Methods of Classifying Costs

The first part of cost accounting involves understanding the various methods in which costs can be classified and, through this classification, defined.

Accounting Function

Costs can be classified by accounting function:

- Financial accounting costs (i.e., accounting costs) are a measurement in monetary terms of the amount of resources used for a certain purpose. Technically, cost is an asset, or a value placed on goods or services. When the value expires, the cost becomes an expense.
- Managerial accounting costs (i.e., financial costs) are present and future costs that help management make better decisions.

Management Function

Costs can be classified by management function:

- Operating costs are associated with producing the product or service.
- Nonoperating costs are associated with supporting the production of a product or service.

Traceability

Costs can be classified by traceability:

- Direct costs are costs that can be traced directly to a department, product, or service.
- Indirect costs (i.e., overhead costs) cannot be traced directly to department, product, or service.
- Full costs include both direct and indirect costs.
- Average costs are full costs that are divided by products or services.

Behavior

Costs can be classified by behavior in relation to volume of products or services:

- Variable costs vary directly and proportionately to changes in volume.
- Fixed costs remain constant in relation to changes in volume.
- Semi-variable costs vary incrementally to changes in volume.
- Marginal costs are the changes in costs related to changes in volume.

Relevance to Decision Making

Costs can be classified by relevance to control and management decision making:

- True costs are hypothetical costs that represent the most accurate representation of full costs.
- Controllable costs are under the manager's influence.
- Uncontrollable costs cannot be influenced by the manager.
- Differential costs (i.e., incremental costs) are the difference in costs between two or more alternatives.
- Sunk costs are costs that have already been incurred and thus will not be affected by future decisions.
- Opportunity costs are foregone by rejecting an alternative.
- Relevant costs are future costs that will differ between alternatives.
- Actual costs are the historic costs incurred.
- Standard costs are estimated or budgeted costs used for comparison purposes.

Methods of Allocating Costs

As is the case with most organizations, healthcare organizations do not generate a separate charge for every product or service they sell. For example, healthcare organizations do not generate a charge for heating/cooling. Instead, the costs of heating/cooling are allocated to a department that generates charges that include the costs of heating/cooling, like radiology and lab.

The process of allocating these indirect costs, and some direct costs, to departments that generate charges is called cost allocation (also called cost finding or cost analysis). The primary purpose of cost allocation is to allocate the indirect costs and some direct costs in a way that ensures that patients are paying for only the costs of the services and products they received. Prior to choosing the best method of cost allocation, healthcare organizations must complete the prerequisite steps (Berman, Kukla, and Weeks 1994):

Organizational Chart

First, the healthcare organization must have an organizational chart and commensurate chart of accounts. The organizational chart identifies who is responsible for each functional area, usually a department, in the organization. The chart of accounts identifies cost centers and revenue centers that correspond to the organizational chart. (Every department is a cost center, but every department is not a revenue center.) This is the basis for responsibility accounting, which means that the organization has identified and holds someone responsible for each revenue and cost center in the organization.

Revenue Center Identification

Second, the healthcare organization must identify and segregate the cost centers that generate revenue from the cost centers that do not generate revenue. The cost centers that do not generate revenue must allocate their costs to the cost centers that generate revenue.

Accounting System

Third, the healthcare organization must have an accounting system that accurately and promptly assigns costs and charges to the appropriate cost and revenue centers.

Workload Statistic

Fourth, the healthcare organization must have a comprehensive information system that generates accurate, nonfinancial statistics for every department. Each department should have a workload statistic that best reflects the work performed in the department. For instance, the workload statistic for the laundry department is usually pounds of laundry; for the personnel department the statistic is usually number of employees in the organization; for the health information department the statistic is usually discharges adjusted for outpatient visits; and for housekeeping the statistic is usually square footage.

Cost Allocation Methods

Fifth, the healthcare organization must have a predetermined cost allocation method. Several methods of cost allocation are used in healthcare organizations.

Direct Apportionment

Direct apportionment is the easiest method of allocation. It involves a one-time allocation of all costs from cost centers of departments that do not generate revenue (NR) to cost centers of departments that do generate revenue (R).

$$\boxed{\text{NR}} \longrightarrow \boxed{\text{R}} \longrightarrow \boxed{\text{Patient}}$$

The main advantage of direct apportionment is its simplicity; the main disadvantage is that it does not take into account the costs of nonrevenue departments doing work for nonrevenue departments. For instance, housekeeping does work for health information management. Because of this disadvantage, most third-party payers do not accept direct apportionment as a method of cost allocation.

Step-Down Apportionment

Step-down apportionment involves a two-time allocation, and takes into account the disadvantage of direct apportionment. It involves a one-time allocation of all costs from cost centers of departments that do not generate revenue to other cost centers of departments that do not generate revenue before a one-time allocation of all costs to cost centers of departments that do generate revenue.

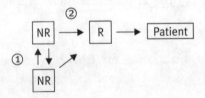

Step-down apportionment has two advantages: (1) it considers the costs of nonrevenue departments doing work for other nonrevenue departments before the final allocation to revenue departments; and (2) although burdensome, it can be performed by hand, without a computer. The disadvantage of step-down apportionment is that it does not consider revenue departments doing work for other revenue departments. For instance, the lab department may take cultures in radiology to determine the source of infections (in most healthcare organizations, this would result in an interdepartment charge).

Double Apportionment

Double apportionment also involves a two-time allocation and takes into account the disadvantage of step-down apportionment. Double apportionment involves a one-time allocation of all costs from cost centers of departments that do not generate revenue to other cost centers of departments that do not generate revenue. It also involves a simultaneous one-time allocation of costs between cost centers that do generate revenue to cost centers of departments that do generate revenue before a one-time allocation of all costs to cost centers of departments that do generate revenue.

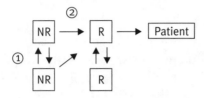

Double apportionment has two advantages: (1) it takes into account the costs of revenue departments doing work for revenue departments before the final allocation to revenue departments; and (2) considering value, or accuracy over cost, double apportionment is the most practical method of cost allocation. The disadvantage of double apportionment is that it requires a computer, which may make it cost-prohibitive for smaller healthcare organizations.

Multiple Apportionment

Multiple apportionment (i.e., algebraic apportionment) also involves a two-step allocation, but takes into account multiple, simultaneous apportionments during the first step.

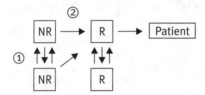

The more allocations the organization makes in the first step, the more accurate will be the costs reflected in the patient's bill. The advantage of multiple apportionment is that it is the most accurate method. The disadvantages are that multiple apportionment requires a computer with significant memory, and requires significant computer time.

Methods of Assembling Costs

After the healthcare organization has allocated the indirect costs and some direct costs by a method that ensures that patients are paying for only the costs of the services and products they received, the organization develops methods of assembling costs in ways that are meaningful for management. Three methods of assembling costs exist; most organizations use more than one method.

Responsibility Costing

Responsibility costing is a method of assembling costs by responsibility center (cost center or department). In this way the healthcare organizations can hold managers responsible for the controllable costs of the organization.[1]

Full Costing

Full costing is a method of assembling direct costs and an allocated share of indirect costs to a product or service for the purpose of determining its profitability.

Differential Costing

Differential costing (sometimes called incremental costing or relevant costing) is a method of assembling costs and sometimes revenues to alternative decisions (Siegel and Shim 1995). Sunk costs (i.e., costs that have already occurred) are not relevant to a decision; incremental or differential costs (i.e., costs that differ between the alternative decisions) are relevant. Generally, such an analysis involves the following steps:

1. Gathering all costs and revenues associated with each alternative;
2. Identifying and dropping all sunk costs;
3. Identifying and dropping all costs and revenues that do not differ between the alternatives; and
4. Selecting the best alternative based on the remaining cost and revenue information.

PROBLEM 6.1
Differential Cost Analysis

Last week the ABC clinic bought a new piece of lab equipment for $100,000. The piece of equipment will perform 100,000 tests over its useful life. Total variable costs are $3 per test, and the clinic is planning to charge $5 per test. This week a competing lab equipment manufacturer introduced a similar piece of equipment for the same price. In effect, the introduction of this piece of equipment made the resale or trade-in value of the existing piece of equipment $0. Total variable costs are $1 per test. Using differential cost analysis, should ABC clinic keep the existing piece of equipment or should the clinic buy the new piece of equipment?

Step 1: Gather all costs and revenues associated with each alternative.

	Keep Old Equipment	Buy New Equipment
Revenue	$500,000	$500,000
Fixed cost		
Old	100,000	100,000
New		100,000
Variable costs	300,000	100,000
Full cost gain/(loss)	$100,000	$200,000

Step 2: Identify and drop all sunk costs (drop the $100,000 fixed cost for old equipment).

	Keep Old Equipment	Buy New Equipment
Revenue	$500,000	$500,000
Fixed cost		
Old		
New		100,000
Variable costs	300,000	100,000

Step 3: Identify and drop all costs and revenues that do not differ between the alternatives (drop the $500,000 revenue from each alternative).

	Keep Old Equipment	Buy New Equipment
Revenue		
Fixed cost		
Old		
New		100,000
Variable costs	300,000	100,000

Step 4: Select the best alternative based on the remaining cost and revenue information.

Differential cost gain/(loss)	($300,000)	($200,000)

Conclusion:
Using differential cost analysis, ABC should buy the new piece of lab equipment because it has a lower differential cost ($200,000) than the old piece of equipment ($300,000).

Methods of Determining Product Costs

After the healthcare organization has assembled costs in ways that are meaningful for management, the organization develops methods of determining product costs, or costs by products like DRGs, patient days, and outpatient visits. Product costs obviously cut across functional (department) lines of responsibility. Product costs are important in determining profitability in prospective payment arrangements like Medicare and managed care, where charges are published before the healthcare organization delivers products and services. Several methods of determining costs exist; organizations may use more than one. The following methods of determining costs are ordered from what are the generally agreed-upon least accurate to most accurate methods.

Ratio of Cost to Charges

Ratio of cost to charges (RCC) is a method of determining product cost by relating its cost to its charge. This is usually calculated by dividing an organization's total operating expenses by the gross patient revenue (obtained from the worksheet for the statement of operations).

The resulting percentage is then applied to any product's charge in the organization to calculate the product's cost. Ratio of cost to charges was the predominant method of calculating product cost during the cost-based reimbursement years prior to 1983. This method has a serious flaw. It assumes a consistent relationship between cost and charge that simply does not exist because of the numerous ways healthcare organizations have set charges over the last 40 years (see Chapter 7). For example, to remain competitive, healthcare organizations may be forced to discount charges below the actual cost of providing the service.

Process Costing

Process costing is a method of determining product cost during a given accounting period. This is usually calculated by dividing the full costs of the organization or department during a given accounting period by the number of products or services produced during the given accounting period. This method of determining product cost might be appropriate in an organization or department that produces products similar in resource consumption. However, assuming similar resource consumption for most products produced in healthcare organizations is inappropriate. For instance, a computed tomographic (CT) scan in the radiology department consumes more resources than a hand x-ray. Process costing would consider each a procedure in the radiology department and therefore assign both procedures the same cost.

Job Order Costing

Job order costing is a method of determining product cost by sampling the product's actual direct costs and developing a relative value unit (RVU)—a measure of resources consumed by each product—in varying amounts for each product. Total direct costs and indirect costs are then assigned to the product based on the relationships established by the RVU. Problem 6.2 demonstrates the process of developing an RVU and determining product costing using the RVU.

PROBLEM 6.2
Job Order Costing

ABC Diagnostic Center is developing an RVU and product cost for the following CT procedures, given the projected volumes and sample direct costs. Projected total costs for the CT department are $10,000,000 ($6,000,000 in direct costs and $4,000,000 in indirect costs). Calculate the cost per procedure using job order costing.

Procedure	Projected Volumes	Labor Expense ($)	Supply Expense ($)
A: CT scan	1,000	60	30
B: Upper GI	2,000	50	20
C: Chest x-ray	4,000	25	10
D: Hand x-ray	5,200	20	05

Stage 1: Calculate the RVU for each procedure.

Divide total sample direct cost (labor expense + supply expense) by either the greatest common denominator (GCD), if there is one, or the average sample direct cost for each procedure.

Procedure	Total Sample Direct Expense	÷	GCD	=	RVU
A	90		5		18
B	70		5		14
C	35		5		7
D	25		5		5

Stage 2: Calculate the total cost for each procedure.

Step 1: Calculate the total projected RVUs by multiplying the RVUs per procedure by the projected volume per procedure.

Procedure	RVU	×	Projected Volume	=	Total RVUs
A	18		1,000		18,000
B	14		2,000		28,000
C	7		4,000		28,000
D	5		5,200		26,000
Total					100,000

Step 2: Calculate the cost per RVU by dividing total costs by total RVUs.

$$\$10,000,000 \div 100,000 = \$100$$

Step 3: Calculate the cost per procedure by multiplying the cost per RVU by the RVUs of each procedure.

Procedure	Cost/RVU	RVU	Cost/Procedure
A	$100	18	$1,800
B	100	14	1,400
C	100	7	700
D	100	5	500

Activity-Based Costing

Activity-based costing is a method of determining product cost by using cost drivers to assign indirect costs to products. Where job order costing assigns indirect costs to products proportionate to direct costs and volumes, activity-based costing uses cost drivers, or activity measures, that cause indirect costs to be incurred. Ideal cost drivers are activities that pertain to each procedure in varying amounts.

In Problem 6.2, labor expense and supply expense, which reflected activities and varied for each procedure, were used to determine both the direct and indirect costs for each procedure. Adding a cost driver that better represents the causal relationship of the indirect costs (like equipment use, which represent a causal relationship to depreciation expense and repair expense) produces the most accurate cost per procedure information available, as demonstrated in Problem 6.3.

The difference in the costs per procedure for job order costing and activity-based costing in Problem 6.3 are a result of the more accurate method of assigning indirect costs using activity-based accounting. Generally speaking, more cost drivers provide a more accurate cost; however, cost-driver information is often expensive to collect. Therefore, only cost drivers that have a high correlation to the consumption of overhead should be used (Siegel and Shim 1995).

PROBLEM 6.3
Activity-Based Costing

ABC Diagnostic Center wants to develop a product cost for the following CT procedures using labor expense and supply expense to assign direct costs, and machine minutes as a cost driver to assign indirect costs. Projected total costs for the CT department are $10,000,000 ($6,000,000 in direct costs and $4,000,000 in indirect costs). Assign costs to each procedure using the following information.

Procedure	Projected Volumes	Labor Expense ($)	Supply Expense ($)	Equipment Use (min.)
A	1,000	60	30	30
B	2,000	50	20	30
C	4,000	25	10	20
D	5,200	20	5	10

Stage 1: Calculate the direct RVU and the indirect RVU for each procedure.

Step 1: Divide total sample direct cost (labor expense + supply expense) by either the greatest common denominator (GCD), if there is one, or the average sample direct cost for each procedure.

Procedure	Total Sample Direct Cost	÷	GCD	=	Direct RVU
A	90		5		18
B	70		5		14
C	35		5		7
D	25		5		5

Step 2: Divide total sample indirect cost by either the GCD or the average sample indirect cost for each procedure. Equipment use in minutes can be used as total sample direct cost because it shows the same relationship as depreciation cost; however, if additional indirect cost drivers, like the number of full-time equivalents (FTEs), are used, then both would be converted to money, added together, and then divided by the GCD.

Procedure	Total Sample Indirect Cost	÷	GCD	=	Indirect RVU
A	30		10		3
B	30		10		3
C	20		10		2
D	10		10		1

Stage 2: Calculate the total cost for each procedure.

Step 1: Calculate the total projected direct RVUs by multiplying the direct RVUs per procedure by the projected volume per procedure.

Procedure	RVU	×	Projected Volume	=	Total Direct RVUs
A	18		1,000		18,000
B	14		2,000		28,000
C	7		4,000		28,000
D	5		5,200		26,000
Total					100,000

Step 2: Calculate the total projected indirect cost Drivers by multiplying the indirect RVUs per procedure by the projected volume per procedure.

Procedure	RVU	×	Projected Volume	=	Total Indirect Cost Drivers
A	3		1,000		3,000
B	3		2,000		6,000
C	2		4,000		8,000
D	1		5,200		5,200
Total					22,200

Step 3: Calculate the direct cost per RVU by dividing direct costs by total direct RVUs.

$$\$6,000,000 \div 100,000 = \$60$$

Step 4: Calculate the indirect cost per cost driver by dividing indirect costs by total indirect cost drivers.

$$\$4,000,000 \div 22,200 = \$180.18$$

Step 5: Calculate the direct cost per procedure by multiplying the direct cost per RVU by the direct RVUs in each procedure.

Procedure	Direct Cost/RVU	Direct RVU	Direct Cost/ Procedure
A	$60	18	$1,080
B	60	14	840
C	60	7	420
D	60	5	300

Step 6: Calculate the indirect cost per procedure by multiplying the indirect cost per cost driver by the indirect cost drivers in each procedure.

Procedure	Indirect Cost/Cost Driver	Indirect Cost Driver	Indirect Cost/Procedure
A	$180.18	3	$540.54
B	180.18	3	540.54
C	180.18	2	360.36
D	180.18	1	180.18

Step 7: Calculate the total cost per procedure by adding the direct cost per procedure and indirect cost per procedure.

Procedure	Direct Cost/Procedure	Indirect Cost/Procedure	Total Cost/Procedure
A	$1,080	$540.54	$1,620.54
B	840	540.54	1,380.54
C	420	360.36	780.36
D	300	180.18	480.18

Standard Costing

Standard costing is not actually a method of determining costs, but is a method of establishing benchmark costs, or usually budget costs, for the purpose of comparing actual costs. This method of comparing standard costs to actual costs produces variances, or differences, that are useful to the manager in controlling costs.

Relationship of Costs to Volume and Revenue

For purposes of determining profit or loss, managers must review costs in relation to associated volumes and revenues. The profit equation is:

$$\text{Profit} = \text{revenues} - \text{expenses}$$

Therefore, the manager first must understand the relationship between costs and expenses. Within this context, cost is the amount spent to acquire an asset, and expense is the amount spent consuming the asset. Therefore, expense is an expired asset. As referenced earlier in this chapter, costs can be classified as fixed costs and variable costs. When classifying these costs in relation to an accounting period, fixed costs remain constant and variable costs change in relation to volume, as demonstrated in Figure 6.1.

FIGURE 6.1
Costs per
Period

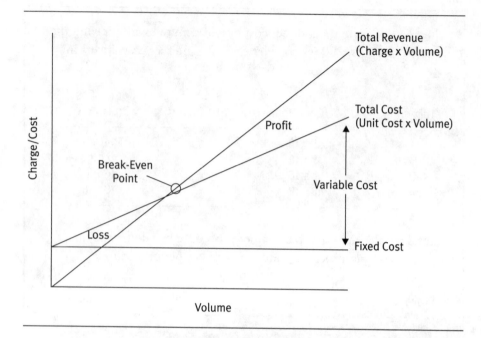

Related to costs per period, the break-even point is the volume in units at which the total revenue line intersects the total cost line, or where total costs equal total revenues, as expressed by the equation

$$\text{Break-even quantity} = \frac{\text{total fixed costs}}{\text{charge} - \text{variable costs per unit}}$$

When classifying these costs in relation to a unit of product or service, fixed costs change in relation to volume, and variable costs remain constant per unit, as shown in Figure 6.2.

FIGURE 6.2
Costs per Unit

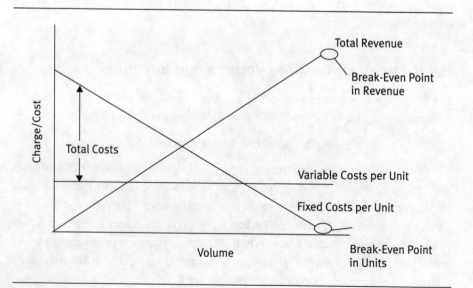

Figure 6.2 is somewhat unorthodox, but it is important to understand the relationship in this way to understand break-even analysis. At any point on the volume axis, total costs equal variable costs per unit, which remain constant, plus fixed costs per unit, which decline as volume increases. Using costs per unit, the break-even point in units or revenues is the point at which fixed costs have been covered. Before that point, each unit sold has not only covered its variable costs, but has also contributed to fixed costs. This is called the contribution margin and can be expressed in dollars with this formula:

$$\text{Contribution margin \$} = \text{charge} - \text{variable costs per unit}$$

It also can be expressed as a percentage,

$$\text{Contribution margin percent} = \frac{\text{charge} - \text{variable costs per unit}}{\text{charge}}$$

and the break-even point in dollars can be expressed with the formula:

$$\text{Break-even point \$} = \frac{\text{total fixed costs}}{\text{contribution margin percentage}}$$

After the break-even point has been reached and fixed costs have been covered, each subsequent unit produced contributes to profit, rather than to fixed costs.

PROBLEM 6.4
Break-Even Analysis

ABC's home health care agency is considering a new product with a fixed cost of $1,000, a charge of $10 per unit, and a variable cost of $5.

What is the break-even point in quantity and in dollars?

What is the contribution margin in dollars and in a percentage?

$$\text{Break-even point quantity} = \frac{1,000}{10-5} = 200 \text{ units}$$

$$\text{Contribution margin \$} = 10 - 5 = \$5$$

$$\text{Contribution margin percent} = \frac{10-5}{10} = 50 \text{ percent}$$

$$\text{Break-even point \$} = \frac{1,000}{.50} = \$2,000$$

Note

1. There is considerable debate regarding which costs and revenues are controllable by department managers and should therefore be reported to department managers. There is no doubt that department managers have some control over direct costs. Assuming that physicians control the volumes and chief financial officers control the charges, department managers have little control over revenues and, in most cases, indirect costs. This information, therefore, is often not reported to department managers.

References

Berman, H. J., S. F. Kukla, and L. E. Weeks. 1994. *The Financial Management of Hospitals, 8th ed.* Chicago: Health Administration Press.

Eastaugh, S. 1987. "Has PPS Affected the Sophistication of Cost Accounting?" *Healthcare Financial Management* 41 (11): 50–53.

Siegel, J. G., and J. K. Shim. 1995. *Accounting Handbook, 2nd ed.* Hauppauge, NY: Barron's Educational Series.

SETTING CHARGES

I n response to a report by ABC's *PrimeTime Live* on how charging practices affected rising healthcare costs, Humana, which at the time was a large for-profit chain of hospitals, responded:

> Hospital charges are inaccurate measurements of the cost of healthcare to patients, since the vast majority of patients and insurers no longer pay them in full. (ABC News 1991)

Essentially, Humana was correct: Few patients or insurers pay what they are charged; most patients and insurers pay charges minus a negotiated discount.[1] Discounting charges and other charging practices have resulted in charges that have little, if any, relationship to costs. How did charges in the healthcare industry arrive at such a nonsensical point? The answer can be found in the history of healthcare charging practices.

Historic Context

Healthcare charging practices have progressed through three distinct eras: consensus-driven charging, financial expediency–driven charging, and competition-driven charging. All of these have had a perverse effect on the relationship between charges and costs.

Prior to Medicare, charging was driven by consensus: healthcare providers set charges consistent with other providers in the community. Providers sought consistent charges for fear that higher than average charges would signal inefficiencies to regulators or drive business to competing providers. Setting charges based on consensus resulted in cost shifting (i.e., the practice of shifting costs to some payers to offset losses from other payers). For instance, a new provider would set charges consistent with other providers in the community, even though the new provider had higher per unit costs resulting from low start-up volumes. To make up for these potential losses, the new provider would shift costs to procedures and the corresponding charges and payers that were not delivered by other providers (Finkler 1982).

With the advent of Medicare and Medicaid, charges became irrelevant for a substantial portion of the provider's business. Medicare—and usually Medicaid—paid hospitals based on reasonable costs, not charges, and paid physicians based on approved charge schedules. Realizing that only patients covered by commercial insurance and patients paying their own way (i.e., charge-based patients) would pay the provider based on charges, most providers set charges based on financial expediency—the financial needs of the provider. The financial needs of the provider included the costs of providing services to charge-based patients; losses to both Medicare or Medicaid; the cost of bad debt; and the cost of charity care. Problem 4.1 demonstrates how these costs are identified and shifted to charge-based patients during the budget process. The actual recovery of shifted costs occurs at the procedural level using charge masters, which are lists of items (i.e., medications, procedures, supplies, and rooms) for which providers generate charges. Providers developed software programs to show each item on the charge master and the item's use by the patient. If the item's use by cost-based payers was high, the charge was set close to allowable cost because allowable cost was the amount the provider would be reimbursed. (Any increase in the charge would result in an increase in contractual allowances and an increase in charges per patient day, but not in collected revenue.) If the item's use by cost-based payers was low, the charge was increased to maximize the collection. Because providers, especially hospitals, set charges in this manner every year, it is easy to understand how some charges, over time, were increased thousands of percent over cost (see Appendix 7.1).

In the early 1980s, the consumer movement complicated charging based on financial expediency. Billing regulations mandated that Medicare patients receive a copy of their bill from the provider, even in cases where patients had no financial liability. In this way, patients could audit the bills to determine whether they had received the items listed on the bill. Patients often complained about high charges for items they could buy for less in their local drugstore (e.g., aspirin, Kleenex, toothbrushes). In response, many providers either reduced the charges for these consumer awareness items or dropped the charges altogether. However, to recover the cost of these items, providers increased the charges for items that patients could not buy in their local drugstore.

Medicare's prospective payment based on DRGs did not change the way providers set charges; however, it did provide the impetus for providers to implement sophisticated cost accounting systems so that providers could determine their profits or losses per DRG. This proved to be an important precursor to the next era—competition-driven charging.

During the competition-driven charging era, which began in the mid-1980s and continues today, providers continued to set charges based on what the market would bear, or what the charge-based patients and their insurers would pay. However, the competition brought about by both managed care, which demanded that providers discount their charges significantly in exchange for business, and the prospective payment system (PPS), which no longer guaranteed cost to providers,[2] resulted in lower effective charges (charges negotiated to include a discount).[3,4]

The practice of charging payers different charges for the same products and services, which could be construed to be a violation of the 1890 Sherman

Antitrust Act, 15 U.S.C. 2, the 1914 Clayton Act, 15 U.S.C. 13, and the 1932 Robinson-Patman Act, 15 U.S.C. 13–13b, 21a, may be thought to be only nominally distinct from the practice of discounting charges to different payers for the same products and services. Third-party payers justified the demands for discounts based on the high volumes of patients they brought to the providers. Based on the fact that the third parties were a sure and predictable source of revenue, product costing became critical during the competition-driven era.[5] Providers needed sophisticated methods of determining product costs so they could negotiate discounts without discounting below cost, or at least below variable costs.[6]

During the early years of competition-driven charging, providers practiced price-driven costing, the practice of determining effective charges, or having effective charges dictated by the insurer, and then cutting costs to break even with the effective charge. However, price-driven costing, even when coupled with aggressive downsizing or reengineering strategies,[7] ultimately arrives at a point at which patients believe additional cost cutting will have a negative effect on quality.[8] But managing costs effectively is only half the strategy for economic survival. The other half is managing revenue effectively by making up for revenue lost as a result of discounting and competition.

Most healthcare organizations have pursued relatively conservative revenue management strategies that have included charging analysis, charge master enrichment, and charge capture assessment (see Murray et al. 1994). Charging analysis ensures that the charge set for a specific item results in maximizing reimbursement related to the payer classification. Charge master enrichment ensures that healthcare organizations charge only for items that third-party payers recognize as legitimate charges. Charge capture assessment ensures that healthcare organizations do not lose charges within the organization. Charge capture assessment compares what patients receive as documented by medical records to what patients are billed as documented in patient bills.

Cross (1997), author of *Revenue Management: Hardcore Tactics for Market Domination,* believes that the healthcare industry is ready for more aggressive revenue management strategies, including charging strategies that have been commonplace in other service industries for a long time. For instance, airlines offer significant discounts to travelers who are willing to travel during off-peak periods and make their reservations in advance. In this way the airlines are better using their fixed costs (i.e., airplanes) while ensuring their variable costs are still met by the discounted charges. The discounted charges have created a new market without hurting the old market. In most cases, business travelers who fly during peak periods are willing to pay the higher charges because their company is reimbursing the cost; vacation travelers who fly during off-peak periods want the lower charges because they pay the cost themselves. Could healthcare organizations enhance their market share by discounting to fill excess capacity, perhaps during the weekends, or create new markets by discounting procedures that patients are likely to pay out-of-pocket? Cross offers seven core concepts of revenue management (Pallarito 1997c):

1. Focus on charges rather than costs when balancing supply and demand.
2. Replace cost-driven charging with competition-driven pricing.
3. Sell to segmented micro markets, not to mass markets.
4. Save your products for your most valuable customers.
5. Make charging decisions based on knowledge, not supposition.
6. Exploit each product's value cycle.
7. Continually reevaluate your revenue opportunities.

In implementing any of these strategies, however, healthcare organizations must be careful not to violate antitrust law or fraud and abuse regulations.

Methods of Setting Charges

Given that many different influences affect the charge-setting decision, the initial charge, before comparisons to other facilities and before discounts, should reflect the healthcare organization's true costs of providing the product or service.[9] Therefore, the following three methods of setting charges based on costs are well established in the literature (Suver, Neumann, and Boles 1992; Berman, Kukla, and Weeks 1994).

RVU Method

The first method of setting charges is called the relative value unit (RVU) method and is used in departments that have an established RVU schedule like laboratory and radiology. RVU schedules are recalculated every three to five years. Costs per RVU and corresponding charges per procedure are calculated more often, usually every year.[10] After full costs per procedure have been established (see Problems 6.2 and 6.3), charges can be set to break even (i.e., charge the full cost) or to realize a gain (i.e., charge the full cost plus a percentage) (see Problem 7.1).

PROBLEM 7.1
RVU Method of Setting Charges

Using job order costing and activity-based costing from Problems 6.2 and 6.3, calculate the charge necessary to realize a 5-percent gain at the diagnostic center.

Using Job Order Costing:

Step 3: Calculate the cost per procedure by multiplying the cost per RVU by the RVUs in each procedure.

Procedure	Cost/RVU	RVU	Cost/Procedure
A	$100	18	$1,800
B	$100	14	$1,400
C	$100	7	$700
D	$100	5	$500

Step 4: Calculate the charge necessary to realize a 5-percent gain at the diagnostic center.

Procedure	Cost/Procedure	+	5 Percent	=	New Charge
A	$1,800		90		$1,890
B	$1,400		70		$1,470
C	$700		35		$735
D	$500		25		$525

Using Activity-Based Costing

Step 7: Calculate the total cost per procedure by adding the direct cost per procedure and the indirect cost per procedure.

Procedure	Direct Cost/Procedure	Indirect Cost/Procedure	Total Cost/Procedure
A	$1,080	$540.45	$1,620.45
B	$840	$540.45	$1,380.45
C	$420	$360.36	$780.36
D	$300	$180.18	$480.18

Step 8: Calculate the charge necessary to realize a 5-percent gain at the diagnostic center.

Procedure	Cost/Procedure	+	5 Percent	=	New Charge
A	$1,620.45		81.02		$1,701.47
B	$1,380.45		69.02		$1,449.47
C	$780.36		39.02		$819.38
D	$480.18		24.01		$504.19

Hourly Rate Method

The second method of setting charges is called the hourly rate method and is used in departments that charge per hour (or per modality or segment of time) for their services. Respiratory therapy, physical therapy, and surgery are three examples of departments that use the hourly rate method for setting charges. Problem 7.2 demonstrates the calculations involved in using the hourly rate method.

PROBLEM 7.2
Hourly Rate Method of Setting Charges

Using the hourly rate method of setting charges, calculate the charge per modality necessary to recover total costs given that at ABC Physical Therapy Clinic:

Total projected cost per year of physical therapy = $800,000
Total projected hours of use per year = 20,000 hours
Modality = 15 minutes

$$\text{Charge per modality} = \frac{\text{total projected cost}}{\text{total projected modality (hour} \times 4)}$$

or

Charge per modality = $800,000 ÷ 80,000 = $10 per modality

Surcharge Method

The third method of setting charges is called the surcharge method and is used in departments that charge for products when the product cost is known and the addition of a surcharge to cover overhead is necessary. Pharmacy and central supply are two examples of departments that use the surcharge method for setting charges. This method is demonstrated in Problem 7.3.

PROBLEM 7.3
Surcharge Method of Setting Charges

Using the surcharge method of setting charges, calculate the charge necessary to cover total costs for 100,000 admission kits given that at ABC Women's Hospital:

Total projected cost of kits and administration = $150,000
Total projected cost of admission kits = $100,000

Step 1: Total cost − cost of kits = total surcharge in dollars

$$\$150,000 - \$100,000 = \$50,000$$

Step 2: Surcharge in dollars ÷ cost of kits = surcharge as percentage

$$\$50,000 \div \$100,000 = .50$$

Step 3: Surcharge as a percentage × cost per kit = surcharge per kit

$$.50 \times \$1 = \$.50$$

Step 4: Surcharge per kit + cost per kit = rate to break even

$$\$.50 + \$1 = \$1.50$$

Future of Setting Charges

According to Eastaugh (1987), increasing competitive pressures will drive healthcare organizations into the same strategic pricing options that other service industries use. Referring to Porter's 1980 book, *Competitive Strategy: Techniques for Analyzing Industries and Competitors*, Eastaugh identifies the competitive pressures as they relate to the healthcare industry:

- Rivalry among existing competitors;
- Potential new entrants to the market;
- Bargaining power of buyers (e.g., Medicare, Medicaid, managed care);
- Bargaining power of suppliers (e.g., physicians); and
- Rivalry from substitute products (e.g., holistic medicine, natural cures, self-care).

These pressures will ultimately force healthcare organizations to accept all of the following strategic pricing options.

- *Predatory pricing*: The practice of pricing products and services low in the short-term to gain market share.
- *Slash pricing*: The practice of pricing products and services low in the long-term by making fundamental changes in the product or service.
- *Follower pricing*: The practice of pricing products and services relative to the market leader.
- *Phase-out pricing*: The practice of pricing products or services high to eliminate poor quality or under-used products and services.
- *Preemptive pricing*: The practice of pricing products and services low to discourage new entrants in the market.

- *Skim pricing*: The practice of pricing products and services high because of high quality or low availability in the market.
- *Segment pricing*: The practice of pricing products and services high relative to their "snob appeal," like high charges for first-class seats on an airplane.
- *Slide-down pricing*: The practice of pricing products and services at different rates for different customers, like high charges for CT scans for charge-based customers and low charges for CT scans for cost-based customers. This type of price discrimination is prohibited by most insurers. Slide-down pricing is different than charging based on financial expediency, which is the practice of setting charges for everyone based on the charge's charge-based use.
- *Loss-leader pricing*: The practice of pricing products and services low to attract customers to complementary products or services that are priced high.

The changes that are occurring in the healthcare environment will require close attention to rate setting and pricing strategies. Sound pricing decisions remain critical to the successful operation of healthcare organizations.

Notes

1. Charge, price, and rate are often used synonymously.
2. Eastaugh (1987) compares the healthcare industry to the airline industry in explaining the competitive pressures brought about by PPS. In the airline industry, routes were deregulated, resulting in airlines competing for the more favorable routes. The competition resulted in inefficient airlines going out of business and efficient airlines gaining market share and reducing prices. In the healthcare industry, the guarantee of reimbursed cost to hospitals ended in 1983 and to physicians ended in 1992; as a result inefficient hospitals and group practices have gone out of business, and the remaining hospitals and group practices have gained market share and reduced charges.
3. Some healthcare organizations and physicians have refused to discount their charges. Reid Hospital in Richmond, Indiana, refuses to discount citing the hospital's pricing policy, which states that "prices should be fair and reflective of the resources used to produce the services performed and uniformly applies" (Pallarito 1997a). Under this policy, the hospital considers it unfair to discount to one payer and shift the costs to another payer.
4. Center for Healthcare Industry Performance Studies (CHIPS) reported that wage-adjusted and case mix–adjusted hospital prices increased only 0.6 percent during 1995, down from 2.4 percent the previous year (Pallarito 1997b).

5. Courts have consistently found that such practices did not lessen competition and therefore were not violations of antitrust law.

6. If fixed costs are covered, effective charges can be negotiated down to variable costs without realizing a relevant loss.

7. Downsizing (i.e., the reduction of resources to meet reduced demand) was an appropriate strategy for healthcare organizations that were losing business or had too many resources. Reengineering, that is, "the fundamental rethinking and radical redesign of business processes to achieve dramatic improvements in critical contemporary measures of performance, such as cost, quality, service, and speed" (Hammer and Champy 1993) was an appropriate strategy for healthcare organizations that were experiencing the same or more demand, but at much reduced effective charges.

8. Anti–managed care laws (i.e., laws designed to control the growth and decision making of managed care organizations, length-of-stay laws, or those that mandate minimum length of stays for certain diagnoses like obstetric delivery), and any-willing-provider laws, or patient protection laws that allow patients to receive care from providers outside a network, are examples of patient reactions to cost-savings endeavors. Opponents of these laws are quick to point out that such laws would increase costs, and, as a result, charges and premiums to patients.

9. True cost is a widely disputed term based largely on the Medicare interpretation of cost during the cost-based reimbursement days. Medicare "disallowed" portions of some costs because the costs were higher than the community standard, and Medicare "unallowed" some costs in their entirety because Medicare did not recognize the nature of the cost (e.g., bad debt in the early days and shift differentials in the latter days of cost-based reimbursement). The term true cost is still important under prospective payment because the payment formulas for DRGs were determined based on Medicare's interpretation of true cost. It is also important to note that true costs could vary considerably between facilities based on volumes in that high-volume healthcare organizations have less fixed cost per unit than low-volume healthcare organizations.

10. For the purpose of setting charges, the use of the same RVU schedule for several facilities or the adoption of a national RVU schedule could constitute price fixing.

Appendix 7.1
Financial Expediency–Driven Pricing

This problem demonstrates how financial expediency–driven pricing works. For the sake of simplicity, this example uses only three procedures and only two types of reimbursement. The projected volume for each procedure is 10.

Procedure A is reimbursed at allowable cost ($100) for all 10 procedures. Five of Procedure B's procedures are reimbursed at allowable cost and five of Procedure B's procedures are reimbursed at the price charged. Procedure C is reimbursed at the price charged for all 10 procedures.

Procedure	Percentage Cost-Based	Projected Volume	Cost/ Procedure	Price/ Procedure	Total Collections
A	100	10	$105	$105	10 × $100 = $1,000
B	50	10	$105	$105	5 × $100 + 5 × $105 = $1,025
C	0	10	$105	$105	10 × $105 = $1,050
Average Price				$105	
Total True Cost		$3,150			
Total Collections				$3,075	

To generate collections that would cover costs without raising the average price, the healthcare organization, using financial expediency–driven charging, could lower the price of the cost-based Procedure A to $100 without affecting collections, could lower the price of Procedure B to $100 with a minimal effect on collections, and could raise the price of procedure C to $115 with a moderate effect on collections.

Procedure	Percentage Cost-Based	Projected Volume	Cost/ Procedure	Price/ Procedure	Total Collections
A	100	10	$105	$100	10 × $100 = $1,000
B	50	10	$105	$100	5 × $100 + 5 × $100 = $1,000
C	0	10	$105	$115	10 × $115 = $1,150
Average Price				$105	
Total True Cost		$3,150			
Total Collections				$3,150	

References

ABC News. 1991. "The Humana Cost." *Prime Time Live.* August 8.

Berman, H. J., S. F. Kukla, and L. Weeks. 1994. "Rate Setting and Pricing Decisions." *The Financial Management of Hospitals,* 8th. ed., 197–213. Chicago: Health Administration Press.

Cross, R. G. 1997. *Revenue Management: Hardcore Tactics for Market Domination.* New York: Broadway Books.

Eastaugh, S. R. 1987. *Financing Health Care: Economic Efficiency and Equity.* Dover, MA: Auburn House Publishing.

Finkler, S. A. 1982. "The Distinction Between Costs and Charges." *Annals of Internal Medicine* 96 (1): 102–109.

Hammer, M., and J. Champy. 1993. *Reengineering the Corporation: A Manifesto for Business Revolution.* New York: Harper Business.

Murray, B. P., R. B. Dwore, R. J. Parsons, P. M. Smith, and L. H. Vorderer. 1994. "Methods of Optimizing Revenue in Rural Hospitals." *Healthcare Financial Management* 48 (3): 52–60.

Pallarito, K. 1997a. "Indiana Hospital Sticks to Guns on 'Fair' Pricing." *Modern Healthcare* 27 (26): 106.

————. 1997b. "Getting in Harmony: As Markets Change, Hospitals Struggle with Pricing." *Modern Healthcare* 27 (26): 100–111.

————. 1997c. "What Airlines Can Teach Hospitals." *Modern Healthcare* 27 (26): 100–101.

Porter, M. 1980. *Competitive Strategy: Techniques for Analyzing Industries and Competitors.* New York: Free Press.

Suver, J. D., B. R. Neumann, and K. E. Boles. 1992. "Pricing Strategies." *Management Accounting for Healthcare Organizations, 3rd ed.* Chicago: Pluribus Press.

Recommended Readings — Part II

Andrianos, J., and M. Dykan. 1996. "Using Cost Accounting Data to Improve Clinical Value." *Healthcare Financial Management* 50 (5): 44–48.

Baker, J. J. 1998. *Activity-Based Costing and Activity-Based Management for Health Care.* Gaithersburg, MD: Aspen Publishers.

Berger, S. 2002. *Fundamentals of Healthcare Financial Management, 2nd ed.* San Francisco: Jossey-Bass.

Canby, J. B. 1995. "Applying Activity-Based Costing to the Healthcare Setting." *Healthcare Financial Management* 49 (2): 50–56.

Chan, Y. L. 1993. "Improving Hospital Cost Accounting with Activity-Based Costing." *Health Care Management Review* 18 (1): 71–77.

Cleverley, W. O. 1997. *Essentials of Health Care Finance, 4th ed.* Gaithersburg, MD: Aspen Publishers.

Conrad, K. A., C. B. Nagle, and R. J. Wunbar. 1996. "Cost Accounting Helps Ensure Group Practice Profitability." *Healthcare Financial Management* 50 (11): 60–64.

Cross, R. G. 1997. *Revenue Management: Hardcore Tactics for Market Domination.* New York: Broadway Books.

Eastaugh, S. R. 1994. *Facing Tough Choices: Balancing Fiscal and Social Deficits.* Westport, CT: Praeger Press.

Feldstein, M. 1988. *Health Care Economics, 3rd ed.* New York: John Wiley & Sons.

Finkler, S. A., and D. M. Ward 1999. *Essentials of Cost Accounting for Health Care Organizations, 2nd ed.* Gaithersburg, MD: Aspen Publishers.

Finkler, S. A., and D. M. Ward. 1999. *Issues of Cost Accounting for Health Care Organizations, 2nd ed.* Gaithersburg, MD: Aspen Publishers.

Finkler, S. A. 2001. *Financial Management for Public Health and Non-Profit Organizations.* Upper Saddle River, NJ: Prentice Hall.

Health Care Financing Administration. 1996. "Overview of the Medicaid Program." *Health Care Financing Review: Medicare and Medicaid Statistical Supplement 1996,* 144–187.

Peterson, P. G. 1996. *Will America Grow Up Before It Grows Old?* New York: Random House.

Petrie, J. T. 1993. "Overview of the Medicare Program." *Health Care Financing Review: Medicare and Medicaid Statistical Supplement*, 1–12.

Porter, M. 1980. *Competitive Strategy: Techniques for Analyzing Industries and Competitors*. New York: Free Press.

Shouldice, R. G. 1991. *Introduction to Managed Care*. Arlington, VA: Information Resources Press.

Tamborlane, T. A. 1996. "Government Launches Major Antifraud Initiative." *Healthcare Financial Management* 50 (5): 38–40.

WORKING CAPITAL

CHAPTER

8

MANAGING WORKING CAPITAL

Every manager in the healthcare organization has either a direct or an indirect effect on working capital. Therefore, understanding working capital, the sources of working capital, and the financing of working capital is important.

Definition of Working Capital

Working capital, properly defined, is the sum of a healthcare organization's investment in current assets, or simply defined as total current assets. Current assets are cash and other short-term assets that the organization expects to convert to cash within one year. Following is a list of what current assets usually include:

- *Cash*: Money on hand, and money that the organization has immediate access to that is deposited in a bank. Cash equivalents are reported as cash and include investments with a maturity of three months or less (e.g., treasury bills and money market funds).
- *Short-term securities*: Investments with a maturity of less than one year.
- *Accounts receivable*: Moneys due to the organization from patients and insurers for services that the organization has already provided.[1]
- *Inventories*: The value of supplies on hand at a given point in time and that are properly presented as a current asset on the balance sheet. When inventories are used, they are presented as a supply expense on the statement of operations.
- *Prepaid expense*: Prepaid expense is money paid in one accounting period for value consumed in a later period. An example of prepaid expense is insurance premiums that are paid in one accounting period for protection in subsequent accounting periods. After the value is consumed, the value is reported as an expense in a similar fashion as inventory.

Current assets are often measured in terms of their liquidity, or their ability to be consumed or converted to cash. Cash is considered the most liquid current asset, followed by cash equivalents, short-term investments, and accounts receivable. Prepaid expense is considered the least liquid current asset; inventories are only slightly more liquid than prepaid expense.

Working capital is often used synonymously with the term net working capital, so it is important to distinguish the difference.[2] While working capital is the organization's total current assets, net working capital is the difference between current assets and current liabilities, and is an important measure of an organization's ability to meet its current liabilities, or its short-term debt-paying capacity.

Current liabilities include accrued wages payable and accounts payable. Accrued wages payable is moneys owed but not yet paid to employees for work already performed for the organization. Accounts payable is moneys owed but not yet paid to vendors for services and products already received by the organization.

Importance of Working Capital

Working capital is important because it is the catalyst that makes fixed or long-term assets productive. For instance, although fixed and long-term assets consist of buildings and equipment, the buildings and equipment cannot be productive or produce revenue unless working capital in the form of employees and inventory are introduced. When introduced, employees, inventory, buildings, and equipment are consumed and converted to accrued wages payable, accounts payable, and depreciation. The costs of this consumption are reflected in the bill to the patient or the patient's insurance company. Until the bill is paid, the amount is carried as an account receivable. When the bill is paid, part of the money is used to start the process again. Healthcare organizations that possess sufficient amounts of working capital also enjoy other benefits. Sufficient amounts of working capital enable organizations to pay their employees and vendors on time, and thus help to ensure good employee and vendor relations. Sufficient amounts of working capital also demonstrate to lenders that organizations have sufficient resources to repay loans and are therefore credit-worthy (Berman, Kukla, and Weeks 1994).

Sources of Working Capital

Sources of working capital include equity, net income, a noncurrent liabilities (i.e., debt) increase, and a noncurrent assets reduction. The sources and methods used to finance working capital, as well as the quantity of working capital to be maintained, are called the working capital policy (Brigham 1992).

Healthcare organizations obtain their permanent working capital (i.e., the minimum amount of working capital that is always on hand) from the owners to cover start-up costs. In the case of governmental organizations, the initial amounts of working capital come from the governmental entity through taxes or bonds. In the case of not-for-profit organizations, the initial amounts of working capital come from the community or religious order through tax-exempt bonds. In some cases, working capital may come from philanthropy. In the case of for-profit organizations, the initial amount of working capital comes from the sale of stock. For-profit organizations not only have greater access to working capital through stock markets, but also have greater flexibility in using the proceeds of stock transactions. Regarding access, for-profit organizations can choose the timing of the sale of stock and the volume of stock necessary to bring about the desired amount of working capital. Regarding flexibility, for-profit organizations have fewer restrictions on how they can use the proceeds of the sale of stock. Governmental and not-for-profit organizations generally have more restrictions from philanthropists and bond issuers (Berman, Kukla, and Weeks 1994). Because healthcare organizations will not generate sufficient working capital from patient revenues for months or even years, depending on the size of the organization and market conditions, it is important that the owners are willing to support start-up working capital needs for an extended period of time.

At some point in a healthcare organization's life cycle, the organization's collected revenues will surpass its expenses. After this point, future working capital needs should be funded by net income. In addition to working capital, other demands on net income will arise. For-profit organizations, for instance, will use portions of net income to pay stockholder's dividends and retain part of the income for future expansion. Not-for-profit organizations will use portions of net income to fund reserves and expansion.

Temporary working capital, which is the additional working capital needed to respond to increases in business that are the result of seasonal fluctuations, should be financed by equity, debt, or trade credit. For instance, unanticipated increases in business may deplete working capital because current liabilities will exceed working capital. Accrued wages payable is typically due every 14 days and accounts payable is typically due every 30 days, and accounts receivable may take as long as 60 days to collect. Figure 8.1 reviews the working capital cycle. Debt should not be used for permanent working capital needs, nor should debt be used for temporary working capital needs unless there is reasonable assurance that the debt can be repaid. For instance, in situations where healthcare organizations lack the working capital necessary to pay employees and vendors because of a decline in business, increasing debt may be a mistake unless alternative sources of funds exist from which the debt can be repaid (see Figure 8.2) (Brigham 1992).

	Day 1	Day 3	Day 14	Day 30	Day 63
Accounts Receivable	Patient seen	Patient billed			Patient pays
Accrued Wages and Accounts Payable	Employees work / Supplies used		Employees paid	Vendors paid	

FIGURE 8.1
Working Capital Cycle

FIGURE 8.2

Sources of
Working
Capital

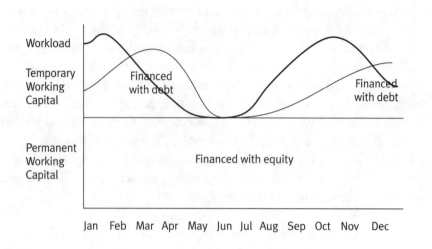

Source: Adapted from Berman, H. J., S. F. Kukla, and L. E. Weeks. 1994. *The Financial Management of Hospitals, 8th ed.*, 261. Chicago:Health Administration Press.

Financing Temporary Working Capital Needs

Temporary working capital needs are generally financed through net assets (owner's wealth), short-term debt, or trade credit.[3] In financing temporary working capital needs, management must determine which method of financing is the least costly to the organization. In the case of using net assets to finance temporary working capital needs, the cost is an opportunity cost: the organization loses the opportunity to invest the net assets in new equipment or income-generating investments. The opportunity cost can be measured in terms of the annual interest rate that such equipment or investments would return (Berman, Kukla, and Weeks 1994).

In the case of using short-term debt to finance temporary working capital needs, most healthcare organizations have a revolving credit agreement, which is a formal line of credit with a commercial bank. The prime rate is the bank's lowest rate of interest on loans afforded to customers with low credit risk. Rates to other customers are generally the prime rate plus, depending on relative credit risk. Interest rates on commercial bank loans are determined using three methods of calculating the effective annual rate: simple interest; discount interest; and add-on interest (Brigham 1992).

- In a simple interest loan, the organization receives the principal and repays the principal plus interest at the end of the loan period. The effective annual interest rate is calculated as:

$$\text{Effective annual interest rate} = \frac{\text{interest}}{\text{principal}}$$

- In a discount interest loan, the organization receives the principal minus the interest at the beginning of the loan period. The effective annual interest rate is calculated as:

$$\text{Effective annual interest rate} = \frac{\text{interest}}{(\text{principal} - \text{interest})}$$

- In an add-on interest loan, or an installment loan, the organization receives the principal and repays the principal plus the interest in monthly installments. The approximate[4] effective annual interest rate is calculated as:

$$\text{Approximate annual interest rate} = \frac{\text{interest}}{(\text{principal}/2)}$$

Problem 8.1 shows the three methods of calculating the effective annual interest rate on a $100,000 loan for one year. In most cases, the bank will determine the interest rate, and the organization may want to calculate the amount of interest owed.

PROBLEM 8.1
Effective Annual Interest Rates on Short-Term Loans

ABC Nursing Home borrows $100,000 for one year and must pay $9,000 in interest. Calculate the effective interest rate using simple interest, discount interest, and add-on interest.

Using Simple Interest

$$\text{Effective annual interest rate} = \frac{\text{interest}}{\text{principal}}$$

$$\text{Effective annual interest rate} = \frac{9,000}{100,000}$$

Effective annual interest rate = .09 or 9 percent

Using Discount Interest

$$\text{Effective annual interest rate} = \frac{\text{interest}}{(\text{principal} - \text{interest})}$$

$$\text{Effective annual interest rate} = \frac{9,000}{(100,000 - 9,000)}$$

Effective annual interest rate = .0989 or 9.89 percent

Using Add-on Interest

$$\text{Effective annual interest rate} = \frac{\text{interest}}{(\text{principal} / 2)}$$

$$\text{Effective annual interest rate} = \frac{9,000}{(100,000 / 2)}$$

Effective annual interest rate = .18 or 18 percent

The same equations can be used with the interest rate and principal as knowns and the amount of interest as the unknown.

In the case of using trade credit to finance temporary working capital needs, in effect the healthcare organization is borrowing money from a vendor by delaying payment to the vendor for goods or services already received by the organization. In using trade credit, the cost involved is either the cost of foregoing an incentive to pay on time or the cost of a late fee. Many vendors offer an incentive, or discount, if the organization pays on time. The term, 2–10, net 30 means the organization receives a 2 percent discount if the organization pays within ten days. Applying 2–10, net 30, to a $100 purchase, it means that if the organization pays within ten days, the vendor will discount the purchase to $98. If the organization pays during days 11–30, the organization must pay $100. Application of a late fee can have the same effect. For instance, the organization purchases a product for $98 and must pay a $2 late fee after day 10. Problem 8.2 (adapted from Berman, Kukla, and Weeks 1994) shows how to calculate the effective annual interest rate for the above referenced situation.

PROBLEM 8.2
Effective Annual Interest Rates on Trade Credit

ABC clinic makes a $98 purchase with a $2 late fee if the clinic pays after five days. What is the effective annual interest rate if the clinic pays on day 6? On day 30?

On day 6:

Step 1: Annual interest paid $= \dfrac{365}{1} = 365 \times \$2 = \$730$

Step 2: Amount borrowed each time $= \$98$

Step 3: Annual interest rate $= \dfrac{\text{annual interest paid}}{\text{amount borrowed each time}}$

$= \dfrac{\$730}{98} = 7.449$ or 744.9%

On day 30:

Step 1: Annual interest paid $= \dfrac{365}{25} = 14.6 \times \$2 = \$29.20$

Step 2: Amount borrowed each time $= \$98$

Step 3: Annual interest rate $= \dfrac{\text{annual interest paid}}{\text{amount borrowed each time}}$

$= \dfrac{\$29.20}{98} = .298$ or 29.8%

Trade credit is usually expensive and should only be used to finance temporary working capital needs if it is the least costly alternative.

Managing Cash Flow

Managing cash flow—the difference between cash receipts and cash disbursements for a given accounting period—is the management of the cash conversion cycle. The cash conversion cycle is defined as the process of converting resources represented by cash outflows into services and products represented by cash inflows. In healthcare organizations, cash outflows consist of employee wages and supply expenses; cash inflows consist of patient revenues. The objective of managing cash flow is to always have the right amount[5] of cash on hand by maximizing and expediting cash inflows and minimizing and delaying cash outflows. The organization must have cash on hand for the following reasons:

- *Transactions*: The expected demand for cash by employees in the form of wages, and suppliers in the form of payments.
- *Precautions*: The unexpected demand for cash in the form of emergencies and other unexpected events.
- *Speculations*: The unexpected demand for cash in the form of price reductions by vendors or other "good deals."

Because cash inflows consist of patient revenues, maximizing and expediting inflows is the primary objective of managing accounts receivable, and will be discussed in detail in Chapter 9. Cash outflows consist of employee wages and supply expenses, and to the extent possible, ethically and legally, they should be minimized and delayed.[6] Minimizing employee wages and supply expenses is a function of the budgeting process where managers should always be exploring new ways to accomplish more work with less resources. In delaying cash outflows, the chief financial officer (CFO) or controller must determine when to pay employees and vendors. Typically, organizations pay employees every two weeks or every month, rather than at the end of each day. In this way, the organization holds and invests money that employees have already earned. Regarding payments to vendors, organizations pay vendors when the money is due, not when the organization receives the supplies or the bill. The organization determines the float period, which is the time difference between the day checks are written and the day checks are presented for payment. The organization uses the float period to transfer money from an interest-bearing account to the checking account as the money is drawn, a process called book overdraft.

Cash Budget

Larger healthcare organizations use a cash budget to help manage cash flows. A cash budget predicts the timing and amount of cash inflows and outflows, and systematically examines the cost implications of various cash management decisions (Berman, Kukla, and Weeks 1994). Basic steps in developing a cash budget for a specific period include the following:

- Prepare a list of all expected sources of cash inflows.
- Estimate the amounts to be received from each source.
- Prepare a list of all expected sources of cash outflows.
- Estimate the amounts to be expended to each source.
- Calculate the period-end cash balance.
- Determine the methods of financing deficit balances (see previous section on Financing Temporary Working Capital Needs) or investing surplus balances.

Short-Term Investments

In the case of investing surplus balances, the organization should have a board-approved investment policy that directs the CFO or controller in making short-term investment decisions. The investment policy should include objectives of investment, authority for investment, and types of investments to be made. Typically, the types of investments to be made include U.S. treasury bills, money market funds, and commercial certificates of deposit, all of which provide both liquidity in the event the organization needs the money invested on short notice, and financial security. Compounding is used to determine the amount of income investments will generate. Compounding is a way of looking at a present amount of money, called present value (PV), and calculating the future amount of money, called future value (FV), using the following formulas:

$FV = PV(1 + i)^n$
where i is the annual interest rate at which the money is invested;
n is the number of years the money is invested; and

$FV = PV(1 + i / m)^{mn}$
where m is the number of times the money is compounded each year.

Problem 8.3 shows how these formulas are used.

PROBLEM 8.3
Calculating the Future Value of an Investment

ABC Physical Therapy Clinic wants to invest $100,000. What is the future value (FV) compounded annually at 7 percent for five years? At 7 percent compounded semiannually for five years?

Compounded annually for five years:
$$FV = \$100,000 (1 + .07)^5$$
$$FV = \$140,300$$
Compounded semiannually for five years:
$$FV = \$100,000 (1 + [.07 / 2])^{2 \times 5}$$
$$FV = \$141,060$$

NOTE: The above referenced answer is formula driven. Use of a calculator or spreadsheet may alter the answer slightly because of rounding or how interest is calculated (at the end of the period versus during the period).

HP 10BII Keys

Key	Store or Calculates
N	The number of payments or compounding periods
I/YR	The annual nominal interest rate
PV	The present value of future cash flows
PMT	The amount of periodic payments
FV	Future value
● P/YR	Store the number of periods per year. The default is 12.
●	Shift key (orange on must models)

HP 10BII Solution to Problem 8.3 compounded annually

Keys	Display	Description
1 ● P/YR	1.00	Sets compounding periods per year to 1
5 N	5.00	Stores the number of compounding periods (1×5)
7 I/YR	7.00	Stores the interest rate
−100,000 PV	−100,000.00	Stores the present value as an anuity (−)
FV	140,255.17	Calculates the future value

HB 10BII Solution to Problem 8.3 compounded semiannually

Keys	Display	Description
2 P/YR	2.00	Sets compounding periods per year to 2
10 N	10.00	Stores the number of compounding periods (2×5)
7 I/YR	7.00	Stores the interest rate
−100,000 PV	−100,000	Stores the present value
FV	141,060	Calculates the future value

Evaluating Working Capital and Cash Performance

Financial analysis, covered in more depth in Chapter 15, is methods used by investors, creditors, and management to evaluate the past, present, and future financial performance of the organization. According to Berman, Kukla, and Weeks (1994), financial analysis includes the following three steps:

1. Establishing the facts in the organization;
2. Comparing the facts in the organization over time and to facts in other similar organizations; and
3. Using perspective and judgment to make decisions regarding the comparisons.

The first step, establishing the facts, usually relates to a review of the organization's financial statements,[7] whose accuracy has been confirmed by independent auditors. The second step, comparing the facts over time and comparing the facts to similar organizations includes ratio analysis, horizontal analysis, and vertical analysis. Ratio analysis is the most common form of comparison and evaluates an organization's performance through computing and showing the relationships of important line items found in the financial statements. Typically, there are four kinds of ratios: liquidity, profitability, activity, and capital structure. Horizontal analysis evaluates the trend in the line items by focusing on the percentage change over time, and vertical analysis evaluates the internal structure of the organization by focusing on a base number and shows the percentages of the relationships of important line items to the base number. For instance, using vertical analysis an organization might want to know what percent of gross revenue is net revenue, bad debt, charity care, or contractual allowance. After ratio analysis, horizontal analysis, and vertical analysis are complete, the organization can make trend and industry comparisons.

Trend comparisons compare the organization's present and past ratios, trends, and percentages to determine the organization's financial performance over time. However, trend comparisons only work with ratios, trends, and percentages that show directionality, meaning that the numbers are always better as they increase in one direction, and always worse as they proceed in the other direction.

Industry comparisons compare the organization's ratios, trends, and percentages to the ratios, trends, and percentages of other similar organizations to determine the organization's financial performance relative to competitors. Several organizations publish key ratios, trends, and percentages: Moody's Investors Service publishes *Health Care Medians*; Dun & Bradstreet publishes *Key Business Ratios*; and Troy publishes the *Almanac of Business and Industrial Financial Ratios*.

The third step of financial analysis, using perspective and judgment to make decisions regarding the comparisons, uses the information obtained in the first two steps, coupled with information derived from the decision maker's unique perspective and judgment, to make the decision. Decisions that may at first be at odds with the information provided in the first two steps may make perfect sense based on pressures from both internal and external constituents including medical staffs, employers, regulators, donors, and others.

When evaluating working capital and cash performance, the following liquidity ratios are important. None of these ratios show directionality: if the ratio is too low, the organization must borrow money to meet its obligations; if the ratio is too high, the organization loses the opportunity to invest in longer-term assets with a higher return.

- **Current Ratio**

$$\frac{\text{total current assets}}{\text{total current liabilities}}$$

The basic indicator of financial liquidity, or an organization's ability to meet its financial obligations. Higher values indicate better debt-paying capacity. The Current Ratio does not take into account the relative liquidity of the different current asset accounts. The Current Ratio median for all hospitals reporting to Ingenix (2004) for 2002 audited financial statements was 2.00—S&P "A" rated hospitals reporting to Ingenix was 1.90.

- **Days Cash on Hand, Short-Term Sources**

$$\frac{\text{cash} + \text{marketable securities}}{(\text{total expenses} - \text{depreciation expense})/365}$$

- **Days Cash on Hand, All Sources**

$$\frac{\text{cash} + \text{marketable securities} + \text{unrestricted long-term investments}}{(\text{total expenses} - \text{depreciation expense})/365}$$

An indicator of how long an organization could meet its obligations if cash receipts were discontinued. The Days Cash on Hand, Short-Term Sources median from all hospitals reporting to Ingenix (2004) for 2002 audited financial statements was 24.8—S&P "A" rated hospitals reporting to Ingneix was 29.7. The Days Cash on Hand, All Sources median from all hospitals reporting to Ingenix for 2002 audited financial statements was 77.5—S&P "A" rated hospitals reporting to Ingenix was 108.6.

- **Average Payment Period**

$$\frac{\text{current liabilities}}{(\text{total expenses} - \text{depreciation expense})/365}$$

An indicator of the average time that passes before a current liability is paid. The Average Payment Period median from all hospitals reporting to Ingenix (2004) for 2002 audited financial statements was 55.4—S&P "A" rated hospitals reporting to Ingenix was 56.0.

The analysis of working capital and cash performance is an important aspect of the financial management of healthcare organizations. The following chapters in Part III take a closer look at the management of two specific current assets: accounts receivable and materials.

Notes

1. Healthcare organizations, like physicians offices, that use cash accounting rather than accrual accounting will not have accounts receivable or bad-debt expense because cash accounting records revenue when paid, whereas accrual accounting records revenue when earned.
2. Net working capital is sometimes confused with cash flow, which is the difference between cash receipts and cash disbursements for a given accounting period.
3. Brigham (1992) also identifies accruals, in which the healthcare organization essentially borrows from its own accrued wages or accrued taxes. However, in both cases, the accounts are likely to be due in two weeks to a month. Brigham also identifies commercial paper, or short-term promissory notes, as having interest rates somewhat below the prime rate; however, the use of commercial paper is restricted to a small number of organizations that are exceptionally good credit risks.

4. The exact effective annual interest rate $= (1 + k_d{}^{12}) - 1$, where k_d equals the cost of debt.
5. The right amount of cash on hand is a function of both the timing and the amount of cash inflows and cash outflows. At a minimum, the right amount of cash on hand is the difference between cash inflows and cash outflows, as expressed in the equation (Berman, Kukla, and Weeks 1994)

Cash outflows − cash inflows = minimum cash balance on hand.

6. Summers (1986) argues that the CFO's primary duty is to the organization; therefore, as long as the implied contract between the organization and its vendors is not violated, paying late is all right.
7. According to the 1996 *AICPA Audit and Accounting Guide for Health Care Organizations*, an organization's financial statements must include a consolidated balance sheet, a statement of operations, a statement of changes in net assets, and a statement of cash flows. Because financial analysis requires an analysis of financial statements, financial analysis is sometimes referred to as financial statement analysis.

References

American Institute of Certified Public Accountants. 1996. *AICPA Audit and Accounting Guide for Health Care Organizations*. New York: AICPA.

Berman, H. J., S. F. Kukla, and L. E. Weeks. 1994. *The Financial Management of Hospitals, 8th ed*. Chicago: Health Administration Press.

Brigham, E. F. 1992. *Fundamentals of Financial Management, 6th ed*. New York: The Dryden Press.

Ingenix. 2004. *Almanac of Hospital Financial and Operating Indicators*. Salt Lake City, UT: Ingenix.

Summers, J. 1986. "Paying Late, Not Paying the Penalty." *Journal of Health Care Materiel Management* 5 (6): 100–102.

Troy, L. 1994. *Almanac of Business and Industrial Financial Ratios*. Englewood Cliffs, NJ: Prentice Hall.

MANAGING ACCOUNTS RECEIVABLE

I n most healthcare organizations, accounts receivable is the largest current asset and deserves special attention. Three factors set the healthcare industry apart from most other industries with regard to accounts receivable: the nature of the services provided, the cost of the services provided, and the method of payment for the services provided. Because many of the services provided by healthcare organizations are provided in an emergent nature, at least in the patient's mind, patients often do not have the time to raise the funds necessary to pay for the services they need or want.

Many of the services provided by healthcare organizations are services requiring highly trained personnel and high-tech equipment available 24 hours a day. Furthermore, many of the services provided by healthcare organizations are services that are reimbursed by third parties; therefore patients rely on the third party to pay for the services they need or want.

Definition of Accounts Receivable

Accounts receivable are moneys due to the organization from patients and third parties for services that the organization has already provided. Accounts receivable is a function of the production and payment cycles, as illustrated in Table 9.1.

During pre-care, the healthcare organization obtains from the patient all the information necessary to both treat and bill (Table 9.2 provides a list of information to be collected during pre-care). HFMA (1998) says that inadequate or incorrect information gathered at this stage is the single greatest reason for not billing or collecting accounts receivable in a timely manner. According to HFMA, unless the care is emergent in nature, treatment should not begin until this stage is completed. From a legal perspective, the organization is not required to initiate treatment—absent an emergency—if the patient is unable to pay.[1] However, after the organization has initiated treatment, the organization cannot terminate treatment solely based on the patient's inability to pay.[2]

During care, the organization should post charges in a prompt and accurate manner. The medical record, which is in the hands of clinicians at this point, should document all phases of the patient's care. The medical record is the primary source of clinical data required for reimbursement from most third parties. Utilization review ensures that the care provided to the patient is appropriate and is care that the patient or third party will reimburse.

TABLE 9.1
Accounts
Receivable
Cycle

Cycle	Patient Activity	Accounts Receivable Activity
Production cycle	Patient seeks care	
	Pre-care	Obtain demographic data Obtain insurance data Verify insurance coverage Obtain authorizations Obtain deductibles Obtain copays
	Care	Record charges Maintain medical record Review utilization
	Care completed	Transfer medical record Analyze medical record Abstract medical record Code medical record Transcribe dictation
Payment* cycle		Print bill Submit bill Follow up bill Collect bill, or Bill resolution

* The payment cycle usually begins when the medical record is complete for billing purposes. However, in organizations where the medical records department reports to the chief financial officer (CFO), the payment cycle may begin at patient discharge owing to the fact that the CFO is responsible for the processing time in medical records.

The organization should conduct utilization review during the care, called concurrent review, as well as after the care, called retrospective review.

During the care-completed phase, sometimes referred to as discharged but not final billed, the medical record is transferred from the clinicians to the medical record department. The patient's record is analyzed for completeness, abstracted, and coded. The medical record department adds transcriptions from the physician including final diagnosis.

On completion of the medical record, the payment cycle begins. In the bill print phase, a claim form is completed. At this time, the gross receivable may be reduced to a net receivable based on previously agreed-upon discounts. In the bill submission phase, a claim is sent from the organization to the patient and/or third-party payer.

In bill collection, the organization makes additional efforts to collect the bill before submitting the patient's account to a collection agency. The organization's credit and collection policy and relevant federal and state laws should cover the extent to which the organization and collection agency should seek payment. The organization's board should decide how aggres-

- Patient name and other identifiers including social security number, gender, date of birth, place of birth, and race;
- Patient address and telephone number;
- Patient occupation, employer, employer address and phone number;
- Resident status of all foreign-born patients;
- Name, address, and telephone numbers of next-of-kin;
- Name, address, and telephone numbers of person responsible for bill;
- Name, address, telephone numbers, and certificate numbers of all third-party payers;
- Benefits to which the patient is entitled;
- Name, address, and telephone number of primary care physician;
- Name, address, and telephone number of attending physician;
- Preliminary diagnosis;
- Date of most recent previous outpatient services or admission;
- Accident information;
- Financial resources information for self-pay patients;
- Authorizations and precertifications;
- Consent for medical treatments and admissions; and
- Assignments of insurance benefits from the patient to the provider.

TABLE 9.2
Patient
Information
Collected
During
Pre-Care

Source: Adapted from Healthcare Financial Management Association. 1998. *HFMA Core Certification Exam Self-Study Manual*, 1–16. White Plains, NY: The MGI Management Institute.

sively the organization should seek payment for services already rendered to patients. In bill resolution, the organization makes a final decision about the bill. At this stage, the organization may decide to write off the bill as a bad debt.

Importance of Accounts Receivable

The amount of current assets tied up in accounts receivable (AR can be as much as 75 percent of the current assets) can vary significantly among organizations, as can the accounts receivable and associated costs. This variance is often attributed to the credit-and-collection policies of the board as well as to management methods used to reduce accounts receivable. Costs associated with accounts receivable include a carrying cost, a routine credit-and-collection cost, and a delinquency cost (Berman, Kukla, and Weeks 1994).

Carrying costs associated with accounts receivable are the costs incurred by the organization for extending credit to the patient after the organization has provided services. If patients paid at the time of service, the organization would have the funds on hand to either invest or pay current liabilities. The costs of carrying patient accounts are therefore opportunity costs in that the organization has lost the opportunity to invest at a given interest rate, or the organization must borrow funds at a given interest rate to pay current liabilities.

Routine credit-and-collection costs associated with accounts receivable are the costs incurred by the organization for billing and collecting during the organization's average payment cycle. If patients paid at the time of service, the organization would generate only one bill per patient. When the organization extends credit, it incurs the cost of sending additional bills and reminders.

Delinquency costs associated with accounts receivable are the costs incurred by the organization for patients or their payers not paying on time, during the organization's average payment cycle, or at all. If patients paid at the time of service, the organization would not incur the costs of a collection agency or the costs of bad debt. When the organization extends credit, it increases the likelihood that some patients or their payers will not pay on time or at all.

Management of Accounts Receivable

The extension of credit for most healthcare organizations is a necessary evil because of the nature and cost of the services provided, and the preponderance of third-party payment. However, the organization's credit-and-collection philosophy should treat the extension of credit as the exception to the rule, and not the rule itself. The rule should be to collect as much money as possible at the time of service, and to extend credit to credit-worthy patients only when necessary. Therefore, the objective of managing accounts receivable is to reduce the collection period, which is the number of days between the time of service and the time of payment, by reducing the amount of receivables.

Policies and Procedures

The first step in managing accounts receivable is to have policies and procedures for the registration/admission of all patients (Berman, Kukla, and Weeks 1994). All patients who are not emergent in nature should go through a pre-registration/preadmission process to obtain the information listed in Table 9.2, as well as to collect deductibles, copayments, and deposits. Organizations are much more likely to obtain information and payments prior to providing services as opposed to obtaining the information after providing services. Organizations cannot hold patients against their will to obtain payment or information (see Showalter 2003 on false imprisonment). The organization should be prepared to preregister/preadmit patients at times most convenient to patients, including evening hours and weekends for larger organizations. In certain cases, preregistration/preadmission can occur over the phone or on the Internet (HFMA 1998). Preregistration/preadmission also expedites the registration/admission of patients, thus avoiding wait times, a key indicator of quality according to patient surveys.

Management Accounting System

The second step in managing accounts receivable is to have an accounting system that provides prompt and accurate recording of charges (Berman, Kukla, and Weeks 1994). Internal auditors often can play a role in determining the effectiveness of the accounting system by verifying the system's internal control. Internal control consists of accounting systems and supporting procedures that provide systematic, automatic safeguards to protect the integrity of the accounting information in the healthcare organizations (Herkimer 1993). Internal controls also (Marrapese and Titera 1989):

- Provides management with information that is up to date, reliable, and accurate;
- Reduces the risk of losing assets through errors or misappropriations;
- Promotes operational efficiency by, among other things, reducing the likelihood of errors; and
- Gives employees direction through policies and procedures.

Table 9.3 provides typical questions that an internal auditor may ask in relation to internal control of accounts receivable.

1.	Do registration/admission procedures exist and ensure that complete and accurate accounts receivable and collection information is gathered, including such documents as signed authorization forms, patient billing information, and insurance assignments?	**TABLE 9.3** Internal Audit of Accounts Receivable Questions
2.	Do procedures exist and ensure that services rendered to patients are medically necessary?	
3.	Is a complete medical record prepared, including physician discharge summaries and physician statements attesting to the principal diagnosis and other clinical information?	
4.	Do procedures exist and ensure that amounts due from third-party payers are properly supported?	
5.	Do procedures exist and ensure that cash receipts are properly recorded?	
6.	Do procedures exist and ensure that charity care balances are identified and deducted from gross revenues?	
7.	Do procedures exist and ensure that detailed accounts receivable records are routinely compared to general ledger control accounts and third-party payer logs?	
8.	Do reviews exist and ensure that allowances for bad debts and contractuals are adjusted periodically to ensure that receivables are reported at estimated net realizable amounts?	
9.	Do procedures exist and ensure that medical records personnel are properly trained and supervised to provide appropriate coding?	
10.	Do procedures exist and ensure prompt coding of Medicare and other similar medical records data?	
11.	Do procedures exist and ensure independent coding reviews, primarily for Medicare patients?	

Source: Adapted from Herkimer, A. G. 1993. *Patient Financial Services*, 288–89. Chicago: HFMA/Probus Press.

Medical Record System

The third step in managing accounts receivable is to have a medical record system that allows for prompt and accurate recording of clinical information. With the advent of Medicare prospective payment in 1983, hospital health information management (HIM) departments had significant pressure to process medical records in a timely fashion so that the physician could attest to the final diagnosis, which was required prior to bill submission. By 1990, to improve medical record turnaround time for billing purposes, almost half of the nation's hospital HIM departments were reporting to the hospital CFO (Gauss 1991). This proved to be a double-edged sword. In most cases, CFOs were responsible for the hospital's information system, which helped HIM departments improve the medical records information system, which in turn improved the turnaround time. However, by inheriting HIM departments, the CFO inherited the physician problems associated with delinquent medical records.

Traditionally, HIM departments were not involved with the medical record until after discharge. With the advent of Medicare prospective payment, hospitals needed a preliminary DRG assignment at patient admission; needed to monitor use during the patient stay; and needed to interface the patient billing system (PBS) with the medical record system (MRS) to determine cost per DRG. The resulting interfaced information systems are shown in Figure 9.1.

Completing the medical record in a timely fashion is still important, particularly for Joint Commission accreditation. The penalty for delinquent medical records—limits on or suspension of medical staff privileges—has always been difficult to enforce because of the financial effect on the hospital caused by limiting physician privileges. St. Elizabeth Medical Center in Granite City, Illinois has initiated fines for physicians with medical records delinquent past 14 days (Rogliano 1997). However, from the accounts receivable perspective, emphasis has changed from medical record promptness to medical record accuracy.

Some of the pressure to complete the medical record in a timely fashion has diminished with the increase in capitation as a method of hospital payment. Also, hospitals are no longer required to have a signed physician attestation before submitting a Medicare claim (HFMA 1995). Finally, as computer-based patient records become more common, medical records turnaround time is expected to improve (Renner 1996).

HIM departments have experienced increased pressure for accuracy in medical records. Coding errors can delay payment until corrected and can initiate federal investigations and resulting fines. Since the passage of the 1986 False Claims Act amendments, the federal government has recovered more than $3 billion in false or erroneous claims to the Medicare program.[3] Unfortunately, accurate coding is less objective than federal investigations and

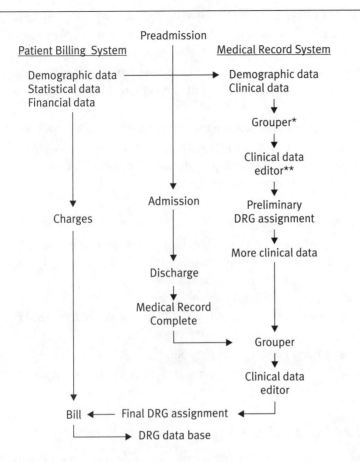

FIGURE 9.1

Patient Billing System/ Medical Record System Interface

---

*Grouper: software package that assigns DRG.
**Clinical data editor: software package that edits clinical data by checking for coding errors.

---

court cases might imply. For instance, current procedural terminology (CPT) codes were developed to identify physician services and often do not work well in hospital outpatient departments, therefore they result in coding problems. Coding problems are often identified by fiscal intermediaries during routine focused medical reviews (FMRs). Recent FMRs have identified the following coding problems (Whitehead and Salcido 1997):

- Different interpretations of national coding standards by fiscal intermediaries and healthcare organizations;
- Improper use of HCFA revenue codes;
- Improper CPT coding of mammography services; and
- Improper use of unlisted CPT codes.

The most effective way for healthcare organizations to avoid fraud and abuse investigations and minimize the effects of investigations if they do occur is to have a comprehensive compliance plan that includes a coding compliance plan (see Chapter 5 for more information on compliance plans). A coding compliance plan provides the framework for effective internal controls. Under the provisions of the False Claims Act, the federal government does not need to prove intent to defraud but only reckless disregard for a claim's validity.

A comprehensive compliance plan that includes a coding compliance plan is one way to defend against charges of reckless disregard (Whitehead and Salcido 1997). A coding compliance plan should ensure that the HIM department is (Russo and Russo 1998):

- Using the right coding resources;
- Documenting all advice from fiscal intermediaries;
- Supplying sufficient coding resources to coders;
- Checking on computerized encoders;
- Requiring periodic training for all coders;
- Staying current on all *International Classification of Diseases, 9th edition,* (ICD-9) and CPT changes;
- Developing and revising coding policies;
- Contracting for and documenting annual external coding audits; and
- Performing and documenting regular internal coding audits.

Credit-and-Collection Policy

The fourth step in managing accounts receivable is to have a board-approved credit-and-collection policy that directs the organization's management in extending credit and collecting accounts. Organizations may vary considerably in how aggressively they collect accounts receivable, but the credit-and-collection policy should address the following issues.

Charity Care   The discussion of charity care (as distinguished from bad debt) should include a discussion on eligibility criteria.

Bad Debt   The discussion of bad debt should include at what point and under what circumstances the organization turns accounts over to a collection agency and at what point and under what circumstances the organization writes off accounts as bad debts.

Self-Pay   Self-pay should include provisions for financial counseling to determine how the services provided will be reimbursed.

Financial counseling is the process of extending credit to self-pay patients. Because of this process, the organization should better understand the patient's ability or inability to pay the organization for services rendered, and the patient should better understand his or her financial responsibilities to the organization. According to HFMA (1998), financial counseling should:

1. Tell the patient about the organization's credit-and-collection policies and how the policies pertain to the patient.
2. Investigate the patient's credit history and determine to what extent the patient can pay for anticipated services.
3. Help the patient evaluate alternative payment options including, but not limited to:
   - credit cards;
   - bank loans, including home equity loans;
   - credit union loans;
   - cash from sale of assets; and
   - extended payment plans, with or without interest.
   Organizations should be willing to significantly discount their charges to obtain payments at time of service.
4. Follow up and resolve any pending financial transactions.

Third-Party Insurance Relationships

The discussion of third-party insurance relationships should include: provisions for coordination of benefits, which is the process of determining the order of insurance company liability when multiple insurance companies are involved; assignment of benefits, which is the process of transferring insurance benefits from patients to the healthcare organization; and third-party audits.

Billing Procedures

The credit-and-collection policy should also discuss billing procedures, including provisions for (Berman, Kukla, and Weeks 1994):

- Bill cutoffs, which is the point at which the organization determines the bill is complete and ready for submission;
- Prompt payment[4] and interest assessment, if any, for late payment; and
- Follow-up billing, including both the format (i.e., how aggressive the language should be) and timing (i.e., how often the organization should mail reminders, called dunning notices).

Deposit Procedures

The section of the credit-and-collection policy on deposit procedures should include provisions for a lock box and electronic data interchange (EDI)[5] to the processing and posting of cash receipts, typically patient revenues. When using a lock box, payers mail the healthcare organization's receipts directly to the bank, which deposits the money and forwards the accompanying paperwork, along with a copy of the check, to the organization for processing. When using EDI, large payers like Medicare wire the check directly to the bank or organization and then Medicare forwards accompanying paperwork either via wire or mail (Berman, Kukla, and Weeks 1994). (For more information, see Moynihan 1996.)

From Accounts Receivable Management to Revenue Cycle Management

The HIPAA transaction standard provides a unique opportunity for health-care organizations to improve their revenue cycle performance. Revenue cycle management conceptualizes the accounts receivable process as a continuum rather than as a set of isolated events (Laforge and Tureaud 2003) and incorporates the use of multidisciplinary teams, including clinicians, to improve performance. Any healthcare organization whose key financial measures lie outside the industry benchmarks should review its revenue cycle practices. Key benchmarks include (Guyton and Lund 2003):

- Outstanding revenues that exceed the industry average of about 50 days;
- More than 15 percent of receivables exceeding 90 days;
- High management turnover in revenue-related areas;
- Evidence of cash flow problems;
- Declining net-to-gross ratios.

Opportunities for improved revenue cycle management are usually found in five key areas:

1. Denials management—virtually all denials are the result of administrative problems or clinical problems;
2. Cash acceleration or follow-up on upaid claims;
3. Patient payments of copays and deductibles at point-of-service and enhanced methods of patient payments;
4. Third-party payment compliance to ensure that payment received was the correct amount (see Lang and Williams 2003 regarding contract management systems)
5. Vendor contract coordination to ensure a broad-based evaluation of contract term in relation to coordination of benefits.

Financing Accounts Receivable

Healthcare organizations employ two methods to receive cash advances on outstanding accounts receivable: factoring receivables and pledging receivables. When an organization factors its accounts receivable, it is selling the accounts at a discount to a bank or other agent to collect. The advantage of factoring is that the organization receives the funds immediately, albeit at a discount. The disadvantage of factoring is that the organization loses control of the collection process, and the collection methods used by the bank or other agent may reflect poorly on the organization.

The second method that healthcare organizations employ to receive cash advances on outstanding accounts receivable is pledging the receivables. When an organization pledges its receivables, it uses the receivables as collateral for a loan. The advantage of pledging accounts receivable is that the organization maintains control of the collection process. The disadvantage of using receivables to secure a loan is that the resulting interest rate on the loan is usually higher than other conventional loans (Zelman, McCue, and Millikan 1998).

Federal Laws Governing Accounts Receivable

Three federal laws govern accounts receivable: the Fair Debt Collection Practices Act, the Truth in Lending Act, and the Fair Credit Reporting Act.

Fair Debt Collection Practices Act

The Fair Debt Collection Practices Act applies only to third-party collectors. As long as the healthcare organization collects its own debts, the act does not apply. If the organization contracts with a collection agency, or operates a collection agency under another name, the act does apply. The act deals with four key bill collecting practices:

1. *Skiptracing*: Governs how the debt collector communicates with consumers owing the debt and under what conditions a debt collector can communicate with others regarding the debt.
2. *Collector communication*: Governs when debt collectors can communicate with consumers.
3. *Harassment*: Identifies certain behaviors and actions by debt collectors that can constitute a claim of harassment by the consumer and that are therefore prohibited.
4. *Deceptive or false representations*: Prohibits misleading representation designed to intimidate the consumer.

Truth in Lending Act

The Truth in Lending Act establishes disclosure rules for consumer credit sales. It provides five criteria for eligibility, including the requirement for a written agreement and four or more installments. If eligible, the lending organization must disclose the following under Regulation Z:

- Annual percentage rate;
- Amount of the finance charge;
- Amount of the principal;

- Amount of payments;
- Number of payments;
- Total of all payments;
- Late charge arrangements;
- Prepayment arrangements; and
- An opportunity for the debtor to receive an itemization of how the payments are to be applied.

Fair Credit Reporting Act

The Fair Credit Reporting Act governs the permissible uses of credit reports. The act lists the ways in which credit reports can be obtained, including by court order, by permission of the consumer, and by legitimate business need. Information that must be removed from credit reports and the time at which that information must be removed follows (HFMA 1998):

- Bankruptcies after ten years;
- Judgments after seven years or when the statute of limitations expires, whichever is longer;
- Paid tax liens after seven years;
- Collection accounts or those charged to profit and loss after seven years;
- Arrests, indictments or convictions after seven years; and
- Other adverse items after seven years.

Evaluating Accounts Receivable Performance

When evaluating accounts receivable performance, Average Collection Period (also called days in accounts receivable) is most often used. Average Collection Period is defined as the number of days of operating revenue that an organization has due from its patient billings after deducting for contractual allowances, bad debt, and charity care. The Average Collection Period median for all hospitals reporting to Ingenix (2004) from 2002 audited financial statements was 59.4—S&P "A" rated hospitals reporting to Ingenix was 59.7.

- **Average Collection Period**

$$\frac{\text{net accounts receivable}}{\text{net patient service revenue}/365}$$

The objective of managing accounts receivable is to reduce the Average Collection Period; the collection period does show direction, meaning that a smaller number is always better. One way to reduce the Average Collection Period is to write off accounts as bad debt. However, writing off accounts prematurely will reduce the days in accounts receivable and may not be in the organization's best interest.

Notes

1. From a legal perspective, the contract between the patient and the healthcare organization does not begin until treatment begins (see *Childs v. Weiss*, 440 S.W.2d 104). The organization's tax status, as well as the organization's ethics as reflected in its credit-and-collection policy, may dictate otherwise, however.
2. Generally speaking, healthcare organizations cannot terminate treatment solely based on the inability to pay (see Holder 1973 on abandonment).
3. See the following cases as reported in Whitehead and Salcido 1997: *Hindo v. University Health Sciences*, 65 F.3d 608 (7th Cir. 1995); *United States ex rel. Stinson v. Prudential Ins.*, 944 F.2d 1149 (3rd Cir. 1991); *United States v. University of Texas M.D. Anderson Cancer Center*, 961 F.2d 46 (4th Cir. 1992); *United States ex rel. Glass v. Medtronic, Inc.*, 957 F.2d 605 (8th Cir. 1992); *United States ex rel. McCoy v. California Medical Review, Inc.*, 723 F.Supp. 1363 (N.D. Cal. 1989); *United States v. Krizek*, 859 F. Supp. 5 (D.D.C. 1994); *United States ex rel. Ramona Wagner and Jeanine Dehner v. Allied Clinical Labs, Medicare & Medicaid Guide* (CCH) 43,142 (S.D. Ohio, 1995).
4. The 1986 Social Security Amendments require fiscal intermediaries (i.e., those that have contracted with the federal government to pay Medicare claims) to pay no less than 95 percent of clean claims, or claims that have no defect, impropriety, or special circumstances, within 24 days of receiving the claim. Effective in 1993, fiscal intermediaries must pay clean claims submitted electronically within 13 days, and clean claims submitted on paper within 26 days (HFMA 1998).
5. The Health Insurance Portability and Accountability Act of 1996 mandates standardized, electronic billing by October, 2002.

References

Berman H. J., S. F. Kukla, and L. E. Weeks. 1994. *The Financial Management of Hospitals, 8th. ed.* Chicago: Health Administration Press.

Childs v. Weiss, 440 S.W.2d 104. 1969. Tex. Civ. App.

Gauss, J. W. 1991. "A Decade of Change: The Emerging Role of the CFO." *Healthcare Financial Management* 45 (5): 54–62.

Guyton, E. M., and Lund, C. 2003. "Transforming the Revenue Cycle." *Healthcare Financial Management* 57 (3): 72–78.

Healthcare Financial Management Association. 1998. *HFMA Core Certification Exam Self-Study Manual.* White Plains, NY: The MGI Management Institute.

———. 1995. "Updata." *Healthcare Financial Management* 49 (10): 5.

Herkimer, A. G. 1993. *Patient Financial Services.* Chicago: HFMA/Probus Publishing.

Holder, A. R. 1973. "Law & Medicine." *The Journal of the American Medical Association* 225 (9): 1157–58.

Ingenix. 2004. *Almanac of Hospital Financial and Operating Indicators.* Salt Lake City, UT: Ingenix.

Laforge, R. W. and Tureaud, J. S. 2003. "Revenue-Cycle Redesign: Honing the Details." *Healthcare Financial Management* 57 (1): 64–71.

Lang, K., and B. Williams. 2003. "Recovering Real Money with a Contract Management System." *hfm* 57 (12): 42–44.

Marrapese, R. L., and W. R. Titera. 1989. *Internal Control of Hospital Finance: A Guide for Management.* Chicago: American Hospital Association Publishing.

Moynihan, J. J. 1996. *Implementation Manual for the 835 Health Care Claim Payment/Advice: Guidelines for Electronic Payment of Healthcare Claims Using the ANSI ASC X12 Electronic Data Interchange (EDI) Standard,* Revised Edition. Westchester, IL: HFMA.

Renner, K. 1996. "Cost-Justifying Electronic Medical Records." *Healthcare Financial Management* 50 (9): 63–70.

Rogliano, J. 1997. "Managing Delinquent Records." *Journal of the American Health Information Management Association* 68 (8): 28–30.

Russo, R., and J. Russo. 1998. "Healthcare Compliance Plans: Good Business Practice for the New Millennium." *Journal of the American Health Information Management Association* 69 (1): 24–31.

Showalter, J. S. 2003. *Southwick's The Law of Healthcare Administration, 3rd ed.* Chicago: Health Administration Press.

Whitehead, T., and R. Salcido. 1997. "Coding Component Important Element of Compliance Plan." *Healthcare Financial Management* 51 (8): 56–58.

Zelman, W. N., M. J. McCue, and A. R. Millikan. 1998. *Financial Management of Health Care Organizations: An Introduction to Fundamental Tools, Concepts, and Applications.* Malden, MA: Blackwell Publishers.

MANAGING MATERIALS

I n most healthcare organizations, materials, including supplies and pharmaceuticals, is the largest nonlabor cost in the operating budget and therefore deserves special attention. Proper management of materials can have a significant effect on operating costs, and as a result, the net income of the organization.

Definition of Materials and Inventory Management

Materials management is defined more broadly than inventory management: Materials management is the management and control of inventory, services, and equipment from acquisition to disposition. Organizations further classify items into two major categories: patient care and administration. Items in patient care include medical supplies, surgical supplies, drugs, linens, and food. Items in administration include housekeeping supplies, office supplies, and other supplies not used for direct patient care.

The primary objective of materials management is to minimize the total cost associated with materials while ensuring that the proper materials, meaning in both quality and quantity, are readily available for patient care and administration.

Inventory management is the management and control of inventory, or items that have an expected useful life of less than 12 months (Suver, Neumann, and Boles 1992).

Importance of Materials Management

Patient Care

Why are materials, and, more specifically, inventory, so important? First and most important, an organization must have the right kind and the right amount of supplies on hand for patient care. The right kind of supplies can be determined by the materials manager, with the help of a user committee. The right amount of supplies can be more difficult to project for three reasons: time, uncertainties, and discontinuities (Berman, Kukla, and Weeks 1994).

Time considers that, for most supplies, a lag time exists between ordering and receiving the supplies.   **Time**

Uncertainties The demand for supplies fluctuates with volume and kind of patient; therefore, the demand for most healthcare supplies is uncertain. Because of uncertain demand, the materials manager must meet with each department manager to determine the actual necessity of every supply item. If the supply item is a life-saving drug used in emergencies, for example, the materials manager will stock the item at a very high level to ensure that the organization never runs out. This procedure is called a stock-out. If the supply in question is a seldom-used office supply, the materials manager will stock the item at a very low level, if at all. This method of classifying inventory, either by cost or by nature (i.e., emergent, routine, seldom used) is the ABC inventory method. If the organization is large or has sufficient influence over its vendors, the organization may use just-in-time (JIT) inventory for some of its inventory items, meaning the supply item is delivered immediately prior to use. JIT means the organization has no, or very little, inventory on hand.

Discontinuities Discontinuities also affect the amount of supplies on hand. Discontinuities means that the inventory process has been disrupted, perhaps by a new model of the supply or a missed delivery, so the organization must have stock on hand to continue the patient care process.

Cost

The second reason materials management is so important is cost. Inventory, like accounts receivable, is a non-productive asset: it does not grow or produce income. In fact, both accounts receivable and inventory lose value over time. For accounts receivable, the more time an account spends in receivables, the more likely it will become an uncollectible. The more time an item spends in inventory, the more likely it will become stolen, expired, or lost. For that reason, organizations want to reduce inventory holdings and increase cash, marketable securities, and other assets that produce income.

Inventory Valuation

Costs related to inventory appear in two places on the healthcare organization's financial statements. First, inventory appears as a current asset on the organization's balance sheet. In this case, inventory, expressed as a dollar amount, represents the unused portion of inventory on hand for a given accounting period.

Second, inventory appears as expense items on the organization's statement of revenues and expenses. In this case, inventory, expressed as supplies, food, and drugs, represents the portion of inventory used for a given accounting period. The value of inventory on the balance sheet is based on the cost paid for the items in inventory. During the year, however, identical items of inventory will be purchased at different prices. Furthermore, some inventory items are expensed as the organization uses them. How does the materials manager determine which inventory items and related costs have been expensed and which inventory items and related costs are still in inventory? There are four commonly accepted methods of valuing inventory: first-in, first-out (FIFO); last-in, first-out (LIFO); weighted average; and specific identification. Each will produce a different value and each has advantages and disadvantages:

- *First-in, first-out (FIFO)*: The first item put into inventory is the first item taken out of inventory. FIFO produces an inventory of newer items. The total cost of inventory is determined by multiplying the unit cost of the newest items in inventory by the number of units in inventory.
- *Last-in, first-out (LIFO)*: The last item put into inventory is the first item taken out of inventory. LIFO produces an inventory of older items. The total cost of inventory is determined by multiplying the unit cost of the oldest items in inventory by the number of units in inventory.
- *Weighted average*: Determines the average cost of items placed in inventory and then multiplies the average cost by the number of units in inventory.
- *Specific identification*: Determines the actual cost of each item in inventory. Specific identification is used when inventory items are easy to identify and when the cost of each inventory item is high.

The organization's management must determine which method is best for the organization (Berman, Kukla, and Weeks 1994). Problem 10.1 demonstrates how each inventory method works.

PROBLEM 10.1
Inventory Valuation

ABC Outpatient Clinic purchased surgical dressing trays at the following dates and amounts.

	Units	Price ($)	Total ($)
January 1 beginning balance	100	10	1,000
March 1 purchase	400	12	4,800
May 1 purchase	400	13	5,200
July 1 purchase	300	14	4,200
September 1 purchase	200	14	2,800
November 1 purchase	100	15	1,500
Total	1,500		$19,500
Ending inventory on Dec. 31	150		

Using FIFO, LIFO, and weighted average, what is the ending cost of inventory?

FIFO (ending inventory is composed of the most recent 150 trays purchased)

	Units	Price ($)	Total ($)
November 1 cost	100	15	1,500
September 1 cost			
(apply 50 trays)	50	14	700
Ending inventory	150		$2,200
			or $14.67 per tray

LIFO (ending inventory is composed of the earliest 150 trays purchased)

	Units	Price ($)	Total ($)
January 1 costs	100	10	1,000
March 1 cost			
(apply 50 trays)	50	12	600
Ending inventory	150		$1,600
			or $10.67 per tray

Weighted average (ending inventory is the average cost per item multiplied by the ending inventory in units)

$$\frac{\$19,500}{1,500} = \$13.00 \text{ per unit} \times 150 = \$1,950$$

Management of Inventory

Costs of Inventory

To minimize the total costs of inventory, the materials manager must have a good understanding of inventory costs.[1] For this reason, this book takes the detailed look necessary to understand the interrelationship of inventory costs. Inventory costs are reflected in the following issues:

- How much of an item to order each time;
- When to order the item; and
- What the cost of the item is.

Purchasing Cost Purchasing cost (PD) is the total cost paid to vendors for a specific item during an accounting period, or year. Purchasing cost is derived by multiplying the price of the item (P) per unit paid to the vendor, by the demand (D) (i.e., the annual amount of the item used).

$$\text{Purchasing cost} = PD$$

Ordering cost (O) is the administrative costs associated with placing a single **Ordering Cost**
order for the inventory item. Ordering cost includes the costs of:

- Writing specifications;
- Soliciting bids;
- Evaluating and awarding bids;
- Preparing and signing the contract;
- Preparing the purchase order;
- Receiving the items; and
- Accounting for and paying the invoice.

Total ordering cost associated with an inventory item is dependent on the number of orders placed for the item, and indirectly on the size of a single order, called quantity (Q). Therefore, total ordering cost for an item in inventory is derived by multiplying the number of orders per year ($\frac{D}{Q}$) by the ordering cost per order (O).

$$\text{Total ordering costs} = \left(\frac{D}{Q}\right) O$$

Carrying cost is the cost of holding an inventory of items. When an organi- **Carrying Cost**
zation holds items in inventory, carrying costs include an opportunity cost at least equal to the average cost of inventory holdings ($[P][\frac{Q}{2}]$), derived by multiplying the price of the item (P) by the average number of items in inventory ($\frac{Q}{2}$), multiplied by the interest rate (I) at which the organization could have invested.

$$\text{Opportunity cost} = IP\,\frac{Q}{2}$$

Carrying cost also includes a holding cost. Holding cost includes the costs of storing, securing, and insuring the items in inventory, and is derived by multiplying the holding cost per unit (H) by the quantity ordered each time (Q).

$$\text{Holding costs} = HQ$$

Therefore, carrying costs can be derived by adding holding costs (HQ) and opportunity costs ($[IP]\frac{Q}{2}$).

$$\text{Carrying costs} = HQ + IP\,\frac{Q}{2}$$

Stock-out cost (S) is the cost associated with having insufficient inventory **Stock-Out Cost**
holdings to meet demand (i.e., running out of the item in inventory). Stock-out cost includes the purchasing costs and ordering costs associated with a

stat (immediate) order, and the intangible costs of loss of goodwill among the organization's medical staff and patients. If the stock-out results in injury or death for the patient, the stock-out cost would include the cost associated with this liability. The stock-out cost is derived on a case-by-case basis.

Overstock Cost   Overstock cost (L) is the cost associated with having more than enough inventory holdings to meet demand. Overstock cost includes the carrying cost associated with stocking items for additional accounting periods until the organization uses and expenses the items.

Total Cost   The total cost (TC) formula produces the minimum costs associated with keeping a specific item in inventory for a period of one year, and is derived by adding purchasing cost (PD), total ordering cost ($[\frac{D}{Q}]O$), carrying cost ($HQ + IP[\frac{Q}{2}]$), stock-out cost (S), and overstock cost (L):

$$\text{Total Costs} = PD + \left(\frac{D}{Q}\right)O + \left(HQ + IP\left[\frac{Q}{2}\right]\right) + S + L$$

The total cost formula can provide a basis for different real-world situations the manager may face. For instance, a vendor offers a manager a 10-percent discount on price if the vendor can reduce the number of deliveries per year to four. In this situation, the total cost formula (TC) changes based on the new information: price (P) becomes $P - 10$ percent, and quantity (Q) becomes $\frac{D}{4}$. After reworking the TC formula, if adjusted total cost is less than the original total cost, the manager should accept the vendor's offer.

If the manager has $10,000 budgeted for an inventory item and must ask the vendor for a discount on price, total cost (TC) is $10,000, and the unknown variable is price (P). Before calculating the total cost formula, the economic order quantity (Q_e) must be calculated.

Economic Order Quantity and Reorder Point

The economic order quantity (EOQ or Q_e) is the quantity of items that should be ordered each time to result in the minimum total inventory costs associated with the item. The Q_e formula is:

$$Q_e = \sqrt{\frac{2DO}{IP + 2H}}$$

The Q_e model makes the following assumptions:

- Demand is fixed and constant during the year.
- Lead time for placing orders is constant.
- No discounts are offered for quantity orders.
- No stock-out or overstock costs exist.

These assumptions may be unrealistic in most healthcare organizations. However, in organizations where demand fluctuates weekly, the fluctuations tend to cancel out so that seasonal demand, or annual demand, appears constant (Siegel and Shim 1995).

Calculation of the reorder point (RP) requires knowledge of the lag time in receiving orders, or how many days occur between ordering an item and receiving the item. Thus, the reorder point in units is the demand during the lag time and the reorder point in days is the lag time.

Problem 10.2 demonstrates the total cost (TC) formula, the economic order quantity (Q_e) formula, and the reorder point.

PROBLEM 10.2
Economic Order Quantity, Total Cost, and Reorder Point

Find the EOQ, the total cost, and the reorder point in units given:

Price (P)	= $10
Annual demand (D)	= 10,000 units with a constant daily demand
Order cost (O)	= $10 per order
Interest (I)	= 7 percent
Holding cost (H)	= $.10 per unit
Lag time	= 5 days

Find the EOQ.

$$Q_e = \sqrt{\frac{2DO}{IP + 2H}}$$

$$Q_e = \sqrt{\frac{2(10,000)(10)}{(.07)(10) + (2)(.10)}}$$

$$Q_e = 471 \text{ units}$$

Find the total cost.

$$TC = PD + \frac{D}{Q}O + \left(HQ + IP\frac{Q}{2}\right)$$

$$TC = (10)(10,000) + \frac{10,000}{471}(10) + \left[(.10)(471) + (.07)(10)\left(\frac{471}{2}\right)\right]$$

$$TC = \$100,424$$

Find the reorder point in units.

$$RP = \frac{D}{365} \times 5, \text{ or } RP = \frac{10,000}{365} \times 5, \text{ or } RP = 137 \text{ units}$$

Find the number of orders to be placed in a year.

$$\text{Orders per year} = \frac{D}{Q}, \text{ or } \frac{10,000}{471}, \text{ or } 21.2$$

Find the number of days between orders.

$$\text{Days between orders} = \frac{365}{\text{orders per year}}, \text{ or } \frac{365}{21.2}, \text{ or } 17.2$$

Find the carrying cost.

$$\text{Carrying cost} = HQ + IP\frac{Q}{2}, \text{ or } \left[(.10)(471) + (.07)(10)\left(\frac{471}{2}\right)\right], \text{ or } \$212.13$$

Find the holding cost.

$$\text{Holding cost} = HQ, \text{ or } \$47.10$$

Find the opportunity cost.

$$\text{Opportunity cost} = IP\frac{Q}{2}, \text{ or } (.07)(10)\frac{471}{2}, \text{ or } \$164.99$$

Find the cost of the average inventory.

$$\text{Average inventory cost} = P\frac{Q}{2}, \text{ or } (10)\frac{471}{2}, \text{ or } \$2,355$$

Find the volume of the average inventory.

$$\text{Volume of the average inventory} = \frac{Q}{2}, \text{ or } \frac{471}{2}, \text{ or } 235.5 \text{ units}$$

The vendor offers a 10-percent discount on price if he can make equal monthly deliveries. Should his offer be accepted?

$$\text{Price (P)} = \$9.00$$

$$\text{Quantity (Q)} = \frac{10,000}{12}, \text{ or } 833 \text{ units}$$

$$TC_2 = (9)(10,000) + \frac{10,000}{833}(10) + (.10)(833) + (.07)(9)\left(\frac{833}{2}\right)$$

$$TC_2 = \$90,467$$

Yes, because \$90,467 is less than \$100,424.

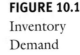

FIGURE 10.1

Inventory
Demand

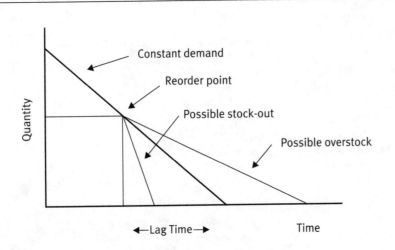

Source: Adapted from Berman, H. J., S. F. Kukla, and L. E. Weeks. 1994. *The Financial Management of Hospitals,* *8th ed.,* 287. Chicago: Health Administration Press.

Managing Inventory When Uncertain Demand Exists

In Problem 10.2, demand was constant. Each day the organization used the same number of the product; daily demand was $10,000 / 365 = 27.4$ units. A constant demand is unlikely in most healthcare organizations. Given an uncertain demand, the probability of stock-outs and overstocks increases, as shown in Figure 10.1. Measuring the costs associated with stock-outs and overstocks is admittedly difficult, but assume that stock-out cost is $7.50 per unit and overstock cost is $2.00 per unit in Problem 10.2.

To determine the reorder point (RP) under conditions of uncertain demand, the organization needs to know the costs associated with stock-outs and overstocks previously given, and the probability of a stock-out based on the history of the inventory item (see Problem 10.3). By multiplying the stock-out or overstock cost by the probability of occurrence, the projected cost can be calculated for each reorder point. For example, at a reorder point of 135 units and a demand of 136 units, one additional unit is needed at a stock-out cost of $7.50, which is then multiplied by the chance of that happening (.25) for a cost in that specific cell of $1.88. In Problem 10.3, the low-cost solution is to establish a reorder point at 138 units, which will minimize the stock-out and overstock costs associated with an uncertain demand (Berman, Kukla, and Weeks 1994).

Evaluating Inventory Performance

The ratio most often used to evaluate inventory performance is the Inventory Turnover, which measures the number of times an organization turns over its inventory relative to operating revenue.

PROBLEM 10.3
Reorder Point Under Conditions of Uncertainty

Find the reorder point under conditions of uncertainty, given the following information:

Stock-out cost = $7.50 per item
Overstocked cost = $2.00 per item

Probability of meeting demand	.10	.25	.30	.25	.10
	135	136	137	138	139

	Potential Demand					
	135	136	137	138	139	
Probability	.10	.25	.30	.25	.10	
Reorder Point						Cost ($)
135	.00	1.88	4.50	5.63	3.00	15.01
136	.20	.00	2.25	3.75	2.25	8.45
137	.40	.50	.00	1.88	1.50	4.28
138	.60	1.00	.60	.00	.75	2.95
139	.80	1.50	1.20	.50	.00	4.00

Source: Adapted from Berman, H. J., S. F. Kukla, and L. E. Weeks. 1994. *The Financial Management of Hospitals, 8th ed.*, 290. Chicago: Health Administration Press.

Answer: The low-cost reorder point under conditions of uncertainty is 138 units at $2.95.

- **Inventory Turnover**

$$\frac{\text{total operating revenue}}{\text{inventory}}$$

Low values indicate overstocking and thus an inappropriate investment in non-productive assets. This ratio does show directionality; higher values are considered to be better. Because of their size, healthcare systems enjoy considerable purchasing power and often receive medical supplies on consignment. This means that the vendors do not charge the system until the supply item is used, so inventory value is very low. The Inventory Turnover median for all hospitals reporting to Ingenix (2004) for 2002 audited financial statements was 59.59—S&P "A" rated hospitals reporting to Ingenix was 63.58.

Note

1. Several formulas are used to determine inventory costs. This book uses the formula and cost descriptions from Berman, Kukla, and Weeks (1994) because of the level of detail.

References

Berman, H. J., S. F. Kukla, and L. E. Weeks. 1994. *The Financial Management of Hospitals, 8th ed.* Chicago: Health Administration Press.

Ingenix. 2004. *Almanac of Hospital Financial and Operating Indicators.* Salt Lake City, UT: Ingenix.

Siegel, J. G., and J. K. Shim. 1995. *Accounting Handbook, 2nd ed.* Hauppauge, NY: Barron's Educational Series.

Suver, J. D., B. R. Neumann, and K. E. Boles. 1992. *Management Accounting for Healthcare Organizations, 3rd ed.* Chicago: HFMA/Pluribus Press.

Recommended Readings — Part III

Brigham, E. F. 1992. *Fundamentals of Financial Management, 6th ed.* New York: Dryden Press.

Cleverly, W. O. 1997. "Working Capital and Cash Management." *Essentials of Health Care Finance, 4th ed.* Gaithersburg, MD: Aspen Publishers.

Herkimer, A. G. 1993. *Patient Financial Services.* Chicago: HFMA/Probus Publishing.

McLean, R. A. 1997. *Financial Management in Health Care Organizations.* New York: Delmar Publishers.

Moynihan, J. J. 1996. *Implementation Manual for the 835 Health Care Claim Payment/Advice: Guidelines for Electronic Payment of Healthcare Claims Using the ANSI ASC X12 Electronic Data Interchange (EDI) Standard*, Revised Edition. Westchester, IL: HFMA.

Suver, J. D., B. R. Neumann, and K. E. Boles. 1992. "Materials Management and Control." *Management Accounting for Healthcare Organizations, 3rd ed.* Chicago: HFMA/Pluribus Press.

Zelman, W. N., M. J. McCue, and A. R. Millikan. "Working Capital Management." *Financial Management of Health Care Organizations.* Malden, MA: Blackwell Publishers.

RESOURCE ALLOCATION

STRATEGIC AND OPERATIONAL PLANNING

Everyone agrees that planning—especially strategic planning—is critical for economic survival in today's turbulent environment. However, planning is a management function often neglected by healthcare managers. In a 1995 survey of over 200 integrated delivery and financing systems (IDFSs),[1] Ernst & Young (1996) found that "strategic planning was incomplete, primarily in terms of goal setting. Only 68 percent of the IDFSs reported setting financial goals. About 10 percent did not have a strategic plan, and only 61 percent had a plan that covered at least three years."

Definition of Planning

Planning as a management function is the process of deciding in advance what must be done in the future. Planning consists of establishing goals, objectives, policies, procedures, methods, and rules necessary to achieve the purposes of the organization. Planning precedes, and serves as a framework for, the other management functions of organizing staffing, influencing, and controlling. Effective planning is a continuous process; managers are responsible for planning for the appropriate use of resources in their areas of responsibility in concert with the operational and strategic direction of the organization. In the absence of effective planning, managers would engage in random activities. In healthcare organizations where customers demand a high degree of predictable outcomes, such random activities on the part of managers would have a disastrous effect (Dunn 2002).

Prerequisites to Planning

Before effective planning can begin, the organization must meet certain requirements. First, the organization must have a sound organizational structure that ensures management accountability for the planning process. Second, the organization must have a well-defined chart of accounts that corresponds with the organizational structure. Third, the organization must have a prompt and accurate accounting system that ensures financial accountability for the planning process. Fourth, the organization must have a comprehensive management information system that captures nonfinancial information for each department (Berman, Kukla, and Weeks 1994).

Types of Planning

Planning can be classified by planning horizon, management approach, and design characteristics.

Planning Horizon

Planning horizon is the length of time management is looking into the future. Strategic plans look three to ten years into the future. Operating plans look one year into the future.

Management Approach

Planning can also be classified by management approach, or top-down versus bottom-up planning. These approaches correspond closely with top-down and bottom-up budgeting as discussed in Chapter 12. In top-down planning, senior management, which includes the division heads or vice presidents, develops the plan with little or no input from subordinates. The advantage of such a design is that senior management may be in the best position to objectively view the future. The disadvantage of the top-down design is that plan implementation may be difficult if subordinates have little or no input.

In bottom-up planning, subordinates develop the plan and submit it to senior management for approval. The advantage to bottom-up planning is the commitment to the plan by those who developed it. The disadvantage is that subordinates may not be in the best position to view the future.[2]

In most cases, a combination of the top-down and bottom-up designs is used, with senior management deciding on plan parameters and subordinates submitting plans within those parameters.

Design Characteristics

Planning can also be classified by design characteristics, which also correspond closely with the design characteristics of budgeting as discussed in Chapter 12.

Incremental Versus Zero-Base Planning

Incremental planning requires planning only for changes like new equipment, new positions, and new programs. Incremental planning assumes that all current operations including positions and equipment are essential to the continued mission of the organization, and that all current operations are working at peak performance. The advantages are the ease of incremental planning, the minimal time commitment required to plan, and the support of a bigger organizational culture. The principle disadvantage of incremental planning is the assumption that all current operations are essential in a healthcare environment that is changing so rapidly. Conversely, zero-base planning takes nothing for granted and requires rejustification for existing equipment, positions, and programs, as well as justification for new equipment, positions, and programs. Therein lies the principle advantage of zero-base planning: in a rapidly changing environment where reimbursement is moving away from cost-based approaches toward prospective payment per case or per enrollee, zero-base planning can eliminate unnecessary programs and improve operations. Disadvantages include the large commitment of time required, employee fear and anxiety, and the significant administrative and communication requirements (Person 1997).

Comprehensive planning integrates the strategic plan and the operational plan into one document. The advantage is the recognition that short-term objectives affect long-term goals. Limited-in-scope planning segregates the plans. Most organizations integrate the plans at the board and executive management level of the organization, but the issue is the level at which the plans should be segregated.

Comprehensive Versus Limited-in-Scope Planning

Fixed plans assume that volumes, and related revenues and variable expenses, remain constant during the year. Fixed plans are easy to project, but they are unrealistic for healthcare organizations whose volumes fluctuate during the year and whose variable expenses, which are dependent on volumes, account for over half of an organization's operating expenses.

Fixed Versus Flexible Planning

Flexible plans take into account fluctuations in volumes, at least within ranges expressed as probabilities, and adjust variable expenses accordingly.

Discrete plans apply to a fixed period of time, usually a year. At the end of the year, a new plan begins. Discrete plans are relatively easy to prepare, but do not take into account certain events that may occur at year end. For instance, department managers who had managed wisely and accomplished their objectives by year end would likely have a new objective in the next planning year.

Discrete Versus Continuous Planning

Continuous plans, sometimes referred to as rolling plans, are updated continuously so that year end never occurs. Department managers who manage wisely roll over their efforts to the next month.

Corporate Planning

Most healthcare organizations have moved away from facility planning—planning based on their own needs—which was popular under retroactive, cost-based reimbursement. They have adopted a business planning approach based on market needs, called corporate planning. Corporate planning consists of four major stages (see Table 11.1):

1. *Strategic planning*: The process used to determine the organization's overall direction in the next three to ten years.
2. *Operational planning*: The process used to convert the strategic plan into next year's objectives.

3. *Budgeting*: The process used to convert the operating plan into budgets for revenues, expenses, and cash.
4. *Capital budgeting*: The process used to convert the operating plan into budgets for capital expenditures.

Strategic Planning

Strategic planning forces managers to anticipate where they want the healthcare organization to be in three to ten years; it forces managers to identify the resources that will be necessary to get there; and it forces managers to preview the provision of healthcare services at the end of the planning horizon. Strategic planning also provides the starting point for the operating plan and budget (HFMA 1998).

The governing board has the overall responsibility for strategic planning for the organization, but it should actively seek input from the organization's stakeholders, which are those constituents with a vested interest in the organization (see Fottler et al. 1989 regarding stakeholders). Certainly the

TABLE 11.1
Planning
Process

STRATEGIC PLANNING	**Planning Horizon**
1. Validate mission and interpretations	3–10 years out,
2. Assess external environment	revised annually
3. Assess internal environment	
4. Formulate vision	
5. Establish strategic thrusts	
6. Identify critical success factors	
7. Develop primary, or core, objectives	
OPERATIONAL PLANNING	1 year out
8. Develop secondary, or department, objectives	
9. Develop policies	
10. Develop procedures	
11. Develop methods	
12. Develop rules	
BUDGETING	1 year out
13. Project volumes	
14. Convert volumes into revenues	
15. Convert volumes into expenses	
16. Adjust revenues and expenses as necessary	
CAPITAL BUDGETING	1–3 years out
17. Identify and prioritize requests	
18. Project cash flows	
19. Perform financial analysis	
20. Identify nonfinancial benefits	
21. Evaluate benefits and make decisions	

community (which may be represented by the board members), the medical staff, and organization employees should provide input (Rakich, Longest, and Darr 1992).

The Planning Process

Step 1: Validate Mission and Strategic Interpretations

The first step in the planning process is for the executive management, which includes the governing body and the chief executive officer (CEO), to validate the organization's mission. The mission is a broad statement of organizational purpose that can be easily communicated throughout both the organization and the community. Because mission statements are broad, organizations should not need to change them frequently; mission statements should survive to the end of the planning horizon. A study of over 200 Fortune 500 companies identified common characteristics of effective mission statements (Pearce and David 1987). The mission statements

- Target customers and markets;
- Indicate the principle services delivered by the organization;
- Specify the geographic area in which the organization intends to operate;
- Identify the organization's philosophy;
- Include confirmations of the organization's self-image; and
- Include the organization's desired public image.

Because organizations want the mission statements to play well to the communities they serve, mission statements do not always accurately reflect the true purposes of the organization. Strategic interpretations, however, should reflect the true purposes of the organization.

Strategic interpretations provide the means for executive management to interpret the mission statement by recognizing the changing character of the healthcare industry and the changing needs of the community. Strategic interpretations may also prioritize organizational purposes when the mission statement includes multiple purposes that might conflict when operationalized. Strategic interpretations are seldom directly stated in any form, and are more often represented in the actions of executive management. For instance, executive management may show a preference for one purpose over another through the budget allocation process.

Step 2: Assess the External Environment

The second step in the planning process is for the governing body or outside consultants[3] to assess the external environment, including factors external to the organization that might have an effect on present or future performance. The first part of the assessment should include a determination on the direction of the industry as a whole by investigating national trends. Some of the national trends for the healthcare industry during the 1990s included (HFMA 1998):

- Decreasing reimbursement from federal and state health programs as government tries to slow rising healthcare costs;
- Increasing popularity of managed care programs, especially among employers;
- Increasing consolidation as a result of competition;
- Continuing expansion into businesses outside the traditional healthcare industry;
- Increasing growth in outpatient care, preventive care, and innovative alternative delivery systems; and
- Declining numbers of rural and public teaching hospitals.

The second part of the external environment assessment should include a determination on the direction of the local market and should include an investigation of the following elements (HFMA 1998):

- Demographic and socioeconomic characteristics of the primary and secondary service areas and their effect on present and future utilization patterns;
- Key economic and employment indicators, and their effect on present and future utilization patterns;
- Patient migration patterns to determine from where patients and potential patients come;
- Market share statistics for key competitors to determine market strengths and weaknesses;
- Competitor profiles including: strengths and weaknesses, use by service, use by payer, exclusive and other managed care contracts, extent of horizontal and vertical integration, potential expansion plans, and cost comparisons;
- Managed care profile to determine present and future managed care penetration; and
- Physician profile to determine numbers, ages, and specialists available in the market.

Any significant difference between national trends identified in the first part of the external environment assessment and the local trends identified in the second part of the external environment assessment should be thoroughly analyzed to determine the reasons for the differences.

Step 3: Assess the Internal Environment

The third step in the planning process is for the governing body or outside consultants to assess the internal environment including factors that might have an effect on performance either now or in the future. The first part of the assessment should include a determination on the direction of the organization by investigating organizational trends. Some of the organizational trends for analysis might include (HFMA 1998):

- Patient composition including historic inpatient and outpatient use patterns (i.e., patient days, outpatient visits, admissions, discharges, length of stays, age, payer, patient origin);
- Medical staff composition including historic use by specialty, age, practice (solo versus group), admissions, length of stays, office locations, and board certification;
- Agreements with payers and managed care organizations;
- Financial ratios including liquidity ratios, profitability ratios, activity ratios, capital structure ratios, and operating ratios (see Chapter 14); and
- Joint Commission status and quality indicators including both rate-based indicators and sentinel event indicators.

Some organizations use a SWOT analysis (strengths, weaknesses, opportunities, and threats) to assess the internal environment. A SWOT analysis forces the organization to identify its strengths and weaknesses during internal assessment. Then the organization identifies opportunities for additional market penetration with existing or new programs and threats from competitors that might reduce the organization's chances for success (Dunn 2002).

Step 4: Formulate the Vision

The fourth step in the planning process is for the executive management to formulate a vision—a view of the future that they think gives the organization the best chance of accomplishing its mission. Executive management bases its vision on the information obtained from assessing the external and internal environments, and management must communicate its vision throughout the organization. Effective vision statements have certain characteristics in common (Peters 1988). They should

- Be inspiring first of all to employees, but also inspiring to customers;
- Be clear, challenging, and about excellence;
- Make sense to the community, be flexible, and stand the test of time;
- Be stable, but change when necessary;
- Provide direction in a chaotic environment;
- Prepare for the future while honoring the past; and
- Be easily translated into action.

Step 5: Establish Strategic Thrusts

The fifth step in the planning process is for executive management to establish strategic thrusts or goals, which are broad statements of significant results that the organization wants to achieve related to the vision. Strategic thrusts should be limited in number, stable and enduring, and, taken together, comprehensive to the point that they provide meaningful end results for all components of the organization's mission (Dunn 2002; Berman, Kukla, and Weeks 1994).

Step 6: Identify Critical Success Factors

The sixth step in the planning process is for executive management to identify critical success factors that will measure progress toward achieving the plan. The assessment of the environment should introduce both strategic thrusts and critical success factors (Dunn 2002). Critical success factors are organization-specific, but most healthcare organizations will include critical success factors from the following areas (HFMA 1998):

- Inpatient use and market share;
- Outpatient use and market share;
- Managed care use and market share;
- Medical staff profiles and activity levels;
- Accessibility indicators;
- Cost-effectiveness indicators; and
- Quality indicators.

Step 7: Develop Core Objectives

The seventh and last step in the strategic planning process is for executive management to develop primary, or core, objectives that support the strategic thrusts or goals. Primary objectives should encompass the entire organization. Organizations have several primary objectives; the real challenge lies in balancing them. See Table 11.2 for a sample strategic plan.

Value of Strategic Planning

The value of strategic planning lies in its systematic approach to dealing with an uncertain future. Many organizations become disillusioned with strategic planning when their plans are not met. These plans often have too narrow a focus—the more narrow the focus the less likely an organization is to accomplish the plan. Strategic planning that establishes the organization's overall direction without attempting to be very specific has the following benefits:

- Integrates missions, visions, strategic thrusts, and primary objectives with the secondary objectives, policies, procedures, methods, and rules of the operating plan.
- Provides a process and time frame for making strategic decisions.
- Provides a framework for the operating plan, budget, and capital budget.

TABLE 11.2

Sample
Not-for-Profit
Nursing Home
Strategic Plan

Mission
- Our mission is to be the nursing home of choice in our community by providing high-quality, competitively priced skilled nursing services.

Interpretation
- To provide a skilled nursing facility to those living in our community in a cost-effective manner to ensure financial survival.

Vision
- Our vision is to expand our services in the next five years to include a residential care facility and a hospice facility while maintaining a high-quality, cost-effective skilled nursing facility.

Strategic Thrusts
1. To provide high-quality skilled nursing care.
2. To provide cost-effective skilled nursing care.
3. To expand service without harming quality or increasing cost.

Critical Success Factors
1. Continued accreditation.
2. Continued licensure.
3. Continued favorable physician relations.
4. Cost increases not to exceed 3 percent per year.
5. Residential care facility and hospice to open within five years.

Primary Objectives
1. Initiate total quality management (TQM) program
2. Initiate patient satisfaction surveys
3. Initiate physician satisfaction surveys
4. Initiate reengineering program to improve processes and reduce cost
5. Build residential care facility
6. Build hospice facility

Operational Planning

For the strategic direction of the organization to be useful, the organization's managers must translate the strategic direction into small, measurable steps to be taken during the next year. Operational planning is the process of translating the strategic plan into a year's objectives. Budgeting is the process of expressing the operating plan in monetary terms and will be covered in Chapter 12. Many organizations have difficulty determining where strategic planning ends and operational planning begins, and where operational planning ends and budgeting begins (Berman, Kukla, and Weeks 1994).

Three characteristics distinguish strategic planning from operational planning:

- *Planning horizon*: Strategic planning is for the next three to ten years, and operational planning is for the next year.

- *Principle participants*: The governing body and executive management develop the strategic plan; the department managers develop or have significant input in the operational plan.
- *Objectives*: Strategic planning lists primary objectives common to the entire organization, and the operating plan lists secondary objectives by division or department.

Step 8: Develop Secondary Department Objectives

In the eighth step in the corporate planning process—the first step in the operational planning process—department managers develop secondary, departmental objectives to support the strategic plan of the organization (Dunn 2002; Berman, Kukla, and Weeks 1994):

- Department objective-setting should be participative. The literature generally agrees that meaningful employee participation in planning improves both morale and the chances of meeting objectives.
- Department objectives should be rigorous but attainable. The department will not progress if the objectives are easily attainable and the department may not attempt objectives that seem too difficult.
- Department objectives should be verifiable and/or measurable to ensure progress and to reward those responsible for the progress. For Joint Commission purposes, the manager and subordinates should discuss desired outcomes and their indicators (see Chapter 1).

One method of developing department objectives is Drucker's management by objectives (MBO) introduced during the 1950s. In a nutshell: (1) the manager provides subordinates a general overview of the work to be accomplished in the coming year; (2) the subordinates propose objectives; and (3) the objectives are negotiated until final agreement. Reported advantages of MBO include directing work activity toward organizational goals; reducing conflict and ambiguity; providing clear standards for control and performance appraisals; and providing improved motivation. MBO is not without disadvantages, including burdensome procedures and paperwork; overemphasis on quantitative objectives at the possible expense of qualitative objectives; suboptimization of performance; and illusionary participation, which means that managers give the perception of participation, but the participation lacks meaningful substance, often because the subordinates sense that decisions have already been made (Berman, Kukla, and Weeks 1994).

Step 9: Develop Policies

The ninth step in the planning process and the second step in the operational planning process is for department managers to develop policies (i.e., broad

guides to thinking) that provide general guidelines for decision making to sub-
ordinates. Policies are the most common type of plan at the department level
(Dunn 2002). Good policies have the following characteristics (Ivancevich,
Donnelly, and Gibson 1989):

- They have been thoroughly discussed in advance and are consistent with
  primary and secondary objectives.
- Policies are flexible so managers can apply them to normal and abnormal
  circumstances.[4]
- Policies are communicated, understood, and accepted by subordinates.
  For subordinates to accept the policy, they must view it as reasonable,
  legitimate, and fair. Subordinates will resist or ignore policies that appear
  to show favoritism to selected groups or appear to be arbitrary with no
  clear purpose. Policy statements should therefore be in writing, and
  should start with a clear statement of purpose or intent.
- Policies are consistent with each other. Inconsistency between policies or
  in the application and enforcement of policies will hurt subordinates'
  morale and will likely detract from accomplishing objectives.
  Inconsistencies frequently occur in the enforcement of organizational
  policies between departments, and can have dire consequences.[5]
- Policies are continuously reevaluated and changed if necessary.

Step 10: Develop Procedures

The tenth step in the planning process and the third step in the operational
planning process is for department managers and supervisors to develop procedures, which are guides to action. Procedures are derived from policies, but
they are considerably more specific. Procedures identify in a step-by-step fashion how to accomplish the policy. Good procedures are the result of a detailed
analysis of how best to accomplish the intent of the policy. Good procedures
provide the manager or supervisor with a consistent and uniform performance
appraisal (Dunn 2002).

Step 11: Develop Methods

The eleventh step in the planning process and the fourth step in the operational planning process is for department managers and supervisors to develop methods (i.e., very detailed, uniform actions, a predictable outcome,
and a work standard for instructions on how to accomplish one step of the
procedure) (Dunn 2002).

Step 12: Develop Rules

The twelfth step in the planning process and the fifth step in the operational
planning process is for department managers to develop rules, which are statements that either require or forbid an action or inaction without deviation.

Policies, procedures, and methods allow the manager or supervisor some flexibility in their application and enforcement, but rules do not. Good rules are those that everyone sees as clearly necessary for the proper order and functioning of the department.

Evaluating Plan Performance

The governing body of the organization should review the strategic plan on an annual basis and evaluate the CEO based on progress in accomplishing primary objectives. Likewise, executive management should review the operating plan, probably on a monthly or quarterly basis. They also should evaluate department managers based on progress in accomplishing secondary objectives, and on compliance with policies, procedures, methods, and rules. The Joint Commission requires that hospitals have a planned, systematic, hospital-wide approach to process design and performance measurement, assessment, and improvement. Four key questions help hospitals to design more effective processes, functions, or services (JCAHO 1998):

1. Is the process, function, or service consistent with the hospital's mission, vision, and other processes, functions, and services?
2. What do the organization's patients, staff, and other customers expect from the processes, functions, and services, and how do they think those processes, functions, and services should work?
3. What do professional experts and other reliable sources say about the design of the processes, functions, and services?
4. What information is available about the performance of similar processes, functions, and services?

Budgeting, the next step in the corporate planning process, begins once the strategic and operating plans have been approved; budgeting consists of converting the operating plan into monetary terms.

Notes

1. Ernst & Young defined IDFSs as provider-controlled organizations that deliver a wide assortment of services and have the capacity to accept a variety of financial arrangements, either directly from employers or indirectly from third-party insurers. Of the over 200 IDFSs referenced, hospitals were majority owners in 76 percent of the IDFSs.
2. Strategic planning for the organization is the responsibility of the governing board, who often contracts the preparation of the plan to outside consultants rather than organization employees. With a planning horizon of three to ten years, employees would be likely to produce plans

with vested interests, rather than a clear picture of where the organization is going. For instance, how many employees would diminish or eliminate their functions in the future if the plan called on them to do so?

3. To maintain objectivity and guard against vested interests, a governing body or outside consultants rather than executive management should be responsible for assessing both the external and internal environments.

4. Managers must be cautious about indiscriminately granting exceptions to policy. Although a manager wants to treat subordinates and patients with mercy, the manager must also seek justice, or fair play. The following two questions may help managers resolve the frequently faced dilemma of mercy versus justice: Can the manager afford to grant everyone with similar extenuating circumstances an exception? How can the manager make sure that the other subordinates or patients know about the exception, are encouraged to apply for the exception if circumstances warrant, and are supportive of the manager's decision to grant the exception? (See Nowicki 1998.)

5. In *St. Mary's Honor Center v. Hicks*, 1993, Melvin Hicks, a black prison guard, sued a Missouri prison for civil rights violations. Mr. Hicks, who had been fired for exceeding the prison's absenteeism policy, claimed other guards who were white had exceeded the absenteeism policy, but had been given exceptions. While Mr. Hicks lost in a 5 to 4 decision (the majority felt that Mr. Hicks had not proven intentional discrimination and the action could have been the result of poor management), the case should have a chilling effect on the indiscriminate granting of policy exceptions.

References

Berman, H. J., S. F. Kukla, and L. E. Weeks. 1994. *The Financial Management of Hospitals, 8th ed.* Chicago: Health Administration Press.

Dunn, R. 2002. *Haimann's Healthcare Management, 7th ed.* Chicago: Health Administration Press.

Ernst & Young. 1996. *Navigating Through the Changing Currents.* Washington, DC: Ernst & Young.

Fottler, M. D., J. D. Blair, C. J. Whitehead, M. D. Laus, and G. T. Savage. 1989. "Assessing Key Stake Holders: Who Matters to Hospitals and Why?" *Hospital & Health Services Administration* 34 (Winter): 530

Healthcare Financial Management Association. 1998. *HFMA Core Certification Exam Self-Study Manual.* White Plains, NY: The MGI Management Institute.

Ivancevich, J. M., J. H. Donnelly, and J. L. Gibson. 1989. *Management Principles and Functions, 4th ed.* 1989. Homewood, IL: Irwin, as cited in *Managing Health Services Organizations, 3rd ed.* by J. S. Rakich, B. Longest, and K. Darr. Baltimore: MD: Health Professions Press.

Joint Commission on the Accreditation of Healthcare Organizations. 1998. *Hospital Accreditation Standards.* Oakbrook Terrace, IL: JCAHO.

Nowicki, M. 1998. "Beware the Slippery Slope of Granting Exceptions." *Journal of Health Care Resource Management* 16 (1): 20–22.

Pearce, J. A. and F. David. 1987. "Corporate Mission Statements and the Bottom Line." *Academy of Management Executives* 1 (2): 109–116.

Person, M. W. 1997. *The Zero-Base Hospital: Survival and Success in America's Evolving Healthcare System.* Chicago: Health Administration Press.

Peters, T. 1988. *Thriving on Chaos.* New York: Alfred A. Knopf.

Rakich, J. S., B. B. Longest, and K. Darr. 1992. *Managing Health Services Organizations, 3rd ed.* Baltimore, MD: Health Professions Press.

St Mary's Honor Center v. Hicks. No. 92-602. 1993.

BUDGETING

In *The Zero-Base Hospital*, Person emphasizes the need for budget skills for every management position in the healthcare organization.

> To function effectively in the healthcare industry in the foreseeable future, managers will need to develop specific financial skills. They will need to acquire an appreciation of volume, expense, and revenue relationships. They will need to become familiar with cost-containment strategies for their particular corner of the market. Most of all they will need to cultivate an intimate knowledge of the details that define their operations and drive their costs, such as utilization statistics, seasonal trends, staffing models, productivity analysis, supply alternatives, inventory management, make/lease/buy options, physician practice patterns, and rate setting. (Person 1997, 67)

In short, healthcare managers must learn how to budget. Considering that most managers in healthcare organizations are specialists in fields other than financial management, and that, as specialists, they have little or no formal education in budgeting, their records of accomplishment to date have been commendable. However, with healthcare costs and rapidly changing demographics at the center of public debate, and with prospective payment limiting the ability of organizations to "just raise rates" to cover expenses, tomorrow's healthcare managers clearly must do more work with less resources.

Definition of Budgeting

Budgeting is the process of converting, or dollarizing,[1] the operating plan into monetary terms. In addition to converting the operating plan into monetary terms for planning purposes, budgets become an important way for managers to exert the control function. Budgets become a control standard against which superiors can easily measure performance of subordinates (Rakich, Longest, and Darr 1992). Budgeting is also an excellent opportunity for the financial staff to educate the nonfinancial department managers regarding the relationship of revenues, expenses, and capital expenditures to the overall financial well-being of the organization.

Sequentially, budgeting occurs after the steps in operational planning have been completed. Budget information therefore does not bias operating information, especially in not-for-profit healthcare organizations. Department managers should prioritize objectives in the operating plan based on community need, not organizational profitability.

Prerequisites to Budgets

Before effective budgeting can begin, the organization must meet several prerequisite requirements, the first four of which were introduced in Chapter 11 related to planning (Berman, Kukla, and Weeks 1994; Herkimer 1988):

1. A sound organizational structure that ensures management accountability for the budgeting process.
2. A well-defined chart of accounts that corresponds with the organizational structure.
3. Prompt and accurate accounting systems that ensure financial responsibility for the budgeting process.
4. A comprehensive management information system that captures nonfinancial information for each department.
5. A budget director who is responsible for coordinating the budget process and who serves as chair of the budget committee.
6. A budget committee that is responsible for establishing a budget manual and a budget calendar, and assisting department managers with the development of their department budgets. Budget committees usually consist of senior managers who represent the department managers in their divisions (e.g., the director of medical services, director of nursing services, director of human resources, director of support services, director of professional services, and the director of financial services).
7. A budget manual that includes necessary strategic planning information; the organizational structure; the chart of accounts; a list of budget committee members who can assist department managers; budget forms and instructions; budget assumptions regarding items such as anticipated growth, inflation, and employee raises; and a budget calendar with important completion dates.
8. Last year's data regarding volumes, revenues, and expenses.

Types of Budgets

Budgeting can be classified by management approach and design characteristics. Many of these classifications also apply to planning and were introduced in Chapter 11.

Management Approach

Budgets can be classified by management approach, either with top-down or bottom-up budgeting. In top-down budgeting, as in top-down planning, senior management develops the budget with little or no input from department managers. The advantage of this design is that senior management may be in the best position to objectively view the future; the disadvantage is that budget implementation may be difficult if subordinates have little or no input.

In bottom-up budgeting, subordinates develop the budget and submit it to senior management for approval. The advantage to bottom-up budgeting, as with bottom-up planning, is the commitment to the budget by those who developed it. The disadvantage is that subordinates may not be in the best position to view the future.

In most cases, a combination of top-down and bottom-up designs is used—senior management decides on budget parameters and subordinates submit plans within those parameters.

Design Characteristics

Budgeting can also be classified by design characteristics; these characteristics also apply to the design characteristics of planning (see Chapter 11).

Incremental Versus Zero-Base Budgeting

Incremental budgeting requires budgeting only for changes like new equipment, new positions, and new programs. Incremental budgeting assumes that all current operations including positions and equipment are essential to the continued mission of the organization and that all current operations are working at peak performance. The advantages are the ease of incremental budgeting, the minimal time commitment required to prepare the budget, and the support of a bigger organizational culture. The principle disadvantage of incremental budgeting is the assumption that all current operations are essential in a healthcare environment that is changing rapidly.

Conversely, zero-base budgeting[2] takes nothing for granted and requires rejustification for existing equipment, positions, and programs, as well as justification for new equipment, positions, and programs. Therein lies the principle advantage of zero-base budgeting: in a rapidly changing environment where reimbursement is moving away from cost-based approaches and moving toward prospective payment per case or per enrollee, zero-base budgeting can eliminate unnecessary costs and improve margins. Disadvantages are numerous and include the large commitment of time, employee fear and anxiety, and the administrative and communication requirements (Person 1997).

Comprehensive Versus Limited-in-Scope Budgeting

Comprehensive budgeting integrates all the budgets into one document. The advantage is the recognition that capital affects operations. Limited-in-scope segregates the budgets. Most organizations integrate the budgets at the executive management level of the organization, but the issue is at what level of the organization the budgets should be integrated. For instance, many healthcare organizations do not show department managers revenue information because they feel that the department managers will not understand the difference between billed revenue and collected revenue, or that the organization uses department revenue to cover expenses in departments that do not generate revenue. Another reason department managers might not be shown revenue information is because department managers cannot affect changes in revenue, which is a function of volumes ordered by the physicians multiplied by rates set by the chief financial officer (CFO). A similar case can be made regarding whether department managers should be shown indirect expenses.

Fixed Versus Flexible Budgeting

Fixed budgets assume that volumes, related revenues, and variable expenses remain constant during the year. Fixed budgets are easy to project, but they are unrealistic for healthcare organizations whose volumes fluctuate during the year and whose variable expenses, which are dependent on volumes, account for over half of an organization's operating expenses.

Flexible budgets take into account fluctuations in volumes, at least within ranges expressed as probabilities, and flexible budgets adjust variable expenses accordingly.

Discrete Versus Continuous Budgeting

A discrete budget applies to a fixed period of time, usually a year. At the end of the year, a new budget begins. Discrete budgets are relatively easy to prepare, but do not take into account certain events that may occur at year end. For instance, department managers who had managed wisely and met their budgets by year end would likely have new, more rigorous budgets for the next budget year.

Continuous budgets, sometimes referred to as rolling budgets, are updated continuously so that year end never occurs. Department managers who manage wisely roll over their efforts to the next month.[3]

Steps in the Budgeting Process

The budgeting process is an extension of the planning process discussed in Chapter 11.

Step 13: Project Volumes

The thirteenth step in the planning process and the first step in the budgeting process is to project volumes for the budget year. This step is often called the statistical budget, and sometimes is part of the operating plan. Typically, the budget committee will give their projections of the organization's production units to department managers in the budget manual. Department managers use the organization's production units to calculate department production units that are specific to each department. For instance, the radiology department manager must be able to determine how many radiology procedures are generated for every 100 admissions.

Production units are the best measures of what an entity is producing. For example, hospitals produce patient days and admissions, but neither production unit reflects severity of illness or the volume of outpatient work produced by the hospital. The unit used to show severity of illness, a factor that affects resource consumption, will vary—many hospitals have adopted DRGs or another severity index.[4] Regarding the volume of outpatient work produced by the hospital, either outpatient work needs to be captured separately as outpatient visits and with the related revenues and expenses, or the inpatient production unit must be adjusted to reflect outpatient work produced.[5] Regardless of which production units are chosen by the organization, the units must be reported by the payer to project both gross and net revenues.

Each department should have a production unit that best measures what the department is producing. Radiology, for example, produces radiology procedures. However, this production unit, like patient days for the hospital, does not reflect the complexity of the procedure and the related resource consumption.[6] To show complexity of the procedure, most departments have developed a relative value unit (RVU) that reflects relative complexity and related resource consumption (refer to Chapter 7 for information on developing RVUs). If the hospital can tell the radiology department manager how many of each DRG they are projecting, the radiology manager should be able to project the number of procedures, and also the type of procedures. In addition to serving as a basis for projecting volumes for budgeting purposes, department production units are used (Herkimer 1988):

- To measure and evaluate department productivity;
- To measure and evaluate employee productivity;
- To serve as the basis for calculating the cost of the procedure (see Chapter 6);
- To serve as the basis for calculating the charge for the procedure; and
- To serve as a basis for determining staffing requirements and staffing schedules.

To project future volumes under conditions of uncertainty, most managers rely on forecasting, which is the process to determine what alternative scenarios are likely to occur in the future, given what managers know about the past and present. To forecast, the manager must first prepare the forecast content, which is a description of the specific situation in question. Next, the manager must prepare the forecast rationale, which is an explanation of how the situation will evolve from its current state to its forecasted state (Reeves, Bergwall, and Woodside 1979).

In preparing the forecast content, the manager first identifies content items, which are descriptions of important occurrences such as admissions, patient days, and outpatient visits. Next, the manager must measure the current status of content items. The final step of the forecast content is to identify the expected state of the content items in the future budget period. Although forecast content often produces quantifiable data, the manager also must consider the effect of the following subjective factors on the forecast content (Reeves, Bergwall, and Woodside 1979):

- Political factors;
- Social factors;
- Economic factors;
- Technologic factors;
- Personal health factors; and
- Environmental health factors.

A manager may use several different forecasting techniques to prepare the forecast content including use of experts, use of causal models, and use of time-series methods.

The use of experts is dependent on the manager's ability to identify and secure the services of appropriate experts. After the manager secures the services of an expert, he or she must consider the advantages and disadvantages of using experts in preparing the forecast. Using experts is usually quick and relatively inexpensive. However, different experts may develop very different, yet valid, opinions about the future. Which expert is correct? To address this disadvantage, the manager can choose a variety of models to obtain their opinion (Reeves, Bergwall, and Woodside 1979):

- A task force brings together several experts who provide collective input into the content of the forecast.
- The Delphi technique gathers information from a group of dispersed experts with limited interaction and anonymity of expert opinions.
- The Delbecq technique, or nominal group process, is similar to the Delphi technique, except that the group of experts meet face-to-face for discussion and present and defend their forecasts.
- Questionnaires are used to gather responses to questions from a large group of experts.
- Permanent panels maintain a group of experts who can be used for several forecasts over time.
- Essay writing obtains opinions from experts in essay format and primarily is used for preparing the forecast rationale.

In addition to relying on expert opinion regarding the future, a manager may apply probability statistics to the expert opinion. Another derivative of using expert opinion is the program evaluation and review technique (PERT). This technique requires estimates of optimistic (O), pessimistic (P), and most likely (ML) future scenarios. These three estimates are weighted to calculate an expected value that equals

$$\frac{(O = P + 4ML)}{6}$$

The manager may use causal models when the forecast variable is dependent on a causal, or independent, variable. The most common statistical method used in causal models is regression analysis, which describes the response of the forecast variable to changes in one or more causal variables. Beyond single-equation regression methods, the manager may use multiple-equation simulation methods, such as multiple regression or econometric methods, which allow the forecast variable in one equation to become the causal, or independent, variable in one or more of the other equations.

Regression analysis mathematically describes an average relationship between a forecast variable and one or more causal variables. The coefficient of determination, symbolized by R^2, indicates the proportion of the variance of the forecast variable that is explained by the regression statistic. When given a choice between two or more regression statistics, the manager should select the statistic that maximizes the coefficients of determination. The causal variables in regression may include time, leading economic indicators, demographic factors, or any other variables that might exhibit a causal relationship with the forecast variable.

A measure of the statistical contribution of a causal variable to regression's causal power is the beta coefficient, which indicates the relative importance of each of the causal variables in explaining or predicting changes in the forecast variable. In multiple regression, the manager can use beta coefficients to decide which causal variables to retain and which to exclude. The manager should be cautioned regarding one flaw in multiple regression: multicollinearity, which is the phenomenon that occurs when causal variables relate to each other in addition to the relationship to the forecast variable.[7]

The manager may use time-series methods when the past behavior of a variable is available to predict the future behavior of the variable. Time-series methods do little to account for causal relationships; rather, they attempt to identify historic patterns that are likely to be repeated in the future. The manager may use regression for long-term forecasts, and time-series methods for forecasts of less than one year.

Many series of data collected over time will exhibit trend, seasonal, cyclical, and random patterns. A trend pattern exists when there is a consistent increase or decrease in the value of the variable over time. A seasonal pattern exists when the value of the variable fluctuates in accordance to a seasonal influence such as hour of the day, day of the week, week of the month, or month of the year. A cyclical pattern is similar to a seasonal pattern; however, the length of each cycle is longer than one year and cycles vary in length. Horizontal patterns exist when there are no changes in the variable's value; random patterns exist when the variable's value changes, but in no predictable way (Bittel and Bittel 1978).

After preparing the forecast content, the manager must prepare the forecast rationale, which is an explanation of how the situation will evolve from its current state to its forecasted state. The forecast rationale clarifies the result of the forecasting process, provides a basis for evaluating the forecasting process, and provides a basis from which future forecasts can be made (Reeves, Bergwall, and Woodside 1979).

Step 14: Convert Volumes into Revenues

The fourteenth step in the planning process and the second step in the budgeting process is to convert volumes into patient revenues. Managers must consider whether the organization should budget revenues before or after the expense budget is completed. Historically, healthcare organizations have determined their expense budgets first and then set rates in their revenue budgets to cover the expenses, which is called cost-led pricing. However, healthcare organizations that are facing increasing proportions of fixed payment arrangements such as prospective payment and premium payment, which essentially dictate the rate to the organization, may be well-advised to calculate revenue first, which is called price-led costing. The organization then must adjust expenses to match the projected patient revenues, or more accurately, the collected patient revenues.

To project gross patient service revenues, projected production units are classified by payer and then multiplied by the projected charge that, at this point, usually includes a projected increase. Next, net patient service revenue is determined by deducting contractual allowances, charity care allowances, and premium revenue (see Problem 4.1 on cost shifting).[8] To project total revenues from operations, net patient service revenue is added to premium revenue, other revenue (i.e., parking, catering, and so on), and net assets released from restrictions and used for operations. Other projected changes in net assets that would be reported at the bottom of the statement of operations may also be available for operations (see Statement of Operations in Chapter 14).

Step 15: Convert Volumes into Expense Requirements

The fifteenth step in the planning process and the third step in the budgeting process is to convert volumes into expense requirements: labor expense with benefits, nonlabor expense, and overhead expense. Department managers should have budget histories that indicate labor expense with benefits per production unit. They should also have budget histories for nonlabor expense per production unit, which includes supplies, travel, and repairs. The budget director should have budget histories for overhead expense for the organization.

Department managers should review the labor expense with benefits per production unit to determine if they can reduce expenses. Senior management determines the benefits package (approximately 32 percent of wages for a full-time employee),[9] but department managers can reduce benefit expenses by using part-time and temporary workers. Part-time employees usually receive benefits in proportion to the number of hours worked (approximately 16 percent of wages for a half-time employee), and temporary workers usually receive only the benefits required by law (approximately 12 percent of wages). Department managers must decide on the appropriate mix of full-time, part-time, and temporary workers. Part-time and temporary workers are less expensive to the department manager, but continuity of patient care may suffer if the manager uses too many part-time and temporary workers. Many department managers staff their minimum needs with full-time workers, moderate needs with part-time workers, and maximum needs with temporary workers (see Figure 12.1).

Staffing mix is the mix of full-time, part-time, and temporary workers and should be reviewed by the department manager; department skill mix, which is the mix of skilled positions, should also be reviewed by managers. Most departments have a variety of tasks requiring a variety of skills performed by a variety of positions paid a variety of wages. The department manager's job is to match the tasks to the positions in the most cost-effective manner possible.

After the department managers have reviewed staffing mix and skill mix and have made any necessary changes, they must consider the effect of employee raises on their expense budget. The budget committee should provide department managers information regarding cost-of-living raises, merit raises, and bonuses. Cost-of-living raises are designed to protect employees from inflation. The use of these raises is declining because inflation has been low and employee spending is not all inflation prone. If the organization uses a cost-of-living raise, however, the raise is administered to all employees at the same time. The effect of cost-of-living raises on the department budget depends on the effective date of the raise. For instance, if the effective date is the first day of the new budget year, the department budget will realize the full effect of the raise. If the effective date of the raise is three months into the new budget year, the department will realize a 75 percent effect of the raise.

Merit raises are designed to motivate employees toward, and reward employees for, meritorious performance. Merit raises as a motivator are dependent on the amount of the raise and the likelihood that superiors will judge performance meritorious. Merit raises are expensive for organizations because the amount of the raise is built into the employee's base pay for future years.

FIGURE 12.1
Staffing Mix

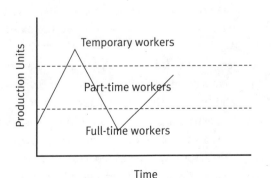

Organizations typically give merit raises in conjunction with employee performance appraisals on employment anniversaries. Assuming that employee employment anniversaries occur in equal distribution throughout the year, the effect on the department budget will be 50 percent of the total amount for merit raises, and the budget should be adjusted accordingly. For instance, if the department manager can give 7 percent raises to meritorious employees on their employment anniversaries, and all the department's employees are meritorious, the annual effect on the department will be 3.5 percent, assuming that 50 percent of the employment anniversaries are in the first half of the budget year and 50 percent of the employment anniversaries are in the second half of the budget year.

Bonuses are designed to motivate employees in much the same way as merit raises. However, using bonuses as a motivator is dependent on the amount of the bonus, the likelihood that superiors will judge performance bonus-worthy, and also the proportion of employees receiving the bonus. For instance, if all employees receive bonuses, motivation resulting from the bonus will be low because everyone receives a bonus. If 1 out of 100 employees receive bonuses, motivation will be low because the chance of being rewarded for bonus-worthy performance is low. However, if one out of seven employees receives bonuses, motivation as a result of the bonus will be maximized because the chances of receiving a bonus are realistic. Organizations typically award bonuses at the end of the budget year, and the funds come from the organization, not the department; budgeting the effect of bonuses, therefore, is relatively easy.

After budgeted department wages have been adjusted for changes in staffing mix, skill mix, and employee raises, department managers multiply the budgeted wages and benefits per production unit by the number of production units projected for the budget year to determine the total budgeted wages and benefits for the department.

Department managers should have budget histories that indicate nonlabor expense per production unit and review the nonlabor expenses per production unit to determine if they can reduce expenses. Managers should review supply use to ensure that generic supplies are used whenever possible. The pharmacy manager should provide information on the use of generic medicines and work with the pharmacy committee to maintain a formulary with as many generics and as few brand-name pharmaceuticals as possible. The pharmacy manager should also establish security measures to ensure that narcotics are secure. Department managers should review travel expenses and bring training programs to the organization whenever possible to reduce travel expense. Department managers should review repair expense and maintenance agreements, and replace equipment when feasible. The manager of materials management should provide department managers with an estimate of anticipated increases in supplies, repairs, and travel as a result of contract renewals or inflation. After department managers have reduced nonlabor expense wherever possible, department managers multiply the nonlabor expense per production unit by the number of production units projected for the budget year to determine the total budgeted nonlabor expense for the department.

Largely, overhead expenses for the organization such as depreciation, heating and cooling, insurance premiums, and so on do not fluctuate with production units. Therefore, the budget committee determines the overhead expenses for the budget year after reviewing historic data to determine if adjustments are necessary.

Step 16: Adjust Revenues and Expenses as Necessary

The sixteenth step in the planning process and the fourth step in the budgeting process is for the budget committee to determine if budgeted net revenues are adequate to cover budgeted expenses. If budgeted expenses exceed budgeted net revenues, the budget committee may recommend to executive management ways to generate additional revenues or ways to reduce expenses. To cover the budget shortfall, executive management must decide whether to generate additional revenues and the possible effect of such action on expenses; whether to reduce expenses and the possible effect on quality and patient access; or whether to release funds from unrestricted net asset accounts to cover the loss.

Evaluating Budget Performance

The governing body of the organization should review the budget on an annual basis and evaluate the CEO based on organizational compliance to the budget. Likewise, the CEO should review senior management on a quarterly basis and evaluate senior managers based on divisional compliance to budget. Senior management should review department managers on a monthly basis and evaluate departmental compliance to budget.

The most common method of evaluating budget performance is variance analysis, which compares budgeted production units, revenues, and expenses to actual production units, revenues, and expenses, typically on a monthly basis. Labor variance analysis including hours and expense may be completed every two weeks in conjunction with payroll. The variance is the amount of the difference between the actual and budgeted:

$$\text{Variance} = \text{actual} - \text{budgeted}$$

For production units and revenue, positive variances are favorable and negative variances are unfavorable.

$$\text{Revenue variance} = \text{actual revenue} - \text{budgeted revenue}$$

For expenses, negative variances are favorable and positive variances are unfavorable.

$$\text{Expense variance} = \text{actual expense} - \text{budgeted expense}$$

Variance analysis ensures accountability by requiring managers responsible for the variances to explain why the variances occurred and what actions are being taken to ensure that favorable variances reoccur and negative variances do not reoccur (Herkimer 1988).

Once the budget has been reviewed and approved, the healthcare organization can begin the capital budgeting process. Problem 12.1 demonstrates the budgeting steps in a Radiology Department.

BUDGETING EXERCISE

The radiology department is developing a budget for DRG 250: Fracture, Sprain, Strain, and Dislocation of Forearm, Hand, and Foot. This year the department saw 1,100 admissions for DRG 250 analyzed in the following way: 50 percent for a hand x-ray (which takes 5 minutes), 20 percent for a foot x-ray (which takes 15 minutes), and 30 percent for a forearm x-ray (which takes 30 minutes). The budget committee is projecting a 9.1 percent increase in DRG 250 for next year analyzed in the same proportions as last year. The controller states that the charges for a hand x-ray will be $75, for a foot x-ray will be $285, and for a forearm x-ray will be $450. The controller also projects the payer analysis for DRG 250 to be 45-percent Medicare (DRG rate is 80 percent of charges), 35-percent Medicaid (DRG rate is 85 percent of charges), 15-percent managed care (discount is 30 percent of charges), and self-pay (self-pay patients pay full charges—10 percent of self-pay result in charity care).

DRG 250 accounts for 25 percent of the radiology department's labor, supply, and overhead expenses. The department's labor expenses are $225,000—labor expenses are expected to increase 5 percent next year due to raises. The department's nonlabor expenses are $185,000—nonlabor expenses are expected to increase 6 percent next year due to inflation. The department's overhead expenses are $375,000—overhead expenses are not expected to increase next year. Using the budgeting steps, calculate the volumes, collected revenues, expenses, and adjustments for DRG 250 in the radiology department.

Step 13: Project Volumes

1. Calculate the current volume for each x-ray procedure.

Procedure	Admissions	Volume
Hand x-ray	1,100 × .50	550
Foot x-ray	1,100 × .20	220
Forearm x-ray	1,100 × .30	330

2. Convert the current volumes to RVU's

Procedure	Minutes	Minutes/ GCD	RVUs/ Procedure	Volume	Total RVUs
Hand x-ray	5	5/5	1	550	550
Foot x-ray	15	15/5	3	220	660
Forearm x-ray	30	30/5	6	330	1,980
					3,190

3. Calculate the projected volume for each x-ray procedure (1,100 DRG 250 × .091 increase = 1,200 DRG 250)

Procedure	Admissions	Volume
Hand x-ray	1,200 × .50	600
Foot x-ray	1,200 × .20	240
Forearm x-ray	1,200 × .30	360

4. Convert the projected volumes to RVUs

Procedure	Minutes	Minutes/ GCD	RVUs/ Procedure	Volume	Total RVUs
Hand x-ray	5	5/5	1	600	600
Foot x-ray	15	15/5	3	240	720
Forearm x-ray	30	30/5	6	360	2,160
					3,480

Step 14: Convert Projected Volumes into Projected Revenues

4. Calculate projected gross and net revenues by payer

MEDICARE

Procedure	Projected Charge	Projected Volume	%	Gross Revenue	Contractual Allowance	Net Revenue
Hand x-ray	$75	600	.45	$ 20,250	.20	$ 16,200
Foot x-ray	285	240	.45	30,780	.20	24,624
Forearm x-ray	450	360	.45	72,900	.20	58,320
				$123,930		$ 99,144

MEDICAID

Procedure	Projected Charge	Projected Volume	%	Gross Revenue	Contractual Allowance	Net Revenue
Hand x-ray	$75	600	.35	$ 15,750	.15	$ 13,388
Foot x-ray	285	240	.35	23,940	.15	20,349
Forearm x-ray	450	360	.35	56,700	.15	48,195
				$ 96,390		$ 81,932

MANAGED CARE

Procedure	Projected Charge	Projected Volume	%	Gross Revenue	Contractual Allowance	Net Revenue
Hand x-ray	$75	600	.15	$ 6,750	.30	$ 4,725
Foot x-ray	285	240	.15	10,260	.30	7,182
Forearm x-ray	450	360	.15	24,300	.30	17,010
				$ 41,310		$ 28,917

SELF-PAY

Procedure	Projected Charge	Projected Volume	%	Gross Revenue	Charity	Net Revenue
Hand x-ray	$75	600	.05	$ 2,250	.10	$ 2,025
Foot x-ray	285	240	.05	3,420	.10	3,078
Forearm x-ray	450	360	.05	8,100	.10	7,290
				$ 13,770		$ 12,393
Total				$275,400		$222,386

Step 15: Convert Projected Volumes into Projected Expenses

1. Calculate current expenses per RVU

$\$225,000 \times .25 = 56,250 \div 3,190 = 17.63$ labor expense/RVU

$185,000 \times .25 = 46,250 \div 3,190 = 14.50$ supply expense/RVU

$375,000 \times .25 = 93,750 \div 3,190 = 29.39$ overhead expense/RVU

2. Calculate projected expenses per RVU

$$\text{Projected labor expense} = 17.63 + 5\% = 18.51$$
$$\text{Projected supply expense} = 14.50 + 6\% = 15.37$$
$$\text{Projected overhead expense} = 29.39 + 0\% = \underline{29.39}$$
$$\text{Total} \qquad\qquad\qquad\qquad\qquad\qquad \$63.27$$

3. Calculate projected expenses per procedure

Procedure	Projected RVUs	Projected Expense/RVU	Total Projected Expense
Hand x-ray	600	$ 63.27	$ 37,962
Foot x-ray	720	63.27	45,554
Forearm x-ray	2,160	63.27	136,663
		Total	$220,179

Step 16: Adjust Revenues and Expenses as Necessary

1. Determine initial gain/loss

Net Revenues	$222,386
Expenses	220,179
Gain/(Loss)	$ 2,207

2. If the adjustment results in a loss, first investigate whether collected revenues can be increased through a rate increase or improvements in collection efforts. If collected revenues cannot be increased, investigate whether expenses can be reduced. Usually this involves investigating variable labor expenses and reviewing both the mix of full-time to part-time to temporary as well as a review of skill mix. If collected revenues cannot be increased and expenses cannot be decreased, then management must decide whether to continue the service at a loss and how that loss is going to be covered by other profitable services.

Source: Neil Dworkin, Ph.D., Assistant Professor of Management, Western Connecticut State University. Used with permission.

Notes

1. A term attributed to Koontz, O'Donnell, and Weihrich (1984) in

Management and picked up by Herkimer (1988) in *Understanding Health Care Budgeting.*

2. For a compelling argument for zero-base planning, see Person's (1997) *The Zero-Base Hospital: Survival and Success in America's Evolving Healthcare System.* Person also provides a historic perspective by identifying the U.S. Department of Agriculture as the first zero-base planner in 1964. Zero-base planning was abandoned at the Department of Agriculture, but it was successfully adopted at Texas Instruments in the late-1960s as related by Pyhrr in a 1970 *Harvard Business Review* article and in a 1973 book. During the 1970s and 1980s, zero-base planning was used by a variety of organizations with a variety of success. Hospitals, according to Person, did not adopt it because of the financial security provided by retrospective, cost-based reimbursement.

3. Continuous budgets avoid the year-end "sucking sound"—the sound of year-end unnecessary spending of budgeted but not-yet-spent funds—that occurs in organizations using discrete budgeting.

4. DRGs measure severity of illness between DRGs, but they do not measure severity of illness within the same DRG. Eastaugh (1987; 1992) discusses several severity of illness (SOI) indices that do measure how ill a patient is within a specific DRG, or condition: Horn's SOI index, Horn's computerized severity index (CSI), Western Pennsylvania Blue Cross patient management categories (PMC), and Brewster's MEDISGRPS.

5. As discussed in Appendix 1.3 after Chapter 1, adjusted patient days is used to reflect outpatient production with the following formula:

$$\text{Inpatient days } + \text{ outpatient visits } \times \frac{\text{outpatient revenue per visit}}{\text{inpatient revenue per day}}$$

6. Even after adopting an RVU schedule for the production unit, most departments maintain a procedure count as a basis for auditing charges (each procedure should generate a charge).

7. Multicollinearity was one of the weaknesses of the Herzlinger and Krasker study on for-profit hospitals, which is referenced in Chapter 3. Arrington and Haddock used discriminate analysis to avoid the multicollinearity problem in their follow-up study, which is also referenced in Chapter 3.

8. For reporting purposes, patient revenue is reported net of contractual allowances, bad debt allowances, and charity care allowances. However, bad debt is reported as an expense based on rates, and charity care is reported in a footnote based on rates, costs, or activity, along with the organization's charity care policy (see Appendix 1.1 after Chapter 1). Premium revenue is reported separately from patient revenue since it is earned by agreeing to provide care, regardless of whether the care was ever provided.

9. Benefits include not only payroll taxes and retirement and health

insurance, but also sick leave (approximately 96 hours, depending on the organization's policy), holiday leave (approximately 84 hours) and vacation (approximately 80 hours). Full-time employees are paid for 2,080 hours per year (52 × 40), but are scheduled (or work, depending on the definition) approximately 1,820 per year.

References

Berman, H. J., S. F. Kukla, and L. E. Weeks. 1994. *The Financial Management of Hospitals, 8th ed.* Chicago: Health Administration Press.

Bittel, L. R., and M. A. Bittel. 1978. "Forecasting Business Conditions." *Encyclopedia of Professional Management.* New York: McGraw-Hill Book Company.

Eastaugh, S. R. 1992. *Health Care Finance: Economic Incentives and Productivity Enhancement.* New York: Auburn House.

Eastaugh, S. R. 1987. *Financing Health Care: Economic Efficiency and Equity.* Dover, MA: Auburn House.

Herkimer, A. G. 1988. *Understanding Health Care Budgeting.* Rockville, MD: Aspen Publishers.

Koontz, H., C. O'Donnell, and M. Weihrich. 1984. *Management, 8th ed.* New York: McGraw-Hill

Person, M. W. 1997. *The Zero-Base Hospital: Survival and Success in America's Evolving Healthcare System.* Chicago: Health Administration Press.

Pyhrr, P. A. 1970. "Zero-Base Budgeting." *Harvard Business Review* 48 (11): 111–21.

Rakich, J. S., B. B. Longest, and K. Darr. 1992. *Managing Health Services Organizations, 3rd ed.* Baltimore, MD: Health Professions Press.

Reeves, P. N., D. F. Bergwall, and N. B. Woodside. 1979. *Introduction to Health Planning, 2nd ed.* Arlington, VA: Information Resources Press.

CAPITAL BUDGETING

apital costs are a relatively small percentage of total organization costs—
in hospitals, they are six to ten percent. However, their importance in
terms of rising healthcare costs and dictating current trends in acquisitions, mergers, joint ventures, and closings cannot be overstated. Under
cost-based reimbursement from 1966 to 1983 (cost-based reimbursement
continued for capital costs until 1990), capital costs for new equipment (38
to 40 percent of capital costs) and plants exploded with very little resistance
from regulation or the market.

Certificate-of-need (CON) legislation passed by the federal government (P.L. 93-641 as the National Health Planning and Resources Development Act of 1974) and Section 1122 of the Social Security Amendments
of 1974 did little to slow capital growth (Eastaugh 1987).

The Social Security Amendments of 1983, which introduced Medicare
prospective payment, did little to slow growth because capital costs were reimbursed based on cost until the Omnibus Budget Reconciliation Act (OBRA)
of 1990 moved capital costs to prospective payment over a ten-year implementation period. The Tax Reform Act of 1986 lowered the tax deductibility
for charitable gifts and restricted or increased the cost of acquiring capital
through tax-exempt bond markets. The Tax Reform Act and OBRA of 1990
slowed capital growth markedly, causing one investment banker to comment:

> Starting in 1988 [1990] the typical hospital should be viewed as
> a more risky venture, and will pay higher interest rates unless they
> can demonstrate DRG profitability. Hospitals shall no longer have
> government as a "Sugar Daddy" paying the interest on their debt
> coupon by coupon. One thousand hospitals may close. We view such
> hospitals as "cross-eyed javelin throwers" in that they will not win
> any rewards, but they will keep the attention of their fearful audience.
> (Eastaugh 1987, 600)

Definition of Capital Expenditures

Capital expenditures are defined by an organization in the capital expenditures policy, and as a result, the definitions vary. Generally speaking, capital
expenditures are purchases of land, buildings, and equipment for operations;
are not for resale; and have a useful life of more than one year, a cost of $500
or more, and are subject to depreciation. Capital expenditures are classified
into the following categories (Herkimer 1988; Person 1997):

- Land including all costs associated with acquiring land and making it ready for use (the cost of the land itself cannot be depreciated);
- Land improvements including all costs associated with sidewalks, parking lots, driveways, and fencing;
- Buildings including all costs associated with constructing or buying buildings;
- Fixed equipment including all costs associated with equipment that is permanently attached to the building, such as the plumbing system, furnace, and air conditioners;
- Major movable equipment including equipment that can be easily moved, has a useful life of three years or more, and has a unit cost of $500 or more; and
- Major repairs that benefit future periods and/or extend the useful life of the building or equipment (ordinary repairs are expensed).

Types of Capital Expenditure Budgets

Healthcare organizations typically divide capital expenditure budgets into two broad categories: replacement and new. Budgets for replacement capital expenditures include requests to replace existing buildings and equipment that are made for a number of reasons:

- For scheduled replacement at the end of the useful life or when fully depreciated[1];
- For improved productivity; and
- For improved quality or because it is required by regulation.

Budgets for new capital expenditures include requests to add buildings and equipment for a number of reasons (Herkimer 1988):

- Expanded services;
- Improved safety conditions;
- Reduced operating expenses; and
- Improved patient care.

Steps in the Capital Budgeting Process

The capital budgeting process is an extension of the budgeting process discussed in Chapter 12. The budgeting process must be concluded to determine funds available for capital expenditures.

Step 17: Identify and Prioritize Requests

The seventeenth step in the corporate planning process and the first step in the capital budgeting process is for the budget committee to identify and prioritize all capital requests. Typically, the budget committee asks department managers including the chief of medical staff services (included with department managers in this chapter discussion) to list the capital equipment and buildings needed, and to justify why the resources are needed. After the department managers have provided a list,[2] the budget committee prioritizes the list using community need and compliance with the strategic plan as initial criteria.[3]

Step 18: Project Cash Flows

The eighteenth step in the planning process and the second step in the capital budgeting process is for the department managers to project, and the budget committee to confirm, cash flows for each capital expenditure request. In cases of replacement equipment, this is a relatively easy step in that revenues (volumes × charge per procedure), and expenses (volumes × expense per procedure), and resulting cash flow (revenues − expenses) already exist.[4] However, the department manager must indicate any changes in revenue or expenses that will occur with the replacement equipment.

For new equipment, or equipment that the organization has never had before, revenues and expenses may be difficult to project. The department manager can obtain volumes in a number of ways. First, if the organization is currently using an outside service that will be replaced by the new equipment, the department manager can obtain volumes from accounts payable. If the organization is not currently using an outside service, the department manager can administer a questionnaire to potential users or complete a medical record review to determine how many patients would have used the new equipment if it had been available. For expensive equipment like computed tomographic scanners, manufacturers will assist in the medical record review; however, the department manager should review manufacturer projections carefully, because manufacturers have a vested interest and may over-project volumes. The department manager can obtain charge information from neighboring facilities or insurance companies. The department manager can also obtain expense information from neighboring facilities or the manufacturer. If he or she obtains the information from the manufacturer, it is a good idea to confirm the information with other organizations that use the same equipment—manufacturers should be willing to provide client lists.

For equipment that does not generate revenue, department managers can still project cash flow by using salary savings, utility savings, and so on.

Previously incurred costs, or sunk costs, and costs that would be incurred regardless of the budget outcome should not be included in cash-flow projections (Berman, Kukla, and Weeks 1994).

Step 19: Perform Financial Analysis

The nineteenth step in the planning process and the third step in the capital budgeting process is for the budget committee or the CFO to perform financial analysis on the requests. Before Medicare stopped reimbursing capital at cost, very few healthcare organizations performed any significant financial analyses on equipment because in the risk-free environment of cost-based reimbursement, healthcare organizations and their lenders were guaranteed a return on capital expenditures, whether they used the equipment or not. In a 1973 study of large hospitals, only 8 percent of the hospitals calculated the net present value of a capital expenditure before purchasing it (William and Rakich 1973). Some hospitals literally had two of everything in case the first one broke (organizations preferred capital expense to labor and repair expenses).

As the Medicare reimbursement for capital costs was folded into the DRG formula during the 1990s as a result of OBRA of 1990, healthcare organizations found themselves competing with other industries for limited capital funds. Healthcare organizations no longer had cost-based reimbursement to put up as collateral, and as a result, lending institutions required financial analysis to ensure that the capital expenditure would generate sufficient revenue to repay the loan.

The typical financial analyses for capital expenditures are payback period analysis, net present value (NPV) analysis, and internal rate of return (IRR) analysis.

Payback Period Analysis

Payback period analysis is the number of years necessary for cash flows to recover the original investment. Payback period analysis is easy to calculate (see Problem 13.1), but it is the least sophisticated of the three analyses because it does not take into account the effects of time on money.

PROBLEM 13.1
Payback Period

ABC Day Surgery Center wants to buy equipment for $10,000 with projected cash flows (net revenues minus expenses) of $3,000 per year during the equipment's five-year useful life. What is the payback period?

Year	Cash Flow ($)	Cumulative Cash Flow ($)
cf_0	(10,000)	($10,000)
cf_1	3,000	(7,000)
cf_2	3,000	(4,000)
cf_3	3,000	(1,000)
cf_4	3,000	2,000
cf_5	3,000	5,000

Initial investment represented by cf_0; cf = cash flow.

The day surgery center will recover the cost of the equipment sometime during year 4. Sometimes when comparing capital equipment requests it might be necessary to use a value more exact than whole years. To determine exactly when during year 4 the equipment will break even, assuming an even distribution of cash flow during the year:

Payback period

$$= \text{year before recovery} + \frac{\text{unrecovered cost at beginning of year}}{\text{cash flow during year}}$$

$$= 3 + (1{,}000 \,/\, 3{,}000)$$

$$= 3.33 \text{ years}$$

The primary disadvantage of payback period analysis is that it does not take into account the effects of time on money. Discounting is used to compare capital expenditures that will generate future cash flows. Discounting is a way of looking at a future amount of money, called future value (FV), and calculating the present value (PV) of the money using the following formula:

$$PV = FV \,/\, (1 + i)^n$$

where i is the discount rate (the annual cost of capital to an organization),[5] and n is the number of years the money is discounted. Problem 13.2 shows how this formula is used.

PROBLEM 13.2
Calculating the Present Value

What is the present value of $100,000, discounted at 5 percent annually for five years?

$$PV = \frac{FV}{(1 + i)^n} = \frac{100{,}000}{(1 + .05)^5} = \frac{100{,}000}{1.2763} = \$78{,}351$$

Note: The above reference answer is formula driven. Use of a calculator or spreadsheet may alter the answer slightly because of rounding or how interest is calculated (at the end of the period versus during the period).

HP 10BII Solution to Problem 13.2

Keys	Display	Description
1 [●] [P/YR]	1.00	Sets compounding periods per year to 1
5 [N]	5.00	Stores the number of compounding periods
5 [I/YR]	5.00	Stores the interest rate
−100,000 [FV]	−100,000.00	Stores the future value as an anuity (−)
[PV]	78,352.62	

After managers understand the concept of discounting, they can apply discounting to payback period analysis, net present value analysis, and internal rate of return analysis. Discounted payback period is similar to payback period except that the manager discounts the projected cash flows by discount factors for the expenditure's discount rate (see Problem 13.3). Managers can find discount factors on a present value table (see Table 13.1).

PROBLEM 13.3
Discounted Payback Period

ABC Day Surgery Center wants to buy equipment for $10,000 with projected cash flows (net revenues minus expenses) of $3,000 per year during the equipment's five-year useful life. What is the discounted payback period at 10 percent?

Year	Cash Flow	Discount Factor	Discounted Cash Flow	Cumulative Discounted Cash Flow
cf_0*	(10,000)	1.000	($10,000)	($10,000)
cf_1	3,000	0.909	2,727	(7,273)
cf_2	3,000	0.826	2,478	(4,795)
cf_3	3,000	0.751	2,253	(2,542)
cf_4	3,000	0.683	2,049	(493)
cf_5	3,000	0.621	1,863	1,370

* Initial investment represented by cf_0

The day surgery center will recover the cost of the equipment sometime during year 5. Sometimes when comparing capital equipment requests it might be necessary to use a value more exact than whole years. The following cycle can be used to determine exactly when during year 5 the equipment will break even (assuming an even distribution of cash flow during the year):

Payback period

$$= \text{year before recovery} + \frac{\text{unrecovered cost at beginning of year}}{\text{cash flow during year}}$$

$$= 4 + \frac{493}{1,863} = 4.265 \text{ years}$$

Note: The above reference answer is formula driven. Use of a calculator or spreadsheet may alter the answer slightly because of rounding or how interest is calculated (at the end of the period versus during the period).

Net Present Value

Net present value (NPV) is a commonly used financial analysis for capital expenditures that relies on discounting cash flows. Where discounted payback period gives the manager an answer in years, NPV gives the manager an answer in dollars. An NPV of zero means that the capital expenditure is generating discounted cash flows just sufficient to repay the original investment. If the NPV is positive, the expenditure is generating discounted cash flows in excess of the amount necessary to repay the original investment. If the NPV is negative, the expenditure is generating discounted cash flows insufficient to

	Discount Rate (%)				
	10	20	30	40	50
Year 1	0.909	0.833	0.769	0.714	0.667
Year 2	0.826	0.694	0.592	0.511	0.444
Year 3	0.751	0.579	0.455	0.364	0.296
Year 4	0.683	0.482	0.351	0.261	0.198
Year 5	0.621	0.402	0.269	0.186	0.132
Year 6	0.564	0.335	0.207	0.133	0.088
Year 7	0.513	0.279	0.159	0.095	0.059
Year 8	0.467	0.233	0.123	0.068	0.039
Year 9	0.424	0.194	0.094	0.048	0.026
Year 10	0.385	0.162	0.073	0.035	0.017

TABLE 13.1

Present Value Table

repay the original investment. NPV can be expressed in the following equation (Brigham 1992):

$$\text{NPV} = cf_0 + \frac{cf_1}{(1+k)^1} + \frac{cf_2}{(1+k)^2} + \cdots \frac{cf_n}{(1+k)^n}$$

where k is the capital expenditures discount rate; cf is cash flow; and n is the number of years the money is discounted.

NPV has some flaws (see Zelman, McCue, and Millikan 1998)—the principle flaw seems to be determining the discount rate. Most theorists agree that NPV is superior to internal rate of return (IRR) as a method of evaluating capital expenditures (Brigham 1992). However, because IRR is a common method of evaluating capital expenditures in the real world, managers should be prepared to calculate both NPV and IRR.

Internal Rate of Return

Internal rate of return (IRR) analysis is the discount rate of a capital expenditure where the discounted cash flows equal the expenditure's original investment, or the discount rate where the NPV is zero. Discounted payback period analysis gives the manager an answer in years and NPV analysis gives the manager an answer in dollars. IRR analysis gives the manager an answer in a percentage. Solving the NPV equation by hand is relatively simple, but solving the IRR is difficult without a calculator. Solving the IRR by hand using the equation necessitates a trial and error methodology—inserting discount factors representing different discount rates until the sum equals zero (Brigham 1992).

$$cf_0 + \frac{cf_1}{(1+\text{IRR})^1} + \frac{cf_2}{(1+\text{IRR})^2} \cdots \frac{cf_n}{(1+\text{IRR})^n} = 0$$

Problem 13.4 shows how the manager can use the calculations from NPV analysis to calculate the IRR using interpolation.

Step 20: Identify Nonfinancial Benefits

The twentieth step in the planning process and the fourth step in the capital budgeting process is for the department manager requesting the capital

PROBLEM 13.4
NPV/IRR Calculation

ABC Day Surgery Center wants to buy equipment for $10,000 with projected cash flows of $3,000 per year during the equipment's five-year useful life. What is the net present value of the equipment at 10 percent? What is the internal rate of return?

HB 10BII Solution to Problem 13.4

Keys	Display	Description
1 P/YR	1.00	Sets compounding periods per year to 1
−10,000 CFj	0 CF	Enters the initial cash flow
3,000 CFj	1 CF	Enters the first cash flow
3,000 CFj	2 CF	Enters the second cash flow
3,000 CFj	3 CF	Enters the third cash flow
3,000 CFj	4 CF	Enters the fourth cash flow
3,000 CFj	5 CF	Enters the fifth cash flow

[In the event that there is a salvage value, enter the value to the last year cash flow.]

10 I/YR	10.00	Stores the interest rate
NPV	1,372.26	Displays NPV in dollars
IRR	15.24	Displays IRR in percent

expenditure to identify nonfinancial benefits for the request. Examples of nonfinancial benefits could include community need or medical staff politics. Even if the organization is buying equipment to please a valuable physician, the organization should still complete a financial analysis to determine the equipment's loss that will need to be subsidized elsewhere.

Step 21: Evaluate Benefits and Make Decisions

The twenty-first and last step in the planning process and the fifth and final step in the capital budgeting process is for the budget committee to evaluate the financial and nonfinancial benefits for each request and make decisions. The budget committee can use a decision matrix with weighted criteria similar to that shown in Table 13.2. Implicit in the decision-making process is an evaluation of the decision. Many healthcare organizations use their internal audit departments to review capital expenditure decisions and the justifications of the department managers to determine their accuracy. Internal auditors can

TABLE 13.2
Decision Matrix
for Capital
Budget

Request	Financial Analysis	Community Need	Cost Containment	Physician Relations	Total
	40	20	30	10	Total
A	30	20	25	10	85
B	40	10	20	05	80
C	35	05	10	10	60
D	20	20	05	10	55

review the actual volumes, revenues, and expenses to determine whether the projections used to support the decisions were accurate.

Financing Capital Expenditures

Healthcare organizations can use cash generated from philanthropy, funded depreciation, operating surpluses, and debt to finance capital expenditures. Generally speaking, the organization should use funded depreciation to finance replacement equipment and philanthropy, operating surpluses, or debt to finance new equipment.

The Tax Reform Act of 1986 limited the tax deduction individuals were able to take for donations; as a result, philanthropy to healthcare organizations has declined from 21 percent of tax-exempt hospital capital financing in 1968 to less than 6 percent since 1984.

The decline in philanthropy parallels an increase in debt financing because of two federal government policies. First, Medicare reduced the risk associated with debt financing by reimbursing 100 percent of the interest on debt (which ended in 1992 when capital and interest associated with capital became part of the DRG formula). Second, the Nixon administration encouraged debt financing by allowing local governments to create taxing authorities that issued tax-exempt bonds. As a result of these two policies, hospitals and many other healthcare organizations have relied on debt financing significantly more than other industries. Private industries finance 40 to 50 percent of their capital needs with debt, and public utilities finance about 60 percent of their capital needs with debt. However, hospitals finance about 80 to 90 percent of their capital needs with debt (Eastaugh 1987).[6]

Facing rising demand for capital caused by aging facilities, the needs for expansion, and the introduction of new technologies, many healthcare organizations may not have the access to the capital they need. Between 2001 and 2002, the percentage of hospitals having broad access to capital declined from 42 percent to 36 percent, while hospitals having limited access to capital increased from 11 percent to 19 percent according to a study conducted by HFMA and PricewaterhouseCoopers LLP (2003). During the same time period, the total amount of capital accessed from traditional sources—tax-exempt and taxable bonds, equity, bank loans, philanthropy, and equipment leases—dropped 29 percent from $51.4 billion to $36.5 billion (HFMA/PricewaterhouseCoopers LLP 2003).

One of the most significant factors affecting any organization's ability to access the capital markets is the organization's credit worthiness. The healthcare industry relies on rating agencies like Standard & Poor to measure credit worthiness using both objective criteria and subjective assessments of organizations and the markets in which they operate.

When issuing bond ratings, rating agencies review the following five factors (HFMA 1998):

1. Legal provisions of the organization including corporate charters, bylaws, and so on;
2. Institutional characteristics and market position including the organization's ability to adapt to changing market conditions;
3. Medical staff characteristics including the number and age relative to the organization's size;
4. Management capability including the depth, education, and experience of management in dealing with medical staff, in providing leadership, in managing budgets, in maintaining financial and human resources, and in defining and striving for the organization's mission and vision; and
5. Financial indicators, including indicators of past performance and indicators of the ability to forecast capacity to pay debt service.

With philanthropy declining and many healthcare organizations at debt capacity, future capital expenditures must be financed through operating surpluses (or joint ventures or acquisitions), which makes the planning and budgeting functions all the more important. Sometimes, leasing might be considered as another method of financing a capital expenditure. In fact, leasing accounts for 20 to 25 percent of all healthcare provider equipment financing (Zelman, McCue, and Millikan 1998).

Lease Versus Purchase Decisions

Lease versus purchase decisions are made after the decision is made to acquire the equipment; therefore, the lease versus purchase decision is in fact a financing decision. Generally, there are two types of leases: operating leases and capital leases. Operating leases are for periods less than the equipment's useful life and are common for copy machines, desk-top computers, and cars. Capital leases are for the equipment's approximate useful life and usually include provisions for the lessee to purchase the equipment at the end of the lease period.

Lease decisions have several advantages over purchase decisions and can provide the lessee with more flexibility, more financing options for other equipment, more protection from unexpected events like changes in technology, and more and better maintenance. In the case of for-profit healthcare organizations, capital leases can provide the same tax advantages as decisions to purchase the equipment.

Lease decisions have several disadvantages over purchase decisions and are generally more expensive than the purchase decision because lessors must make a profit and cover their risks of loss.

Problem 13.5 gives a simple way of analyzing the costs associated with a non-profit facility purchasing or leasing a $1.3 million MRI by applying a present value of 10 percent to both decisions (a for-profit facility would have tax shields, or reductions in the amount of income taxes paid, due to the tax deductibility of depreciation and interest expense).

Evaluating Capital Budgeting Performance

When evaluating capital budgeting performance, several ratios are used to determine how much debt an organization can incur.

LEASE VERSUS PURCHASE DECISION EXERCISE

Purchase considerations	Lease considerations
Borrow $1.3 million at 10 percent on declining balance	Lease payments of $26,000 per month for 60 months (includes maintenance)
Depreciate straight line over five years	
Trade-in value of $130,000 at end of useful life	
Maintenance expense of $12,000 per year	

[Revenues, as well as labor and supply expenses, are the same for both decisions, and therefore are not included in the analysis.]

PURCHASE

Year	Principal Payment	Interest Payment	Maintenance Expense	Total Expense	PV Factor at 10%	PV Expense
1	260,000	130,000	12,000	402,000	0.909	365,418
2	260,000	104,000	12,000	376,000	0.826	310,576
3	260,000	78,000	12,000	350,000	0.751	262,850
4	260,000	52,000	12,000	324,000	0.683	221,292
5	260,000	26,000	12,000	298,000	0.621	185,058
Trade-in (130,000)					0.621	(80,730)
						1,264,464

LEASE

Year	Lease Payment	PV Factor at 10%	PV Expense
1	312,000	0.909	283,608
2	312,000	0.826	257,712
3	312,000	0.751	234,312
4	312,000	0.683	213,096
5	312,000	0.621	193,752
			1,182,480

Because the present value expense of the lease decision is less than the present value expense of the purchase decision, the financial merit supports the lease decision. However, other criteria mentioned in the advantages and disadvantages of the lease decision mentioned above should also be considered before making a final decision.

- **Debt-to-Capitalization Ratio**

$$\frac{\text{long-term debt}}{(\text{long-term debt} + \text{net assets})}$$

Debt-to-Capitalization, or long-term debt to capitalization, is an indicator of the long-term debt divided by the long-term debt plus net assets. Higher values imply a greater reliance on debt financing as a percentage and may imply a reduced ability to carry additional debt. The Debt-to-Capitalization median for all hospitals reporting to Ingenix (2004) for 2002 audited financial statements was 27.4—S&P "A" rated hospitals reporting to Ingenix was 33.8.

- **Capital Expense Ratio**

$$\frac{(\text{interest expense} + \text{depreciation expense})}{\text{total expense} \times 100}$$

Capital Expense Ratio provides an important indicator of operating leverage. Since both interest expense and depreciation expense are considered fixed, a high capital expense ratio as a percentage would imply greater sensitivity to changes in volume. The Capital Expense median for all hospitals reporting to Ingenix (2004) for 2002 audited financial statements was 6.6—S&P "A" rated hospitals reporting to Ingenix was 7.6.

- **Average Age of Plant**

$$\frac{\text{accumulated depreciation}}{\text{depreciation expense}}$$

Average Age of Plant provides an indicator in years of the healthcare organization's fixed assets. Higher values reflect an older plant and equipment and indirectly may imply a difficulty in competing with "newer" healthcare organizations while lower values reflect a newer plant and equipment. The Average Age of Plant median for all hospitals reporting to Ingenix (2004) for 2002 audited financial statements was 9.77—S&P "A" rated hospitals reporting to Ingenix was 9.08.

Notes

1. Useful life is part of the depreciation controversy between providers and insurers regarding allowable cost for reimbursement purposes. The issues include what the useful life should be; whether the amount to be depreciated should be based on historic cost or replacement cost; and what method of computing depreciation (i.e., straight line, sum-of-the-years digits, or double declining balance—the latter two of which are accelerated) should be used (Berman, Kukla, and Weeks 1994).

2. In some cases, the budget committee may ask the medical staff or chief of the medical staff to prioritize the list of chief-of-service requests before submitting it to the budget committee. This avoids the problem of nonphysician department managers making decisions on physician-generated requests.

3. Most organizations prioritize replacement equipment that is fully depreciated ahead of new requests to avoid the snowball effect of not replacing assets on schedule. Doing so is easy to justify because the need for the equipment is supportable with procedure logs; if the organization funded the equipment's depreciation properly, funds exist for the replacement. Some organizations prioritize new equipment ahead of replacement equipment to generate new streams of revenue. However, this strategy could result in long-term problems for the organization, especially if the organization uses funded depreciation to acquire the new equipment.

4. Usually the budget committee, CFO, or designee is responsible for converting gross revenue to net revenue by subtracting contractual adjustments, charity care adjustments, and bad debt adjustments. This can be accomplished in a fashion similar to that shown in Problem 4.1, Step 1, in Chapter 4.

5. Three common sources of discount rates include costs of a specific financing source such as debt; yield achievable from other investments;

and the weighted cost of capital (percent debt × cost of debt) + (percent equity × cost of equity). The actual discount rate used is not of critical importance to most healthcare organizations because criteria in addition to discounted cash flow analyses will be used. If the same discount rate is used for all capital requests, relative rankings will not change (Cleverly 1997).

6. Health economists agree that organizations with this kind of excessive debt have great difficulty with cyclical recessions or downturns in the economy. This helps explain the growing trend of not-for-profit organizations joint-venturing or being acquired by for-profit organizations that have access to different capital markets.

References

Berman, H. J., L. E. Kukla, and S. F. Weeks. 1994. *The Financial Management of Hospitals, 8th ed.* Chicago: Health Administration Press.

Brigham, E. F. 1992. *Fundamentals of Financial Management, 6th ed.* New York: Dryden Press.

Cleverly, W. O. 1997. *Essentials of Health Care Finance, 4th ed.* Gaithersburg, MD: Aspen Publishers.

Eastaugh, S. R. 1987. *Financing Health Care: Economic Efficiency and Equity.* Dover, MA: Auburn House.

Healthcare Financial Management Association. 1998. *HFMA Core Certification Exam Self-Study Manual.* White Plains, NY: The MGI Management Institute.

HFMA/PricewaterhouseCoopers LLP. 2003. "How Are Hospitals Financing the Future? Access to Capital in Healthcare Today—Part I." [Online retrieval, 03/18/04.] http://www.hfma.org.

Herkimer, A. G. 1988. "Capital Expenditure Planning." *Understanding Health Care Budgeting.* Rockville, MD: Aspen Publishers.

Ingenix. 2004. *Almanac of Hospital Financial and Operating Indicators.* Salt Lake City, UT: Ingenix.

Person, M. W. 1997. *The Zero-Base Hospital: Survival and Success in America's Evolving Healthcare System.* Chicago: Health Administration Press.

William, J., and J. Rakich. 1973. "Investment Evaluation in Hospitals." *Hospital Financial Management* 23 (2): 30–35.

Zelman, W. N., M. J. McCue, and A. R. Millikan. 1998. "Technical Concerns Regarding Net Present Value." *Financial Management of Health Care Organizations.* Malden, MD: Blackwell Publishers.

Recommended Readings — Part IV

Cleverly, W. O. 1997. *Essentials of Health Care Finance, 4th ed.* Gaithersburg, MD: Aspen Publishers.

Fottler, M. D., J. D. Blair, C. J. Whitehead, M. D. Laus, and G. T. Savage. 1989. "Assessing Key Stake Holders: Who Matters to Hospitals and Why?" *Hospital & Health Services Administration* 34 (Winter): 530.

Herkimer, A. G. 1988. *Understanding Health Care Budgeting.* Gaithersburg, MD: Aspen Publishers.

Ingenix. 2004. *Almanac of Hospital Financial and Operating Indicators.* Salt Lake City, UT: Ingenix.

Koontz, H., C. O'Donnell, and H. Weihrich. 1984. *Management, 8th ed.* New York: McGraw-Hill Publishers.

McLean, R. A. 1997. "Budgeting and Variance Analysis." *Financial Management in Health Care Organizations.* New York: Delmar Publishers.

Nowicki, M. 1998. "Beware the 'Slippery Slope' of Granting Exceptions." *Journal of Healthcare Resource Management* 16 (1): 20–22.

Person, M. W. 1997. *The Zero-Base Hospital: Survival and Success in America's Evolving Healthcare System.* Chicago: Health Administration Press.

Pyhrr, P. A. 1973. *Zero-Based Budgeting: A Practical Management Tool for Evaluating Expenses.* New York: John Wiley & Sons Publishers.

———. 1970. "Zero-Base Budgeting." *Harvard Business Review* 48 (11): 111–121.

Reeves, P. N., D. F. Bergwall, and N. B. Woodside. 1979. *Introduction to Health Planning.* Arlington, VA: Information Resources Press.

Zelman, W. N., M. J. McCue, and A. R. Millikan. 1998. *Financial Management of Health Care Organizations.* Malden, MA: Blackwell Publishers.

FINANCIAL ANALYSIS

FINANCIAL ANALYSIS AND MANAGEMENT REPORTING

Financial analysis and management reporting are integral parts of both the management functions of control and financial management. As introduced in Chapter 8, financial analysis includes methods used by investors, creditors, and management to evaluate the past, present, and future financial performance of the healthcare organization. On completion of the analysis, the information is reported to the appropriate parties both inside and outside the organization, at which time the parties take corrective action in the form of decisions.

Steps in Financial Analysis

Financial analysis includes the following three steps (Berman, Kukla, and Weeks 1994):

1. Establishment of the facts in the organization;
2. Comparison of the facts in the organization over time and to facts in similar organizations; and
3. The use of perspective and judgment to make decisions regarding the comparisons.

Financial analysis by management can occur at any level—departmental, divisional, or organizational—within the organization.

At the organizational level, establishing the facts (the first step), usually relates to a review of the organization's key financial statements, including the balance sheet, statement of operations, statement of changes in net assets, and statement of cash flows. Healthcare organizations with permanent controlling financial interests in other healthcare organizations should prepare consolidated financial statements to properly report the relationship (AICPA 1996). Financial analysis by investors and creditors may require that independent auditors review the financial statements first to confirm their accuracy.

The second step, comparing the facts in the organization over time and to facts in other similar organizations, includes ratio analysis, horizontal analysis, and vertical analysis. Ratio analysis evaluates an organization's performance by computing the relationships of important line items found in the financial statements. There are four kinds of ratios: liquidity, profitability, activity, and capital structure.

Horizontal analysis evaluates the trend in the line items by focusing on the percentage change over time. Vertical analysis evaluates the internal structure of the organization by focusing on a base number and showing percentages of important line items in relation to the base number. Once ratio analysis, horizontal analysis, and vertical analysis are complete, the organization can develop trend comparisons that compare the organization's present ratios, trends, and percentages to the organization's past ratios, trends, and percentages. The organization can also develop industry comparisons that compare the organization's present ratios, trends, and percentages to ratios, trends, and percentages of other, similar organizations to determine the organization's financial performance relative to competitors.[1]

The third step of financial analysis, using perspective and judgment to make decisions, uses the information obtained in the first two steps, in addition to information derived from the decision maker's unique perspective and judgment, to make the decision. Decisions that may at first appear to be contrary to the information provided in the first two steps may make perfect sense based on pressures from both internal and external constituents, including medical staffs, employers, regulators, donors, and others.

Balance Sheet

The balance sheet shows the organization's financial position at a specific point in time, typically at the end of an accounting period (see Figure 14.1). The balance sheet presents the organization's assets, liabilities, and net assets (or shareholders' equity in for-profit organizations) and their relationships, which are reflected in the accounting equation:

$$\text{Assets} = \text{liabilities} + \text{net assets}$$

Assets are economic resources that provide or are expected to provide benefit to the organization. *Current assets* are economic resources that have a life of less than one year (i.e., the organization expects to consume them within one year). Current assets are listed on the balance sheet in order of liquidity. *Cash* is money on hand and in the bank that the organization can access immediately. *Cash equivalents* is money placed in instruments with high liquidity and safety, such as treasury bills. *Short-term investments* is money placed in securities with maturities up to one year, such as commodities and options. *Assets limited as to use* is money set aside for specific purposes, such as debt repayment, during the next year. *Patient accounts receivable*, or the net of allowance for doubtful accounts, is money due to the organizations from patients and third parties for services already provided, minus an estimate of how much money the organization will not collect. *Other current assets* is money and other economic resources that the organization expects to consume and expense within one year, such as inventories and prepaid expenses.

Long-term assets are economic resources that have a life of more than one year. *Assets limited as to use* is money set aside for specific purposes, such as

	20X7	20X6
Assets		
Current assets:		
Cash and cash equivalents	$ 4,758	$ 5,877
Marketable securities	15,836	10,740
Assets limited as to use	970	1,300
Patient accounts receivable, net of allowance for doubtful accounts of $2,500 in 20X7 and $2,400 in 20X6	15,100	14,194
Other current assets	2,670	2,856
Total current assets	39,334	34,967
Assets limited as to use:		
Internally designated for capital acquisition	12,000	12,500
Held by trustee	6,949	7,341
	18,949	19,841
Less amount required to meet current obligations	(970)	(1,300)
	17,979	18,541
Long-term investments	4,680	4,680
Long-term investments restricted for capital acquisition	320	520
Property and equipment, net	51,038	50,492
Other assets	1,695	1,370
Total assets	$115,046	$110,570
Liabilities and Net Assets		
Current liabilities:		
Current portion of long-term debt	$ 1,470	$ 1,750
Accounts payable and accrued expenses	5,818	5,382
Estimated third-party payer settlements	2,143	1,942
Other current liabilities	1,969	2,114
Total current liabilities	11,400	11,188
Long-term debt, net of current portion	23,144	24,014
Other liabilities	3,953	3,166
Total liabilities	38,497	38,368
Net assets:		
Unrestricted	70,846	66,199
Temporarily restricted	2,115	2,470
Permanently restricted	3,588	3,533
Total net assets	76,549	72,202
Total liabilities and net assets	$115,046	$110,570

FIGURE 14.1

Sample Not-for-Profit Hospital Balance Sheets December 31, 20X7 and 20X6 (in thousands of dollars)

See accompanying notes to financial statements in Appendix 14.1, items 1–4.
Source: Reprinted with permission from the AICPA. 2003. *AICPA Audit and Accounting Guide: Health Care Organizations*, 165–166. New York: AICPA. Copyright by the American Institute of Certified Public Accountants, Inc.

debt repayment, minus the amount needed for the current accounting period referenced above. *Long-term investments* is money placed in securities with maturities of more than one year such as stocks and bonds. *Property and equipment, net* is economic resources such as land, buildings, and equipment, minus the amount that has been depreciated over the life of the buildings and equipment, which is accumulated depreciation. *Other assets* is money and other economic resources not previously referenced.

Liabilities are economic obligations, or debts, of the organization. *Current liabilities* are economic obligations, or debts, that are due in less than one year. *Current portion of long-term debt* is money due within one year on a long-term debt. *Accounts payable and accrued expenses* is money due within one year to vendors and employees (sometimes called accrued wages). *Estimated third-party settlements* is an estimate of money due within one year to third parties for overpayment of claims. *Other current liabilities* are other economic obligations that are due in less than one year. These may include deferred revenue, which is revenue received but not yet earned such as premium revenue from managed care organizations.

Long-term liabilities are economic obligations, or debts, that are due in more than one year. *Long-term debt, net of current portion* is an economic obligation, or debt, that is due in more than one year, minus the amount that is due within one year referenced above. *Other liabilities* are economic obligations, or debts, not previously referenced.

Net Assets[2] is the current American Institute of Certified Public Accountants (AICPA)–approved terminology for the difference between assets and liabilities in not-for-profit healthcare organizations. *Unrestricted net assets* includes net assets that have not been externally restricted by donors or grantors, such as the excess of revenues to expenses from operations. Unrestricted net assets includes net assets that are contractually limited by the governing body such as proceeds of debt issues, funds deposited with a trustee and limited to use by an indenture agreement, and funds set aside under self-insurance arrangements and statutory reserve requirements. *Temporarily restricted net assets* includes donor-restricted net assets that the organization can use for the donor's specific purpose once the organization has met the donor's restriction, such as the passage of time or an action by the organization. *Permanently restricted net assets* includes donor-restricted net assets with restrictions that never expire, such as endowment funds.

Shareholders' equity is the current AICPA-approved terminology for the difference between assets and liabilities in for-profit healthcare organizations and represents the ownership interest of stockholders in the organization. Shareholders' equity is also called stockholders' equity, owners' equity, and net worth and is comprised of common stock and retained earnings. *Common stock* is money invested in the organization by its owners. *Retained earnings* is income earned by the organization from operations minus dividends (which are distributions of earnings paid to stockholders based on the number of shares of stock owned).

Explanatory notes for the balance sheet and the other financial statements should identify extraordinary events as well as certain required provisions, and should be presented following the financial statements.

Statement of Operations

The statement of operations, called the income statement for for-profit organizations, summarizes the organization's net revenues, expenses, and excess of net revenues over expenses, or income before taxes in a for-profit organization, over a period of time (see Figures 14.2 and 14.3). The relationship of the statement of operations to the balance sheet can be best expressed by the expanded accounting equation:

$$\text{Assets} = \text{liabilities} + \text{net assets} + (\text{net revenue} - \text{expenses})$$

where the permanent accounts of the balance sheet, which are accounts that carry balances forward to the next year, relate to the temporary accounts of the statement of operations, which are accounts that zero out at the end of each year. To zero out the net results of the statement of operations at the end of the year, the net results are transferred to unrestricted net assets on the balance sheet, or to retained earnings on the balance sheet of a for-profit organization.

Unrestricted revenues, gains, and other support include four categories of revenue. *Net patient service revenue* is money generated by providing patient care minus an estimate of how much money the organization will not collect as a result of discounting charges per contractual agreement and providing charity care. For financial reporting purposes, patient service revenue does not include provisions for charity care because charity care was never intended to result in cash flow. The organization's policy for providing charity care, in addition to the amount of charity care provided based on revenues, costs, or units, must be in the notes to the financial statements.

Premium revenue is money generated from capitation arrangements that must be reported separately from patient service revenue since premium revenue is earned by agreeing to provide care, regardless of whether care was ever delivered. *Other revenue* is money generated from services other than health services to patients and enrollees. These revenues may include revenue from rental equipment and office space, sales of supplies and pharmaceuticals to employees, cafeteria and gift shop sales, and so on. *Net assets released from restrictions used for operations* is money previously restricted by donors that has become available for operations.

Five expenses are categorized on the statement of operations. *Operating expenses* is money spent on operations to generate revenue. These expenses

FIGURE 14.2

Sample Not-for-Profit Hospital's Statement of Operations Year End December 31, 20X7 and 20X6 (in thousands of dollars)

	20X7	20X6
Unrestricted revenues, gains, and other support:		
Net patient service revenue	$85,156	$78,942
Premium revenue	11,150	10,950
Other revenue	2,601	5,212
Net assets released from restrictions used for operations	300	
Total operating revenues, gains, and other support	99,207	95,104
Expenses:		
Operating expenses	88,521	80,585
Depreciation and amortization	4,782	4,280
Interest	1,782	1,825
Provisions for bad debts	1,000	1,300
Other	2,000	1,300
Total expenses	98,055	89,290
Operating income	1,152	5,814
Other income: Investment income	3,900	3,025
Excess of revenues over expenses	5,052	8,839
Change in net unrealized gains and losses on other than trading securities	300	375
Net assets released from restrictions used for purchase of property and equipment	200	
Change in interest in net assets of Sample Hospital Foundation	283	536
Transfers to parent	(688)	(3,051)
Increase in unrestricted net assets, before extraordinary item	5,147	6,699
Extraordinary loss from extinguishment of debt	(500)	
Increase in unrestricted net assets	$ 4,647	$ 6,699

See accompanying notes to financial statements in Appendix 14.1, items 1–4.
Source: Reprinted with permission from the AICPA. 2003. *AICPA Audit and Accounting Guide: Health Care Organizations*, 167. New York: AICPA. Copyright by the American Institute of Certified Public Accountants, Inc.

include employee wages and benefits, supplies, pharmaceuticals, and so on, and are often itemized on the statement of operations.

Depreciation and amortization is the expensing of long-term assets over time to reflect their declining value. *Interest* is the expense incurred with borrowed money. *Provisions for bad debt* is an estimate of how much money the organization will not collect as a result of bad debt, and the amount reported must be based on charges. Provisions for bad debt should not be confused with provisions for charity care. Bad debt amounts reflect that the

	20X7	20X6
Unrestricted net assets:		
Excess of revenues over expenses	$ 5,052	$ 8,839
Net unrealized gains on investments, other than trading securities	300	375
Changes in interest in net assets of Sample Hospital Foundation	283	536
Transfers to parent	(688)	(3,051)
Net assets released from restrictions used for purchase of property and equipment	200	
Increase in unrestricted net assets before extraordinary item	5,147	6,699
Extraordinary loss from extinguishment of debt	(500)	
Increase in unrestricted net assets	4,647	6,699
Temporarily restricted net assets:		
Contributions for charity care	140	966
Net realized and unrealized gains on investments	5	8
Net assets released from restrictions	(500)	
Increase in temporarily restricted net assets	(355)	1,004
Permanently restricted net assets:		
Contributions for endowment funds	50	411
Net realized and unrealized gains on investments	5	2
Increase in permanently restricted net assets	55	413
Increase in net assets	4,347	8,116
Net assets, beginning of year	72,202	64,086
Net assets, end of year	$76,549	$72,202

FIGURE 14.3
Sample Not-for-Profit Hospital's Statement of Changes in Net Assets Year End December 31, 20X7 and 20X6 (in thousands of dollars)

See accompanying notes to financial statements in Appendix 14.1, items 1–4.
Source: Reprinted with permission from the AICPA. 2003. *AICPA Audit and Accounting Guide: Health Care Organizations*, 169. New York: AICPA. Copyright by the American Institute of Certified Public Accountants, Inc.

organization provided services with the expectation of payment. Charity care amounts reflect that the organization provided services with no expectation of payment. *Other expenses* is miscellaneous expenses that have not been reported above such as utilities, travel, telephone, and so on.

Operating income is the money earned from providing patient care services and includes the total revenue, gains, and other support minus the total expenses; *other income* is the money earned from non–patient care services such as investment income. *Excess of revenues over expenses* (or net income in for-profit organizations) is the operating income plus the other income minus total expenses. For not-for-profit organizations, AICPA requires excess of revenues over expenses to be reported as the performance indicator that reflects the results of operations. Not-for-profit organizations must report the performance indicator in a statement of operations that also presents the total changes in unrestricted net assets. The notes to the financial statements should provide a description of the nature and composition of the performance indicator (AICPA 2003).

Change in net unrealized gains and losses on other than trading securities is money reflecting the change in the fair market value of stocks other than security trades. *Net assets released from restrictions used for purchase of property and equipment* is money that was temporarily restricted by donors that is now available for property and equipment. *Changes in interest in net assets of Sample Hospital Foundation* is money released from the Foundation.

Transfers to parent is money transferred to Sample Hospital from a subsidiary corporation. *Extraordinary loss from extinguishment of debt* is money reflecting an unusual loss or gain in net assets. *The increase in unrestricted net assets* presents the total changes in unrestricted net assets during the statement period.

Statement of Changes in Net Assets

The statement of changes in net assets, called equity in a for-profit organization, shows the reasons why net assets changed from the beginning of the statement period to the end of the statement period as reported in summary fashion on the balance sheet (see Table 14.3). Because AICPA requires not-for-profit organizations to report changes of unrestricted net assets on the statement of operations, many organizations also include changes in temporarily restricted and permanently restricted net assets on the statement of operations, which eliminates the need for a separate statement of changes in net assets. This statement is important in showing how the changes in the excess of revenues over expenses affect the net asset, or equity, position of the organization.

Unrestricted net assets comes directly from the statement of operations and has already been explained in that section. *Temporarily restricted net assets* presents the changes in temporarily restricted net assets during the statement period. *Contributions for charity care* is money donated to Sample Hospital for the provision of charity care. *Net realized and unrealized gains on investments* is an increase in the value of the investment (unrealized until sold) and an increase in cash (realized through dividends or interest). *Net assets released from restrictions* is money previously restricted by donors that has become available for use. *Increase (decrease) in temporarily restricted net assets* presents the total changes in temporarily restricted net assets during the statement period.

Permanently restricted net assets presents the changes in permanently restricted net assets during the accounting period. *Contributions for endowment funds* is money received from donors with permanent restrictions on the principal and interest. *Net realized and unrealized gains on investments* is an increase in value of the investment and an increase in cash. The increase in net assets is the difference between total net assets at the beginning of the year and total net assets at the end of the year.

Statement of Cash Flows

The statement of cash flows shows the organization's cash flow, which is the amounts of cash receipts and where they came from and the amounts of cash disbursements and where they went during the statement period (see Figure 14.4). In a not-for-profit organization, the statement is divided into cash flows from operations, cash flows from investments, and cash flows from financing including restricted income and contributions. For-profit organizations do not divide the cash flows into categories, but the bottom line is the same— net increase (decrease) in cash.[3]

Cash flows from operating activities begins with the change in net assets from the statement of changes in net assets or computed from the difference in total net assets between statement periods on the balance sheet and then includes the changes in cash between statement periods for providing patient care services. Using the indirect method of computing cash flows, information from the statement of operations was prepared using accrual accounting as required by generally accepted accounting principles (GAAP). This means that revenues were recorded when the services were billed, not when the bills were paid. Expenses were recorded when they contributed to operations, not when they were paid. Revenues and expenses must be adjusted as well as noncash events such as depreciation. The remainder of this section of the statement of cash flows makes the necessary adjustments (Prince 1992).

Cash flows from investing activities includes the changes in cash between statement periods for investing in fixed assets such as property and equipment and for selling fixed assets. Cash flows from financing activities includes the changes in cash between statement periods for financing activities such as debts, endowments, grants, and transfers to and from parent organizations. Net increase (decrease) in cash and cash equivalents is computed by adding the net cash from operating, investing, and financing activities.

Cash and cash equivalents, beginning of year corresponds with the cash and cash equivalents, end of year for the previous year. Cash and cash equivalents, end of year is computed by adding the net increase (decrease) in cash and cash equivalents to the cash and cash equivalents, beginning of year, and corresponds to cash and cash equivalents on the balance sheet for the same statement period.

Ratio Analysis

Financial statements report an organization's financial position at a point in time, and its financial operations over a period of time. Financial statements are analyzed to predict the organization's financial performance. Investors and

	20X7	20X6
Cash flows from operating activities:		
Change in net assets	$ 4,347	$ 8,116
Adjustments to reconcile change in net assets to net cash provided by operating activities:		
Extraordinary loss from extinguishment of debt	500	
Depreciation and amortization	4,782	4,280
Net realized and unrealized gains on investments, other than trading	(450)	(575)
Undistributed portion of change in interest in net assets of Sample Hospital Foundation	(48)	(51)
Transfer to parent	688	3,051
Provisions for bad debts	1,000	1,300
Restricted contributions and investment income received	(290)	(413)
(Increase) decrease in:		
Patient accounts receivable	(1,906)	(2,036)
Trading securities	215	
Other current assets	186	(2,481)
Other assets	(277)	(190)
Increase (decrease) in:		
Accounts payable and accrued expenses	436	679
Estimated third-party payer settlements	201	305
Other current liabilities	(145)	(257)
Other liabilities	787	(128)
Net cash provided by operating activities	10,026	11,600
Cash flows from investing activities:		
Purchase of investments	(3,769)	(2,150)
Capital expenditures	(4,728)	(5,860)
Net cash used in investing activities	(8,497)	(8,010)
Cash flows from financing activities:		
Transfers to parent	(688)	(3,051)
Proceeds from restricted contributions and restricted investment income	290	413
Payments on long-term debt	(24,700)	(804)
Payments on capital lease obligations	(150)	(100)
Proceeds from issuance of long-term debt	22,600	500
Net cash used in financing activities	(2,648)	(3,042)
Net (decrease) increase in cash	(1,119)	548
Cash and cash equivalents, beginning of year	5,877	5,329
Cash and cash equivalents, end of year	$ 4,758	$ 5,877

Ratio	S&P "A" Rated	Sample Hospital 20X7	Sample Hospital 20X6	Evaluation Standard	Evaluation Trend
Liquidity					
Current	1.90	3.45	3.13	Good	Good
Collection Period	59.7	64.72	65.62	Fair	Fair
Days Cash-on-Hand, All Sources	108.6	98.90	89.21	Fair	Good
Days Cash-on-Hand, Short-Term	29.7	80.59	91.44	Fair	Fair
Average Payment Period	56.0	44.61	48.04	Good	Good
Profitability					
Operating Margin (%)		1.20	6.10	Not reported by S&P	
Total Margin (%)	2.10	5.10	9.30	Good	Poor
Return on Net Assets (%)	3.90	6.60	12.20	Good	Poor
Asset Efficiency					
Total Asset Turnover	.89	.90	.89	Good	Good
Age of Plant	9.08	7.30	7.16	Good	Good
Fixed Asset Turnover	2.15	2.02	1.94	Good	Good
Current Asset Turnover	3.40	2.62	2.81	Good	Good
Inventory Turnover	63.58			Not reported by Sample	
Capital Structure					
Net Asset Financing (%)	53.5	66.50	65.3	Fair	Fair
Long-Term Debt-to-Net Assets		.30	.33	Not reported by S&P	
Debt Service Coverage	2.91	.44	6.68	Poor	Good
Cash Flow-to-Debt (%)	16.8	28.5	37.3	Good	Fair

FIGURE 14.5
Selected
Financial Ratios

Source: Reprinted with permission from Ingenix. 2004. *2004 Almanac of Hospital Financial and Operating Indicators*. Salt Lake, Utah: Ingenix. Copyright by Ingenix.

creditors analyze the information to predict future earnings and the ability to service debt. Managers analyze financial statements to predict the future and to plan strategies that will influence the future. Ratio analysis is often the most important step in comparing the facts over time in the organization and comparing the facts to facts in similar organizations (Brigham 1992). Financial statement analysis concentrates on four classifications of ratios: liquidity; profitability; activity; and capital structure (see Figure 14.5).

Liquidity Ratios

In reference to organizations, liquidity ratios are measures of an organization's ability to meet short-term obligations. Measuring an organization's liquidity is important in evaluating an organization's financial performance.

- **Current Ratio**

$$\frac{\text{total current assets}}{\text{total current liabilities}}$$

Current Ratio is the basic indicator of financial liquidity, which is an organization's ability to meet its obligations. Higher values mean better debt-paying capacity; however, a ratio that is too high will result in opportunity costs in that the organization could invest excess current assets more wisely. The primary disadvantage of the Current Ratio is that it does not take into account the relative liquidity of the different current assets.

- **Average Collection Period**

$$\frac{\text{net receivables}}{\text{net patient service revenue}/365}$$

The Average Collection Period is also called days in accounts receivable and is a measure of how long the average patient (or payer) takes to pay the bill after discharge. Lower values indicate liquidity.

- **Days Cash-On-Hand, Short-Term Sources**

$$\frac{\text{cash} + \text{marketable securities}}{(\text{total expenses} - \text{depreciation expenses})/365}$$

- **Days Cash-On-Hand, All Sources**

$$\frac{\text{cash} + \text{marketable securities} + \text{unrestricted long-term investments}}{(\text{total expenses} - \text{depreciation expenses})/365}$$

Days Cash On Hand is a measure of how long an organization could meet its obligations if cash receipts were discontinued. Higher values indicate liquidity.

- **Average Payment Period**

$$\frac{\text{total current liabilities}}{(\text{total expenses} - \text{depreciation expenses})/365}$$

Average Payment Period is a measure of how long the organization takes to pay its obligations. Lower values indicate liquidity.

Profitability Ratios

Profitability ratios reflect an organization's ability to exist and grow by measuring the relationship of revenues to expenses. Profitability is a two-edged sword for not-for-profit healthcare organizations in that too much profit brings criticism from the community (and possibly the IRS) and too little profit brings criticism from the governing body.

- **Operating Margin**

$$\frac{\text{operating income}}{\text{total operating revenue}}$$

Operating Margin is operating income divided by total operating revenue net of allowances and uncolllectibles and therefor reflects profits from only operations. Higher values indicate profitability.

- **Total Margin**

$$\frac{\text{excess of revenues over expenses}}{\text{total revenue}}$$

Total Margin is the excess of revenues over expenses divided by total revenues net of allowances and uncollectibles and therefore reflects profits from both operations and nonoperations (typically investment income). Higher values indicate profitability.

- **Return on Net Assets**

$$\frac{\text{excess of revenues over expenses}}{\text{net assets}}$$

Return on Net Assets is the basic measure of profit in relationship to investment. Higher values reflect profitability.

Asset Efficiency Ratios

Asset efficiency ratios reflect an organization's ability to be efficient by measuring the relationship between revenue and assets. For purposes of these ratios, total revenue includes net nonoperating gains.

- **Total Asset Turnover**

$$\frac{\text{total operating revenue} + \text{other income}}{\text{total assets}}$$

Total Asset Turnover is the basic measure of how efficiently an organization is using its assets in relation to making revenue. Higher values usually indicate higher efficiency; however, older facilities with assets that are mostly depreciated may appear to be efficient because of a low numerator. Cleverly (1997) recommends calculating the age of plant ratio to determine whether efficiency or an older facility is causing a high total asset turnover ratio. The formula to determine the average age of a facility is:

$$\frac{\text{accumulated depreciation}}{\text{depreciation expense}}$$

Lower values are preferable. Note: accumulated depreciation is found in the footnotes to the financial statements.

- **Fixed Asset Turnover**

$$\frac{\text{total operating revenue} + \text{other income}}{\text{net fixed assets}}$$

Fixed Asset Turnover is a subset of the total asset turnover in that it measures how efficiently an organization is using its fixed assets in relation to generating revenue. Higher values indicate higher efficiency.

- **Current Asset Turnover**

$$\frac{\text{total operating revenue} + \text{other income}}{\text{current assets}}$$

Current Asset Turnover measures how efficiently an organization is using its current assets in relation to generating revenue. Higher values indicate higher efficiency and can be obtained by increasing revenue proportionately more than current assets or decreasing current assets proportionately more than total revenue.

- **Inventory Turnover**

$$\frac{\text{total operating revenues and other income}}{\text{inventory}}$$

Inventory Turnover measures the number of times an organization turns over its inventory relative to total operating revenue and other income. Low values usually indicate overstocking.

Capital Structure Ratios

Capital structure ratios reflect the organization's long-term liquidity by measuring a variety of relationships to capital. Capital structure ratios are used by banks and bond rating agencies to determine credit-worthiness.

- **Net Asset Financing**

$$\frac{\text{net assets}}{\text{total assets}}$$

Net asset (equity) Financing measures the relationship between assets owned by the organization and total assets. Higher values are preferable.

- **Long-Term Debt to Net Assets**

$$\frac{\text{long-term debt}}{\text{net assets}}$$

Long-Term Debt to Net Assets measures the relationship between long-term debt and assets owned by the organization. Lower values are preferable.

- **Debt Service Coverage**

$$\frac{\text{excess of revenues over expenses} + \text{depreciation} + \text{interest}}{\text{principal payment} + \text{interest}}$$

Debt Service Coverage measures the ability to meet long-term debt obligations. Higher values indicate an organization's ability to meet long-term debt obligations. Note: principal payments are found as payments on long-term debt on the statement of cash flows.

- **Cash Flow to Debt**

$$\frac{\text{excess of revenues over expenses} + \text{depreciation}}{\text{current liabilities} + \text{long-term debt}}$$

Cash Flow to Debt measures the ability to meet both short-term and long-term obligations. Higher values indicate an organization's ability to meet both short-term and long-term obligations, and lower values indicate a possible problem in meeting long-term obligations. Cleverly (1997) indicates that the cash flow to debt ratio is one of the best predictors of financial failure in organizations.

Operating Indicators

In addition to ratio analysis using information found in the financial statements, management may also analyze the following operating indicators that are an important measure of financial performance in relation to operations. Operating indicator information is not usually found on the financial statements, but should be readily available on a variety of reports used by management.

- **Average Length of Stay (ALOS)**

$$\frac{\text{patient days}}{\text{discharges}}$$

The Average Length of Stay measures how long patients stay in the hospital on the average. Because a high percentage of hospital patients reimburse the hospital either per case or are on a capitated arrangement, lower ALOSs that hold down costs are preferable. However, hospital management should be aware of the incremental costs associated with keeping patients longer before developing rigorous discharge policies to lower their ALOS. Median ALOS for all hospitals reporting to Ingenix (2004) for 2002 was 4.23—S&P "A" rated hospitals was 4.66. Hospital management should also be aware that ALOS varies for a variety of reasons including case mix. Adjusted ALOS usually means that ALOS has been adjusted for case mix. Median ALOS adjusted for case mix for all hospitals reporting to Ingenix (2004) for 2002 was 3.71—S&P "A" rated hospitals was 3.77.

- **Occupancy Rate**

$$\frac{\text{patient days}}{365 \times \text{licensed beds}}$$

Occupancy Rate measures capacity, or the percentage of the hospital that is being used. Higher values are typically preferable unless a large portion of the hospital's business is represented by capitation agreements. Median ALOS for all hospitals reporting to Ingenix (2004) for 2002 was 43.84. Hospital management should also be aware that Occupancy Rate varies for a variety of reason including the difference between licensed beds in the the facility and staffed beds in the facility. Median Occupancy Rate for staffed beds for all hospitals reporting to Ingenix (2004) for 2002 was 57.74—S&P "A" rated hospitals was 61.82.

- **Outpatient Revenue as a Percentage of Total Patient Revenue**

$$\frac{\text{outpatient revenue}}{\text{total revenue}}$$

Outpatient Revenue as a Percentage of Total Revenue measures the proportion of outpatient operations to total operations. Higher values are typically preferable as the healthcare industry shifts the focus from acute care to preventive care. Median Outpatient Revenue as a Percentage of Total Revenue for all hospitals reporting to Ingenix (2004) for 2002 was 45.18—S&P "A" rated hospitals was 44.51.

- **Full-Time Equivalents (FTEs) per Occupied Bed**
FTEs per Occupied Bed measures the overall staffing levels of the organization and like LOS, FTEs per Occupied Bed can also be adjusted for case mix. Sometimes another adjustment is made to account for variances in outpatient activity. Lower values are preferable. Median FTEs per Occupied Bed for all hospitals reporting to Ingenix (2004) for 2002 was 5.05 (S&P does not use this indication) and median FTEs per Occupied Bed adjusted for case mix was 4.10.

- **Salary per FTE**

$$\frac{\text{salaries}}{\text{FTEs}}$$

Salary per FTE measures the average direct labor expense per employee. Lower values are preferable. Hospital management should be aware that Salary per FTE varies for a variety of reasons including cost of living (wage index). Median Salary per FTE for all hospitals reporting to Ingenix (2004) for 2002 was $39,761—S&P "A" rated hospitals was $41,388, and median Salary per FTE adjusted for wage index was $42,423—S&P "A" rated hospitals was $43,686.

- **Compensation Costs per Discharge**

$$\frac{\text{inpatient salary costs} + \text{inpatient benefit costs}}{\text{discharges}}$$

Compensation Costs per Discharge measures the proportion of operating expenses attributable to labor expense, including salary and fringe benefits. Lower values are preferable. Hospital management should be aware that Compensation Costs per Discharge varies for a variety of reasons including wage index, case mix, and facility size. While Compensation Costs per Discharge can be adjusted for wage index and case mix, generally the measure is not adjusted for size. One might assume that compensation costs would decrease proportionately (based on economies of scale) as facility size increases, but actually just the opposite is true. Median Compensation Costs per Discharge for all hospitals reporting to Ingenix (2004) for 2002 was $2,948.77—S&P "A" rated hospitals was $3,359.50 and median Compensation Costs per Discharge adjusted for wage index and case-mix index for all hospitals reporting to Ingenix (2004) for 2002 was $2,844.81—S&P "A" rated hospitals was $2,926.50.

Financial Analysis and Annual Reports

For-profit organizations prepare annual reports, which report financial and other information, and send them to their stockholders. Only recently have not-for-profit organizations begun preparing annual reports as a vehicle of communication and accountability to the community.

There are several principles for preparing good reports, including annual reports (Berman, Kukla, and Weeks 1994).

- *Audience and Purpose*: Management should prepare reports with the audience and purpose as the central focus. It is always dangerous to prepare reports that readers will not understand. For instance, executive management should use a different level of detail in preparing a report for department managers and preparing a report for the governing body. In addition to audience, management should always keep in mind the primary reason for the report. For instance, annual reports for for-profit organizations that have selling stock as a primary purpose will attract attention by using lots of color. Not-for-profit organizations, which must be more concerned about costs incurred, will provide an austere, yet functional, annual report.
- *Timeliness*: Reports designed to provide control within the organization, such as budget reports, must be prepared and distributed in a timely manner to maximize the effects of corrective action.
- *Accuracy*: Accuracy in reporting information is more important than timeliness. Reports with mistakes are detrimental to the organization because such reports create credibility problems.
- *Clarity*: Reports should be clear and concise to the audience, and leave little room for misinterpretation.

- *Comparability*: Reports should maintain formats to accommodate easy comparisons from statement period to statement period and among different organizations.
- *Commentary*: Reports should provide explanations when necessary. Even financial statements should provide explanations in the form of notes to the financial statements.
- *Meaningfulness*: Reports should be used for better decision making, which can only happen if the information is needed by the decision maker.

Annual reports provide accountability of the organization to the stockholders, and act as a vehicle to sell more stock.

Appendix 14.1
Sample Not-for-Profit Hospital Notes to Financial Statements December 31, 20X7 and 20X6

1. **Description of Organization and Summary of Significant Accounting Policies**

Organization. The Sample Not-for-Profit Hospital (the Hospital), located in Tulsa, Oklahoma, is a not-for-profit acute care hospital. The Hospital provides inpatient, outpatient, and emergency care services for residents of northeastern Oklahoma. Admitting physicians are primarily practitioners in the local area. The Hospital was incorporated in Oklahoma in 20X1 and is affiliated with the ABC Health System.

Use of estimates. The preparation of financial statements in conformity with GAAP requires management to make estimates and assumptions that affect the reported amounts of assets and liabilities and disclosure of contingent assets and liabilities at the date of the financial statements and the reported amounts of revenues and expenses during the reporting period. Actual results could differ from those estimates.

Cash and cash equivalents. Cash and cash equivalents include certain investments in highly liquid debt instruments with original maturities of three months or less. The Hospital routinely invests its surplus operating funds in money market mutual funds. These funds generally invest in highly liquid U.S. government and agency obligations.

Investments. Investments in equity securities with readily determinable fair values and all investments in debt securities are measured at fair value in the balance sheet. Investment income or loss (including realized gains and losses on investments, interest, and dividends) is included in the excess of revenues over expenses unless the income or loss is restricted by donor or law. Unrealized gains and losses on investments are excluded from the excess of revenues over expenses unless the investments are trading securities.

Assets limited as to use. Assets limited as to use primarily include assets held by trustees under indenture agreements and designated assets set aside by the Board of Trustees for future capital improvements, over which the Board retains control and may at its discretion subsequently use for other purposes. Amounts required to meet current liabilities of the hospital have been reclassified in the balance sheet at December 31, 20X7 and 20X6.

Property and equipment. Property and equipment acquisitions are recorded at cost. Depreciation is provided over the estimated useful life of each class of depreciable asset and is computed using the straight-line method. Equipment under capital lease obligations is amortized on the straight-line method over the shorter period of the lease term or the estimated useful life of the equipment. Such amortization is included in depreciation and amortization in the financial statements. Interest cost incurred on borrowed funds during the period of construction of capital assets is capitalized as a component of the cost of acquiring those assets.

Gifts of long-lived assets such as land, buildings, or equipment are reported as unrestricted support, and are excluded from the excess of revenues over expenses, unless explicit donor stipulations specify how the donated assets must be used. Gifts of long-lived assets with explicit restrictions that specify how the assets are to be used and gifts of cash or other assets that must be used to acquire long-lived assets are reported as restricted support. Absent explicit donor stipulations about how long those long-lived assets must be maintained, expirations of donor restrictions are reported when the donated or acquired long-lived assets are placed in service.

Temporarily and permanently restricted net assets. Temporarily restricted net assets are those whose use by the Hospital has been limited by donors to a specific time period or purpose. Permanently restricted net assets have been restricted by donors to be maintained by the Hospital in perpetuity.

Excess of revenues over expenses. The statement of operations includes excess of revenues over expenses. Changes in unrestricted net assets that are excluded from excess of revenues over expenses, consistent with industry practice, include unrealized gains and losses on investments other than trading securities, permanent transfers of assets to and from affiliates for other than goods and services, and contributions of long-lived assets (including assets acquired using contributions that by donor restriction were to be used for the purposes of acquiring such assets).

Net patient service revenue. The Hospital has agreements with third-party payers that provide for payments to the Hospital at amounts different from its established rates. Payment arrangements include prospectively determined rates per discharge, reimbursed costs, discounted charges, and per diem payments. Net patient service revenue is reported at the estimated net realizable amounts from patients, third-party payers, and others for services rendered, including estimated retroactive adjustments under reimbursement agreements with third-party payers. Retroactive adjustments are accrued on an estimated basis in the period the related services are rendered and adjusted in future periods as final settlements are determined.

Premium revenue. The Hospital has agreements with various health maintenance organizations (HMOs) to provide medical services to subscribing participants. Under these agreements, the Hospital receives monthly capitation payments based on the number of each HMO's participants, regardless of services actually performed by the Hospital. In addition, the HMOs make fee-for-service payments to the Hospital for certain covered services based upon discounted fee schedules.

Charity care. The Hospital provides care to patients who meet certain criteria under its charity care policy without charge or at amounts less than its established rates. Because the Hospital does not pursue collection of amounts determined to qualify as charity care, they are not reported as revenue.

Donor-restricted gifts. Unconditional promises to give cash and other assets to the Hospital are reported at fair value at the date the promise is received. Conditional promises to give and indications of intentions to give are reported at fair value at the date the gift is received. The gifts are reported as either temporarily or permanently restricted support if they are received with donor stipulations that limit the use of the donated assets. When a donor restriction expires, that is, when a stipulated time restriction ends or purpose restriction is accomplished, temporarily restricted net assets are reclassified as unrestricted net assets and reported in the statement of operations as net assets released from restriction. Donor-restricted contributions whose restrictions are met within the same year as received are reported as unrestricted contributions in the accompanying financial statements.

Estimated malpractice costs. The provision for estimated medical malpractice claims includes estimates of the ultimate costs for both reported claims and claims incurred but not reported.

Income taxes. The Hospital is a not-for-profit corporation and has been recognized as tax-exempt pursuant to Sec.501(c)(3) of the Internal Revenue Code.

2. Net Patient Service Revenue

The Hospital has agreements with third-party payers that provide for payments to the Hospital at amounts different from its established rates. A summary of the payment arrangements with major third-party payers is as follows:

- Medicare. Inpatient acute care services rendered to Medicare program beneficiaries are paid at prospectively determined rates per discharge. These rates vary according to a patient classification system that is based on clinical, diagnostic, and other factors. Inpatient nonacute services, certain outpatient services, and defined capital and medical education costs related to Medicare beneficiaries are paid based on a cost reimbursement methodology. The Hospital is reimbursed for cost reimbursable items at a tentative rate with final settlement determined after submission of annual cost reports by the Hospital and audits thereof by the Medicare fiscal intermediary. Beginning in 20X3, the Hospital claimed Medicare payments based on an interpretation of certain "disproportionate share" rules. The intermediary disagreed and declined to pay the excess reimbursement claimed under that interpretation. Through 20X6, the Hospital has not included the claimed excess in net patient revenues pending resolution of the matter. In 20X7, the intermediary accepted the claims and paid the outstanding claims, including $950,000 applicable to 20X6 and $300,000 applicable to 20X5 and prior, which has been included in 20X7 net revenues.
- Medicaid. Inpatient and outpatient services rendered to Medicaid program beneficiaries are reimbursed under a cost reimbursement methodology. The Hospital is reimbursed at a tentative rate with final settlement determined after submission of annual cost reports by the Hospital and audits thereof by the Medicaid fiscal intermediary.

The Hospital also has entered into payment agreements with certain commercial insurance carriers, HMOs, and preferred provider organizations. The basis for payment to the Hospital under these agreements includes prospectively determined rates per discharge, discounts from established charges, and prospectively determined daily rates.

3. Investments

Assets Limited as to Use

The composition of assets limited as to use at December 31, 20X7 and 20X6, is set forth in the following table. Investments are stated at fair value.

Internally designated for capital acquisition:	20X7	20X6
Cash	$ 545,000	$ 350,000
U.S. Treasury obligations	11,435,000	12,115,000
Interest receivable	20,000	35,000
	12,000,000	12,500,000
Held by trustee under indenture agreement:		
Cash and short-term investments	352,000	260,000
U.S. Treasury obligation	6,505,000	7,007,000
Interest receivable	92,000	74,000
	6,949,000	7,341,000
	$18,949,000	$19,841,000

Other investments

Other investments, stated at fair value, at December 31, 20X7 and 20X6, include:

Trading:	20X7	20X6
U.S. Corporate Bonds	$ 1,260,000	$ 1,475,000
Other:		
U.S. Treasury obligations	$19,266,000	$14,233,000
Interest receivable	310,000	232,000
	20,836,000	15,940,000
Less:		
Long-term investments	4,680,000	4,680,000
Long-term investments restricted for capital acquisitions	320,000	520,000
Short-term investments	$15,836,000	$10,740,000

Investment income and gains for assets limited as to use, cash equivalents, and other investments are comprised of the following for the years ending December 31, 20X7 and 20X6.

Income:	20X7	20X6
Interest income	$ 3,585,000	$ 2,725,000
Realized gains on sales of securities	150,000	200,000
Unrealized gains on trading securities	165,000	100,000
	$ 3,900,000	$ 3,025,000

Other changes in unrestricted assets:		
Unrealized gains on other than trading securities	$ 300,000	$ 375,000

4. Property and Equipment

A summary of property and equipment at December 31, 20X7 and 20X6, follows:

	20X7	20X6
Land	$ 3,000,000	$ 3,000,000
Land improvements	472,000	472,000
Buildings and improvements	46,852,000	46,636,000
Equipment	29,190,000	26,260,000
Equipment under capital lease obligations	2,851,000	2,752,000
	82,365,000	79,120,000

Less accumulated depreciation and amortization	34,928,000	30,661,000
	47,437,000	48,459,000
Construction in progress	3,601,000	2,033,000
Property and equipment, net	$51,038,000	$50,492,000

Depreciation expense for the years ended December 31, 20X7 and 20X6 amounted to approximately $4,782,000 and $4,280,000. Accumulated amortization for equipment under capital lease obligations was $689,000 and $453,000 at December 31, 20X7and 20X6, respectively. Construction contracts of approximately $7,885,000 exist for the remodeling of Hospital facilities. At December 31, 20X7, the remaining commitment on these contracts approximated $4,625,000.

5. Long-Term Debt

A summary of long-term debt and capital lease obligations at December 31, 20X7 and 20X6, follows:

	20X7	20X6
7.25 percent 20X7 Tax-Exempt Revenue Bonds, principal maturing in varying annual amounts, due November 1, 20XX, collateralized by a pledge of the Hospital's gross receipts	$21,479,000	
8.50 percent 20X2 Tax-Exempt Revenue Bonds, principal maturing in varying annual amounts, due June 1, 20XX		$22,016,000
7.75 percent mortgage loan, principal maturing in varying annual amounts, due January 1, 20XX, collateralized by a mortgage on certain property and equipment	2,010,000	2,127,000
7.75 percent note payable, payable in monthly installments of $12,000, including interest, due March 20XX, unsecured	125,000	671,000
Capital lease obligations, at varying rates of imputed interest from 6.8 percent and 9.3 percent collateralized by leased equipment	1,000,000	950,000
	26,614,000	25,764,000
Less current portion	1,470,000	1,750,000
	$23,144,000	$24,014,000

Under the terms of the 20X7 and 20X6 revenue bond indentures, the Hospital is required to maintain certain deposits with a trustee. Such deposits are included with assets limited as to use. The revenue note indenture also places limits on the incurrence of additional borrowings and requires that the Hospital satisfy certain measures of financial performance as long as the notes are outstanding.

Scheduled principal repayments on long-term debt and payments on capital lease obligations are as follows:

Year Ending December 31	Long-Term Debt	Capital Leases Obligations
20X8	$ 970,000	$ 550,000
20X9	912,000	260,000
20Y0	983,000	260,000
20Y1	1,060,000	45,000
20Y2	1,143,000	—
Thereafter	18,546,000	—
	$23,614,000	$ 1,115,000
Less amount representing interest under capital leases obligations	115,000	
		$ 1,000,000

A summary of interest cost and investment income on borrowed funds held by the trustee under the 20X7 and 20X2 revenue bond indentures during the years ended December 31, 20X7 and 20X6, follows:

	20X7	20X6
Interest cost:		
Capitalized	$ 740,000	$ 700,000
Charged to operations	1,752,000	1,825,000
Total	2,492,000	2,525,000
Investment income:		
Capitalized	$ 505,000	$ 663,000
Credited to other revenue	330,000	386,000
Total	$ 835,000	$ 1,049,000

6. Temporarily and Permanently Restricted Net Assets

Temporarily and restricted net assets are available for the following purposes or periods at December 31, 20X7 and 20X6.

	20X7	20X6
Healthcare services		
Purchase of equipment	$ 320,000	$ 520,000
Indigent care	840,000	950,000
Health education	350,000	400,000
For periods after December 31, 20X9	605,000	600,000
Total	$ 2,115,000	$ 2,470,000

Permanently restricted net assets at December 31, 20X7 and 20X6, are restricted to:

	20X7	20X6
Investments to be held in perpetuity, the income from which is expendable to support healthcare services (reported as operating income)	$ 2,973,000	$ 2,923,000
Endowment requiring income to be added to original gift until fund value is $1,500,000	615,000	610,000
	$ 3,588,000	$ 3,533,000

During 20X7, net assets were released from donor restrictions by incurring expenses satisfying the restricted purposes of indigent care and healthcare education in the amounts of $250,000 and $50,000, respectively.

7. Medical Malpractice Claims

The Hospital purchases professional and general liability insurance to cover medical malpractice claims. These are known claims and incidents that may result in the assertion of additional claims, as well as claims from unknown incidents that may be asserted arising from services provided to patients. The Hospital has employed independent actuaries to estimate the ultimate costs, if any, of the settlement of such claims. Accrued malpractice losses have been discounted at seven percent and, in management's opinion, provide an adequate reserve for loss contingencies.

On March 15, 20X7, a patient filed a suit against the Hospital for malpractice during care received as an inpatient. The Hospital believes it has meritorious defenses against the suit; however, the ultimate resolution of the matter could result in a loss. The patient has claimed $16 million in actual damages. Under state law, punitive damages are determined at trial. The Hospital maintains insurance coverage for malpractice claims. The coverage does not include punitive damages awards. Trial is scheduled to occur within the next year.

8. Pension and Other Postretirement Benefit Plans

The Hospital has a defined benefit pension plan covering substantially all of its employees. The plan benefits are based on years of service and the employees' compensation during the last five years of covered employment. Contributions are intended to provide not only for benefits attributed to service to date but also for those expected to be earned in the future.

[*The following paragraph is encouraged but not required.*]

The Hospital also sponsors two defined benefit postretirement plans that cover both salaried and nonsalaried employees. One plan provides medical and dental benefits, and the other provides for the payment of life insurance premiums. The postretirement health care plan is contributory, with retiree contributions adjusted annually; the life insurance plan is noncontributory. The accounting for the healthcare plan anticipates future cost-sharing changes to the written plan that are consistent with the Hospital's expressed intent to increase retiree contributions each year to 50 percent of the excess of the expected general inflation rate over 6 percent. Beginning in 20X7, the Hospital adopted a funding policy for its postretirement health care plan similar to its funding policy for its life insurance plan—an amount equal to a level percentage of the employees' salaries is contributed to the plan annually. For 20X7, that percentage was 4.25, and the aggregate contribution for both plans was $34,000.

The following table sets forth the changes in benefit obligations, changes in plan assets and components of net periodic benefit cost for both the pension plan and the other postretirement benefit plans:

	Pension Benefits		Other Benefits	
	20X7	20X6	20X7	20X6
Change in benefit obligations:				
Benefit obligation at beginning of year	$ 9,710	$9,700	$585	$500
Service cost	905	770	14	15
Interest cost	700	650	50	44
Plan participants' contributions			34	34
Actuarial gain	(20)		(7)	
Benefits paid	(375)	(1,410)	(66)	(8)
Benefit obligation at end of year	10,920	9,710	610	585
Change in plan assets:				
Fair value of plan assets at beginning of year	9,800	9,610	89	40
Actual return on plan assets	759	810	4	4
Employer contribution	866	790	39	19
Plan participants' contributions			34	34
Benefits paid	(375)	(1,410)	(66)	(8)
Fair value of plan assets at end of year	11,050	9,800	100	89
Funded status	130	90	(510)	(496)
Unrecognized net actuarial gain	(30)	(40)	(30)	(40)
Unrecognized prior service cost	50	55	16	19
Unrecognized transition obligation			445	470
Unrecognized transition asset	(15)	(20)		
Prepaid (accrued) benefit cost	$ 135	$ 85	$ (79)	$ (47)
Weighted-average assumptions as of December 31:				
Discount rate	7.00%	7.00%	7.00%	7.00%
Expected return on plan assets	8.00%	8.00%	6.60%	6.60%
Rate of compensation increase	6.00%	6.00%		

For measurement purposes, a 7-percent annual rate of increase in the per capita cost of covered healthcare benefits was assumed for 20X8. The rate was assumed to decrease gradually to 5 percent over the next five years.

	Pension Benefits		Other Benefits	
	20X7	20X6	20X7	20X6
Components of net periodic benefit cost:				
Service cost	$ 905	$ 770	$14	$15
Interest cost	700	650	50	44
Expected return on plan assets	(784)	(769)	(6)	(3)
Amortization of prior service cost	5	7	3	2

Recognized net actuarial (gain)	(5)	(2)	(15)	(1)
Amortization of transition obligation			25	25
Amortization of transition asset	(5)	(1)	—	—
Net periodic benefit cost	$ 816	$ 655	$71	$82

Assumed healthcare cost trend rates have a significant effect on the amounts reported for the healthcare plans. A one-percentage-point change in assumed healthcare cost trend rates would have the following effects:

	1-Percentage-Point Increase	1-Percentage-Point Decrease
Effect on total of service and interest cost components	$13	$(11)
Effect on postretirement benefit obligation	73	(67)

9. Concentrations of Credit Risk

The Hospital grants credit without collateral to its patients, most of whom are local residents and are insured under third-party payer agreements. The mix of receivables from patients and third-party payers at December 31, 20X7 and 20X6, was as follows:

	20X7	20X6
Medicare	51%	53%
Medicaid	17%	14%
Blue Cross	18%	17%
Other third-party payers	7%	9%
Patients	7%	7%
	100%	100%

10. Commitments and Contingencies

Operating leases. The Hospital leases various equipment and facilities under operating leases expiring at various dates through April 20Y2. Total rental expense in 20X7 and 20X6 for all operating leases was approximately $859,000 and $770,000, respectively.

The following is a schedule by year of future minimum lease payments under operating leases as of December 31, 20X7, that have initial or remaining lease terms in excess of one year.

Year End December 31,	Amount
20X8	$517,000
20X9	506,000
20Y0	459,000
20Y1	375,000
20Y2	343,000

Litigation. The Hospital is involved in litigation and regulatory investigations arising in the course of business. After consultation with legal counsel, management estimates that these matters will be resolved without material adverse effect on the Hospital's future financial position or results from operations.

Allowance for doubtful accounts. Beginning in 20X5, the Hospital has provided care under an agreement with Associated HMO. The HMO currently owes the Hospital $950,000, substantially all of which is overdue. The Hospital has notified the HMO that further services under the contract cannot be provided without payment on the outstanding balance. The HMO has assured the Hospital that additional funds are being obtained to pay the overdue balance and continue service under the agreement, however, if the HMO is unable to make payments, additional allowances for bad debts would need to be accrued.

11. Extraordinary Loss

In 20X7, the Hospital advance refunded its 20X2 Revenue Bonds in the amount of $22 million by issuing 20X7 Revenue Bonds. As a result of this in-substance defeasance transaction, an extraordinary loss totaling $500,000 was recorded. As of December 31, 20X7, $21 million of advance refunded bonds, which are considered extinguished, remain outstanding.

12. Related Party Transactions

During the years ending on December 31, 20X7 and 20X6, the Hospital contributed capital to ABC Health System, an affiliate with some board members in common with the Hospital, in the amounts of $640,000 and $3 million, respectively.

The Sample Hospital Foundation (the Foundation), which is controlled by Sample Health System, was established to solicit contributions from the general public and to support the Hospital. Funds are distributed to the Hospital as determined by the Foundation's Board of Directors. A summary of the Foundation's assets, liabilities, net assets, results of operations, and changes in net assets follows.

At December 31,	20X7	20X6
Assets, principally cash and cash equivalents	$ 521,000	$ 472,000
Liabilities	11,000	10,000
Net assets	510,000	462,000
Total liabilities and net assets	$ 521,000	$ 472,000
Support and revenue	$ 269,000	$ 535,000
Expenses		
Distributions to Sample Hospital for property acquisitions	235,000	485,000
Other	13,000	16,000
Total expenses	248,000	501,000

Excess of support and revenue over expenses	21,000	34,000
Other changes in net assets	27,000	17,000
Net assets, beginning of year	462,000	411,000
Net assets, end of year	$ 510,000	$ 462,000

Liabilities include $10,000 payable at the end of each year to Sample Hospital. These amounts were paid after the end of each year.

13. Functional Expenses

The Hospital provides general healthcare services to residents within its geographic location. Expenses related to providing these services are as follows (in thousands of dollars):

At December 31,	20X7	20X6
Healthcare services	$ 86,000	$ 78,647
General and administrative	12,055	10,643
	$ 98,055	$ 89,290

14. Fair Value of Financial Instruments

The following methods and assumptions were used by the Hospital in estimating the fair value of its financial instruments:

Cash and cash equivalents: The carrying amount reported in the balance sheet for cash and cash equivalents approximates its fair value.

Investments: Fair values, which are the amounts reported in the balance sheet, are based on quoted market prices, if available, or estimated using quoted market prices for similar securities.

Assets limited as to use: These assets consist primarily of cash and short-term investments and interest receivable. The carrying amount reported in the balance sheet is fair value.

Accounts payable and accrued expenses: The carrying amount reported in the balance sheet for accounts payable and accrued expenses approximates its fair value.

Estimated third-party payer settlements: The carrying amount reported in the balance sheet for estimated third-party payer settlements approximates its fair value.

Long-term debt: Fair values of the Hospital's revenue notes are based on current traded value. The fair value of the Hospital's current incremental borrowing rates for similar types of borrowing arrangements.

The carrying amounts and fair values of the Hospital's financial instruments at December 31, 20X7 and 20X6, are as follows (in thousands of dollars):

	20X7		20X6	
	Carrying Amount	Fair Value	Carrying Amount	Fair Value
Cash and cash equivalents	$ 4,758	$ 4,758	$ 5,877	$ 5,877
Short-term investments	15,836	15,836	10,740	10,740
Assets limited as to use	18,949	18,949	19,841	19,841
Long-term investments	4,680	4,680	4,680	4,680
Long-term investments restricted for capital acquisition	320	320	520	520
Accounts payable and accrued expenses	5,818	5,818	5,382	5,382
Estimated third-party payer settlements	2,143	2,143	1,942	1,942
Long-term debt	24,614	23,980	25,764	24,918

15. Promises to Contribute

At December 31, 20X7, the Hospital had received $1,500,000 of conditional promises to contribute to the building of a new facility for outpatient services. These contributions will be recorded as temporarily restricted support, when received. The Hospital had no material outstanding unconditional promises of support at December 31, 20X7.

16. Charity Care

The amount of charges foregone for services and supplies furnished under the Hospital's charity care policy aggregated approximately $4,500,000 and $4,100,000 in 20X7 and 20X6, respectively.

17. Subsequent Event

On February 9, 20X8, the Hospital signed a contract in the amount of $1,050,000 for the purchase of certain real estate.

Sample Hospital notes to financial statements is reprinted with permission from the AICPA. 1996. *AICPA Audit and Accounting Guide: Health Care Organizations.* New York: AICPA. Copyright by the American Institute of Certified Public Accountants, Inc.

Notes

1. Acquiring ratio, trend, and percentage data on specific competitors may be impossible. However, several services sell data in the aggregate for comparable organizations, and some data is published by Moody's Investors Service, Dun and Bradstreet, and Troy.
2. In the 1996 *AICPA Audit and Accounting Guide for Health Care Organizations,* the term net assets replaced the term fund balance in not-for-profit healthcare organizations for external reporting purposes. Prior

to 1996, not-for-profit organizations established numerous self-balancing funds consisting of assets, liabilities, and fund balances. AICPA, and more specifically Financial Accounting Standards Board (FASB) Statement No. 117, concluded that some not-for-profit organizations did not always present information about the fund balances on external reports. Although the AICPA and FASB Statement No. 117 does not preclude not-for-profit healthcare organizations from using fund accounting for internal reporting purposes, those organizations are now required to classify all fund balances into three broad categories and report the categories on the balance sheet.

3. Statements of cash flow can be prepared using either the indirect method or the direct method. The indirect method of computing cash flows is based on accrual accounting changes in various assets and liabilities. The direct method of computing cash flows is based on the actual changes in cash accounts for revenues and expenses. The direct method, which is recommended by FASB Statement No. 95, focuses on the primary sources of cash such as patients and third-party payers and uses of cash such as salaries and supplies. The computation of the direct method is a complex process because of the number of accruals in each line item. It is difficult to determine what proportion of healthcare organizations have adopted the direct method of computing cash flows; Prince (1992) reported that less than 5 percent of the major industrial firms had adopted the direct method in the first four years of the FASB recommendation.

References

American Institute of Certified Public Accountants (AICPA). 2003. *AICPA Audit and Accounting Guide for Health Care Organizations*. New York: AICPA.

———. 1996. *AICPA Audit and Accounting Guide for Health Care Organizations*. New York: AICPA.

Berman, H. J., S. F. Kukla, and L. E. Weeks. 1994. *The Financial Management of Hospitals, 8th ed*. Chicago: Health Administration Press.

Brigham, E. F. 1992. Fundamentals *of Financial Management, 6th ed*. New York: Dryden Press.

Cleverly, W. O. 1997. "Financial Statements" and "Analyzing Financial Statements." *Essentials of Health Care Finance, 4th ed*. Gaithersburg, MD: Aspen Publishers.

Ingenix. 2004. *Almanac of Hospital Financial and Operating Indicators*. Salt Lake, UT: Ingenix.

Prince, T. R. 1992. *Financial Reporting and Cost Control for Health Care Entities*. Chicago: Health Administration Press.

Recommended Readings — Part V

Baker, J. J., and R. W. Baker. 2000. *Health Care Finance: Basic Tools for Nonfinancial Managers.* Gaithersburg, MD: Aspen Publishers.

Brigham, E. F. 1992. "Analysis of Financial Statements." *Fundamentals of Financial Management, 6th ed.* New York: Dryden Press.

Gapenski, L. C. 2002. *Healthcare Finance: An Introduction to Accounting and Financial Management, 2nd ed.* Chicago: Health Administration Press.

Cleverly, W. O. 1997. *Essentials of Health Care Finance, 4th ed.* Gaithersburg, MD: Aspen Publishers.

Finkler, S. A. 2001. *Financial Management for Public, Health, and NonProfit Organizations.* Upper Saddle River, NJ: Prentice Hall.

McLean, R. A. 1996. "Organizational Diagnostics: Financial Statement Analysis." *Financial Management in Health Care Organizations.* New York: Delmar Publishers.

Prince, T. R. 1992. "Financial Statement Analysis." *Financial Reporting and Cost Control for Health Care Entities.* Chicago: Health Administration Press.

Zelman, W. N., M. J. McCue, and A. R. Millikan. 1998. "Health Care Financial Statements." *Financial Management of Health Care Organizations.* Malden, MA: Blackwell Publishers.

HEALTHCARE'S FUTURE

FUTURE TRENDS

Past Prediction

Berman, Kukla, and Weeks

It became a tradition that Berman, Kukla, and Weeks would conclude each edition of their book *The Financial Management of Hospitals* (eight editions in all) with a philosophic look at the future. Their final edition published in 1994 was no exception. They anticipated that healthcare spending would continue to increase and that:

> . . . the entire shape and operation of the health care financing and delivery system will change [as a result]. The initial changes will, in retrospect, be relatively modest, e.g., insurance reform, beginning at the small-group level. However, as each step falls short of its goal— universal affordability and accessibility—the subsequent measures will be more intrusive, and will involve government in a larger and larger role. In fact, it is likely that, before the cost increase curve is tamed, the federal government will have expanded its role to the point where the country has adopted a uniquely American national health insurance system (Berman, Kukla, and Weeks 1994, 669–670).

With laws like HIPAA of 1996, BBA of 1997, BBRA of 1999, BIPA of 2000, and MMA of 2003, one could certainly argue that the federal government has expanded its role in the delivery of healthcare in an attempt to make healthcare more affordable and accessible to the American people. Expansions of both Medicare eligibility and Medicaid eligibility as well as substantial improvements in benefit packages will certainly bring the country closer to a national health insurance system (in 2002, the federal government funded 32.5 percent of all healthcare spending)..

Berman, Kukla, and Weeks believed that five factors were shaping their view of the future: changing demographics, emerging technologies, public expectations, limits on resources, and ethical issues. Policy reaction could take three forms: a public system of healthcare, a private system of healthcare, or a private/public system of healthcare. Berman, Kukla, and Weeks opted for a private/public system of healthcare that could be enriched if each system realized the need for the other. For instance, the private system must realize that it cannot meet the entire needs of the nation, and the public system must realize that healthcare delivery and finance are local affairs and cannot be managed by a central authority.

The response of management to the rapidly changing environment would be threefold, according to Berman, Kukla, and Weeks:

1. *Regulation and competition*: Regulation dominated the 1970s and competition dominated the 1980s, but it was apparent in the 1990s that both were needed.
2. *Strategic alliances*: The 1970s and 1980s provided the background for another experiment—diversification. Berman, Kukla, and Weeks contend that diversification, even in the form of vertical integration, failed and was replaced with strategic alliances with groups that share common goals.
3. *Reinventing the hospital*: Central to both regulation/competition and strategic alliances is the role of hospitals. Hospitals will need to change not only their focus, but also their relationships with the communities they serve.

While Berman, Kukla, and Weeks were certainly prophetic regarding the need for continuing the private/public partnership and the need for hospitals to change their focus and relationships, it may be too early to declare vertical integration dead. Zelman (1996) sees fully integrated organized delivery systems (ODSs) competing for managed care contracts and premiums as inevitable. Strategic alliances will continue, but they appear to have less control over costs than their fully integrated counterparts.

Healthy People 2010

Another view of the future that merits a review is *Healthy People 2010: Healthy People in Healthy Communities* published by the U.S. Department of Health and Human Services in 2001. A strategic plan for the nation's health, *Healthy People 2010* builds on initiatives pursued over the last 20 years. The 1979 Surgeon General's Report, *Healthy People* and then *Healthy People 2000: National Health Priorities and Disease Prevention Objectives* both established national health objectives and served as the basis for the development of state and community health plans. Nearly all states have developed their own Healthy People plans. Most states have built on *Healthy People 2000* health objectives while tailoring the objectives to meet their own specific needs. A 1993 National Association of County and City Health Officials survey showed that 70 percent of local health departments used at least some of the *Healthy People 2000* objectives.

Healthy People 2000 was developed as a national initiative involving 22 expert working groups and 300 national organizations; receiving testimony from more than 750 individuals; and including over 10,000 people in the preparation of the final report.

According to the report, the primary health goals for the nation were:

- To increase the span of healthy life for Americans;
- To reduce health disparities among Americans; and
- To achieve access to preventive services for all Americans.

These goals would be met by establishing health priorities and objectives in the areas of health promotion, protection, and prevention, and with improved surveillance and data systems. To promote health, the authors of the report proposed the increase in physical activity and fitness; improvement of nutrition; reduction of tobacco use; reduction of alcohol and drug abuse; improvement of facility planning; improvement of mental health; reduction in violent and abusive behavior; and enhancement of health education.

The following objectives were suggested to protect the health of the nation: reduce unintentional injuries; improve occupational safety; improve environmental health; ensure food and drug safety; and improve oral health.

Preventive services could be enhanced by: improvement in maternal and child health; reduction in heart disease and stroke; prevention and control of cancer; reduction of diabetes and chronic disease; prevention and control of HIV infection; reduction in sexually transmitted diseases; an increase in immunizations; and expanding access to preventive services. Finally, surveillance and data systems could be improved.

Each objective in *Healthy People 2000* included the status, as of 1990, of the objective and the proposed status of the objective by the year 2000. For instance, the 1990 status and the proposed 2000 status of physical activity and fitness include:

- increasing the number of Americans who participate in moderate daily physical activity (30 minutes or more at least five times a week) from 22 percent of adults to 30 percent of adults (a 36 percent increase); and
- reducing the number of Americans with sedentary lifestyles (no leisure-time physical activity) from 25 percent of adults to 15 percent of adults (a 38 percent decrease).

In addition to presenting the nation's strategic plan for health, *Healthy People 2000* also identified specific responsibilities in order of priority.

Personal Responsibility

The individual is both the starting point and the ultimate target of the campaign toward *Healthy People 2000*. An individual fills many roles in daily life, and is afforded numerous opportunities for promoting health and preventive disease. With these opportunities comes responsibility; the first role that must be undertaken is responsibility for personal health habits. Improving personal health behavior can count among the most potent means to prevent disease and promote health. Measurable decreases in risks to health can result from changes in diet, exercise, tobacco use, alcohol and other drug use, injury prevention behavior, and sexual habits, but each individual must choose to make changes a personal priority (USDHHS 1990, 85).

Family Responsibility

The family is the primary context in which health-promoting activities occur and is therefore potentially the most immediate source of health-related support and education for the individual. It is in the context of the family that attitudes and behaviors regarding diet, physical activity, hygiene, smoking, and alcohol and other drug use are often learned and maintained. Therefore, the family offers the primary opportunity for change in these areas. Parents can teach children healthy habits and offer the supportive environment necessary to sustain them. In addition, parents can ensure that their children receive needed preventive services—immunizations, screening tests, and counseling and education about health risks and behaviors (DHHS 1990, 85).

Community Responsibility

In today's society, a supportive community can make a vital difference in the well-being of its members, Accordingly, there is evidence that community-based health programs can play a strong role in improving the health status of a community's citizens. Multiple opportunities exist for community health-promotion efforts on the part of government, voluntary and self-help groups, businesses, and schools. Such local community programs are often more efficient than centralized programs managed far from the point of delivery. Furthermore, indigenous programs maintain the sensitivity to family and neighborhood values that is vital to successfully encouraging change toward healthier lifestyles within the community (DHHS 1990, 86).

Health Professionals Responsibility

Responsibility also falls to physicians and other healthcare providers, who are for many Americans the primary sources of health information. Professional training gives providers the skill to translate science into practice. Practice can take the form of partnerships with nonprofessionals in the pursuit of individual, family, and community healthcare. The effectiveness and efficiency of preventive services—screening tests, immunizations, and counseling—will be enhanced by such partnerships. America's physicians, dentists, nurses, pharmacists, medical technicians, and other health professionals must be knowledgeable in the basic clinical sciences; but they also must be life-long learners, excellent communicators, good team players, managers of scarce resources, healthcare visionaries, and community leaders. The day of the solo practitioner, dealing with the patient in isolation from other professionals, is past (DHHS 1990, 87).

Media Responsibility

The day of print and electronic media is, however, very much here, and these media can contribute to the exchange of health information between health professionals and the public, as well as among health professionals.

The average American is exposed to many different kinds of health-related messages, some explicit in news, public affairs, and documentaries, and some buried in the plots and characters seen in entertainment programs through the mass media. In partnerships with the media, voluntary and professional organizations can expand the reach of their programs while performing an important community service (DHHS 1990, 87).

Government Responsibility

Policy decisions that can assist health professionals and the public in reaching our national health goals are made regularly. These decisions range from healthcare legislation to legislation that bears on the environment, business, farming, production, energy, housing, information dissemination, education, and the economy. The health interests of Americans are directly and indirectly shaped by such policy decisions. Local, state, and federal governments can ensure that health promotion and disease prevention activities receive adequate attention and support. The accomplishment of this task can be effectively bridged through partnerships with each other and with the private sector (DHHS 1990, 88).

Like its predecessor plan, *Healthy People 2010* was developed through a broad consultation process, building on the best scientific knowledge and designed to measure actual performance compared to objectives over time. *Healthy People 2010* has two primary goals for the nation:

1. To increase the quality and years of healthy life; and
2. To eliminate health disparities.

These goals would be met by addressing leading health indicators (LHIs) in four primary objectives: to promote healthy behaviors; to promote healthy and safe communities; to improve systems for personal and public health; and to prevent and reduce diseases and disorders. Ten LHIs support the primary objectives:

1. Physical Activity
2. Overweight and Obesity
3. Tobacco Use
4. Substance Abuse
5. Responsible Sexual Behavior
6. Mental Health
7. Injury and Violence
8. Environmental Quality
9. Immunization
10. Access to Healthcare

Congress has specified that *Healthy People* objectives be used as the measure for assessing the progress of the Indian Health Care Improvement Act, the Maternal and Child Health Block Grants to the states, and the Preventive Health and Health Services Block Grants to the states (HHS 2001).

Healthcare Reform

Need for Healthcare Reform

In the current healthcare system the need for national healthcare reform has focused on two problems: access and cost.

Access Proponents of healthcare reform to ensure access argue that 15 percent of Americans, or approximately 40 million Americans, are without health insurance. Many proponents feel that healthcare is the right of every American. Opponents of healthcare reform argue that while 15 percent of Americans are without insurance, 85 percent of Americans have insurance. Opponents also argue that insurance coverage is available for many Americans in need: Medicare for the elderly, Medicaid for the poor and disabled, Aid to Families with Dependent Children (AFDC), and SCHIP for children. Opponents argue that most of the uninsured represent the young (see Table 15.1) whose risk for serious illness and resulting large healthcare expenditures is small (see Table 15.2). Opponents also argue that many of the uninsured are employed (85 percent) and earn more than the federal poverty level for Medicaid eligibility, but refuse to purchase health insurance (74 percent) because it is too expensive (Scalise and Thrall 2002).

TABLE 15.1
Uninsured by Age Group, 1996

Age Group	% Uninsured
Under 18	19%
19–24	34%
25–34	19%
35–44	15%
45–64	13%

Source: Center for Cost and Financing Studies, Agency for Health Care Policy and Research, as reported in Feldstein, P. J. 2003. *Health Policy Issues: An Economic Perspective, 3rd ed.* Chicago: Health Administration Press, page 395.

TABLE 15.2
Health Expenditures by Age Group, 1996

Age Group	% of Persons with Health Expenditures During Year	Mean Annual Health Expenditures for Persons with Health Expenditures
Under 6 years	87.9	$995
6–17 years	81.5	1,022
18–44 years	78.9	1,855
45–64 years	88.9	3,125
65+	95.3	6,229

Source: Center for Cost and Financing Studies, Agency for Health Care Policy and Research. *Health, United States, 2003*, Table 117.

Year	Health Expenditures (in $ billions)	Per Capita ($)	Percent GDP
1950	12.7	82	4.4
1960	26.9	146	5.3
1970	73.2	341	7.1
1980	247.3	1,052	8.9
1990	699.5	2,691	12.2
2000	1,310.0	4,670	13.3
2010 (projected)	2,702.2	8,885	17.1
2013 (projected)	3,358.1	10,709	18.4

TABLE 15.3
Growth in Healthcare Expenditures, Total Expenditures, Per Capita, and Percent of GDP

Source: Centers for Medicare and Medicaid Services, Office of the Actuary, 2004. [Online retrieval, 02/16/04]. http://www.cms.hhs.gov/statistics/nhe/projections.htm.

Cost

The argument for healthcare reform to reduce costs is far more compelling; employers, employees, tax payers, and patients are seemingly all in agreement that healthcare costs are too high. Table 15.3 shows the growth in healthcare expenditures, per capita healthcare expenditures, and healthcare expenditures as a percent of GNP since 1950 and projected through 2013.

The federal government is now the single largest payer of healthcare expenditures, accounting for 32.5 percent of the total expenditures in 2002, while state and local government account for an additional 13.4 percent of total expenditures. Considering the size of the government's financial commitment to healthcare, it is easy to understand the government's growing interest in reducing the growth of healthcare expenditures. Because professional providers and hospitals are the largest recipients of healthcare dollars (32.3 percent and 31.3 percent, respectively, in 2002), it is easy to understand the government's growing emphasis on reducing the rate of growth for expenditures for hospital and physician care (HCFA 2001). However, data suggests that additional attention is needed regarding increasing drug costs, which account for 44 percent of the 6.6 percent cost increase from 1998 to 1999, while 32 percent of the increase was attributable to physician fees, 21 percent of the increase was attributable to hospital outpatient spending and 3 percent of the increase was attributable to hospital inpatient spending (HFMA 2001).

Early Healthcare Reform

Until the defeat of President Clinton's healthcare proposal, the American Health Security Act of 1993, during the summer of 1994, it was unclear whether healthcare reform would be market-based, legislation-based, or both. Healthcare reform prior to 1994 could best be characterized as reactionary, meaning that policy and resulting legislation reacted to each problem without overall guiding principles.

Surplus physicians, created in part by federal support to medical schools, increased in number from 88 medical schools producing 7,409 graduates per year in 1965 to 126 medical schools producing 15,135 graduates per year in 1980. This rapid increase in physicians coincided with a slow growth in population, making physician-to-population ratios grow from 148 physicians per 100,000 population in 1960 to 202 physicians per 100,000 population in 1980 (Starr 1982).[1]

In 1973, Congress passed legislation to facilitate HMO development and growth. In addition to allocating seed money to develop HMOs, the law also required employers of 25 or more employees to offer HMO coverage, if available, as a competitive alternative to traditional indemnity coverage.

Legislation that ended Medicare cost-based reimbursement for hospitals and initiated a competitive environment under prospective payment where hospitals could either lose money or make money on Medicare business was passed by Congress in 1983. Eastaugh (1987) compared prospective payment in the healthcare industry to the deregulation in the airline industry. When routes were deregulated in the airline industry, excess capacity was diminished and prices fell markedly (and some would say quality improved). By deregulating payment methods in healthcare, or by eliminating the guaranteed return provided by cost-based reimbursement, excess capacity should be diminished and prices should fall as a result of increased competition.

In 1984, Congress passed legislation that limited the amount an employer could deduct for health benefits for employees, and because costs beyond the limits were absorbed by employees and through employees the employers, employers became sensitive to the costs of health benefits. Managed care became an alternative for many employers seeking to reduce health benefit costs.

Congress passed legislation in 1992 that ended Medicare charge-based reimbursement for physicians and initiated a competitive environment under prospective payment where physicians could either lose money or make money on Medicare business.

Unsuccessful Legislative Attempts at Reform

During the late 1980s and early 1990s, a variety of healthcare reform bills circulated through Congress. While none of these bills were passed into law, it is useful to review them in broad classifications to better understand the Clinton Plan's demise and subsequent legislation.

Incremental proposals assumed that the current healthcare system was working well and needed only minor changes. The advantages of the incremental proposals were that they attempted to build on the current public/private healthcare system, spent fewer federal dollars, and enjoyed bipartisan support. The disadvantages included the assumption that the private sector would be able to control costs, the continuance of patching healthcare coverage, and the provision of solutions to symptoms of healthcare problems and not to the problems themselves. Examples of incremental proposals included the Affordable Health Care Now Act of 1993 by Senator Robert Michel (R-IL) and the Health Equity and Access Reform Today Act by Senator John Chafee (R-RI).

Single-payer proposals assumed that the current healthcare system was broken and needed a radical change—the provision of near-universal coverage from a single payer, presumably the federal government. Advantages of the single-payer proposals included eliminating cost shifting, providing near-universal coverage, reducing administrative costs by billing one payer, and accommodating spending limits through global budgeting. Disadvantages included shifting resources from the relatively efficient private sector to the relatively inefficient public sector, allowing financing and management by the federal government, and forcing queuing up for elective procedures. Proponents of single-payer proposals pointed out the successes of Canadian-type models, and opponents pointed out their failures and the differences between Canada and the United States. Examples of single-payer proposals included the American Health Security Act by Representative James McDermott (D-WA) and the Mediplan Health Care Act of 1993 by Representative Peter Stark (D-CA).

Employer-based proposals assumed that businesses were responsible for providing health insurance coverage to their employees. Advantages included building on the current public/private system, provision of increased access, and a decrease in the government cost burden. Disadvantages included placing an unfair burden on business and encouraging businesses to dump high-risk workers. An example of an employer-based proposal was Health America of 1993 by Elizabeth Mitchell (D-ME).

Managed competition proposals assumed that the advantages of government regulation, including improved access, could be integrated with the advantages of free market competition, including lower prices. Advantages included the fixing and provision of community rating of health insurance premiums, which requires that the fortunate healthy subsidize the unfortunate sick; encouraging competition based on quality; providing portable coverage that employees could transfer from one employer to another; and prohibiting insurers from canceling or declining insurance coverage based on illness, pre-existing illness, or high risk for illness. Disadvantages included mandating participation; requiring management of the system by the federal government; establishing community rating of premiums that discourages incentives for leading healthy lifestyles; limiting physician and hospital choice; and limiting access to certain procedures. An example of a managed competition proposal was the Managed Competition Act of 1993 by Senator James Cooper (D-TN).

The Clinton Plan

In early 1992, presidential candidate Bill Clinton seemed to be favoring employer-based proposals while promising to lower healthcare costs to win support from businesses. During the early presidential primaries, the Jackson Hole Group received phone calls from the Clinton campaign regarding the Jackson Hole theory to expand the cost efficiencies of managed care into a national system that would cover all Americans. Since early in the 1970s, a group of health economists had been meeting each year in Jackson Hole, Wyoming, to discuss and recommend health policy. The group's founders, Paul Ellwood of InterStudy and Alain Enthoven of Stanford University had developed a theory called managed competition, which was simple in principle but had never been practiced. The theory called for a government-guided system of private health plans and insurance companies competing to enroll large pools of employees. Competition to win contracts with employers would drive down the cost of healthcare; the savings then could be used to enroll the uninsured. President Clinton's proposed Health Security Act of 1993, the result of Hillary Rodham Clinton's much criticized secret task force, was sold as managed competition. However, Alain Enthoven, considered by many to be the father of the managed competition theory, disagreed, calling the Clinton proposal a "grotesque" interpretation of his theory (Kilborn 1998). For the detailed description of the Clinton proposal, see Appendix 15.1.

After the Clinton Plan

With the defeat of the Clinton plan without a congressional vote, no one in Congress or the White House was willing to introduce the massive legislation necessary for managed competition, single-payer, or employer-based healthcare reform. In the absence of such legislation, it appeared, almost by de facto, that the country was willing to let Congress address the access problem with incremental legislation and to let the free market control healthcare costs with competition.

Regarding incremental legislation, it seemed safe to predict that bipartisan legislation addressing the concerns identified in most of the early proposals could be enacted if the legislation was deficit-friendly and supported by the public. Some of these common concerns included (Nowicki 1996a, 1994):

- delivery reform to provide improved access;
- insurance reform to provide improved coverage;
- finance reform to reduce cost shifting;
- tort reform to reduce defensive medicine costs;
- paperwork reform to reduce administrative costs associated with billing;
- Medicare/Medicaid reform to reduce fraud and abuse; and
- IRS reform to clarify the distinction between for-profit and not-for-profit organizations.

The first major piece of health-related legislation enacted by Congress after the Clinton plan defeat was the Health Insurance Portability and Accountability Act of 1996, which included the following provisions:

- insurance reform, to protect currently insured people from losing coverage as a result of job change or family illness and to require insurance companies who offer small group insurance coverage to make policies available to all small groups.[2]
- medical savings accounts (MSAs), which allow a four-year pilot study of 750,000 MSA policies available to the self-employed and small employers.
- administrative simplification, which mandated the development of standardized electronic billing, claims, and remittance within 42 months.
- healthcare tax rule changes, which allowed the self-employed to increase their deduction for healthcare costs and insurance premiums from 30 percent in 1996 to 80 percent by 2006, and made long-term care costs and insurance premiums and costs tax deductible.
- Medicare fraud and abuse changes that appropriated a new trust fund to pay for expanded investigations; broadened the authority of the FBI in fraud and abuse investigations; expanded the Medicare Integrity Program, in which the HHS contracts with private organizations that are charged with decreasing fraud and abuse; established a whistle-blower initiative that includes qui tam provisions (i.e., cash awards); and allowed advisory opinions on safe harbors (see Feldor 1998).

The Balanced Budget Act of 1997, in addition to cutting Medicare expenditure over a five-year period, also included provisions for increasing access. It allowed provider-sponsored organizations (PSOs) to bid on Medicare and Medicaid business and states the option to require Medicaid beneficiaries to enroll in managed care plans (which effectively eliminated the previous requirement for a waiver). The act also adopted Kids Care, a Kennedy (D-MA)/ Hatch (R-UT) proposal to provide $23.4 billion over five years to expand health coverage for children whose parents' income is too high to qualify for Medicaid but too low to afford private insurance. Kids Care was predicted to effectively insure about 50 percent of the nation's uninsured children.

After significant evidence that the Balanced Budget Act (BBA) of 1997 was cutting more than the projected $115 billion from the budget (some estimate that BBA was cutting two to three times more than the $115 billion originally intended), Congress passed and the president signed the Balanced Budget Refinement Act (BBRA) in November of 1999. The plan provided an estimated $16 billion in Medicare relief over five years. BBRA, also known as the Balanced Budget of 1997 Amendments, was passed as part of the Consolidated Appropriations Act of 2000.

In December of 2000, the Congress passed and the president signed Medicare, Medicaid, and SCHIP (State Children's Health Insurance Program) Benefits Improvement and Protection Act (BIPA) of 2000. BIPA provided about $35 billion in Medicare relief over five years and increases Medicare and Medicaid healthcare provider payments; added preventive benefits and reduces beneficiary cost sharing under Medicare; and improved insurance options for low-income children, low-income families, and low-income seniors. This BBA relief legislation was part of a $109 billion appropriations bill which also included $2.5 billion in additional funding for the National Institutes of Health (NIH), $800 million in additional funding for the Centers for Disease Control (CDC), $213 million in additional funding for the Ryan White CARE Act, and $235 million in additional funding to independent children's hospitals to train pediatricians.

In late November 2003, Congress passed the Medicare Prescription Drug, Improvement, and Modernization Act (MMA) of 2003 which President Bush signed in early December. Heralded as the most significant expansion of the Medicare program since its inception, the Act was a compromise between Republicans who wanted to privatize Medicare and Democrats who wanted to expand Medicare benefits. In addition to the increased payments to healthcare providers, MMA provided a Medicare-endorsed prescription drug discount card; a Medicare prescription drug benefit beginning in 2006; more rapid delivery of generic drugs to market; possible drug importation from Canada; savings and subsidies for state governments and employers related to their prescription drug costs; new preventive benefits; funding for modernizing drug delivery systems; an 18-month moratorium on the development of new and the expansion of existing specialty hospitals; the introduction of health-related savings accounts; and Medicare Advantage to replace Medicare+Choice;

Early criticism of MMA has focused on its cost (the White House projected a ten-year cost of $534 billion in its 2004/05 budget) and its popularity with Medicare beneficiaries, many of whom already have prescription drug coverage provided by employers after the beneficiaries retired or through Medigap policies. A well-respected study indicated that 73 percent of Medicare beneficiaries had some drug coverage in 1998 (Poisal and Murray 2001). MMA prohibits Medicare beneficiaries from possessing insurance coverage that would cover the beneficiary's share of drug costs under the new benefit. Congress cited two reasons for this controversial provision: to prevent duplication of coverage and ensure that beneficiaries would bear some of the cost out-of-pocket to help reduce overutilization (Pear 2003).

Regarding the free market controlling costs with competition, after the defeat of the Clinton plan in 1994, managed care began to dominate the marketplace, having evolved on its own in response to economic pressures. Eighty-five percent of all workers were covered by some form of managed care in 1998, which was up from 50 percent in 1994. Managed care, although still plagued with complaints regarding limited choice,[3] slowed soaring healthcare costs. While the nation's spending for healthcare reached $1 trillion in 1996, the amount was only $50 billion more than that spent in 1995, for an increase of 4.4 percent, which was the smallest percent increase in 37 years (Kilborn 1998). In 1997, the American Association of Health Plans released a study by the Lewin Group that credited managed care with between $116 billion and $181 billion in healthcare savings from 1990 to 1996. If employers passed on the healthcare savings to their employees, the average worker would take home an additional $228 per year—even more in states with higher HMO penetration like California, where the savings could mean an additional $770 per year. Unfortunately, few employees associate healthcare savings to their paycheck (Brink 1998).

The most recent research (Smith et al. 1998) indicates that the health-care savings that occurred during the 1990s was a one-time phenomenon that cannot be expected to continue in the new millennium. Analysts at the CMS (2004) project healthcare spending to nearly double between 2000 and 2010 (as shown in Table 15.3). Private sector health insurance premiums increased 10.4 percent in 2003, the third consecutive year of double-digit increases. The rate of growth in private sector insurance premiums is expected to slow to 7.1 by 2003 (Heffler et al. 2004).

Hospitals will experience slower growth in spending in 2003, with a 6.5-percent increase over 2002 with further decreases to 6.2 percent annual increase in 2005. Physicians, however, will experience faster growth in 2003, averaging 7.3 percent growth, while prescription drugs will average 13.4 percent growth (Heffler et al. 2004).

Regarding clinical quality, there is growing evidence that managed care provides better healthcare than the previous fee-for-service plans. For example, HMO patients are 25 percent less likely to endure futile, painful, degrading, unwanted care during the last six months of a terminal illness. Such care accounts for 21 percent of all Medicare spending (Cher and Lenert 1997). Because of the emphasis on prevention and early detection, managed care should detect cancers at an earlier stage than fee-for-service plans and, as a result, reduce the need for surgical intervention. Regarding patient satisfaction, enrollees continue to complain about managed care limiting the number of providers patients can choose and about waiting times for elective procedures.

The Future of Healthcare

If Americans really are not satisfied with either the quality of managed care or the procedural hoops they have to jump through to receive care, then the savings achieved by managed care will have been a pyhrric victory. A majority of working Americans are not being provided with a choice of health plans by their employers. This means that for most individuals, the free market in medicine is not a free market at all. Is it any wonder that consumers are turning to the government for protection because they are not getting it from the marketplace?

> If we fail both to control costs and to provide care for most
> Americans using private-sector initiatives—and the enthusiasm for
> the consumer bill of rights implies that we have—then government
> intervention is inevitable (see Brink 1998). It will be up to our
> nation's policy leaders to find the proper method of satisfying the
> electorate without destroying the real cost savings and healthcare
> delivery gains that have been and can be attained (Scott 1998a, 25).

The year 1998 began with a flurry of anti–managed care proposals at the federal level that were often labeled as "patients' bill of rights" legislation. Forty-three states have already passed consumer protection legislation related to managed care (Kilborn 1998). Responding to a 34-member Advisory Commission on Consumer Protection and Quality in the Health Care Industry, President Clinton introduced his "Consumer Bill of Rights and Responsibilities" in January, a proposal that Republican leaders quickly dubbed "ClintonCare II," even though as many as 100 Republicans indicated support for Clinton's proposal or similar legislation.[4]

Clinton's proposal included the following provisions:

- Information should be disclosed to help patients choose plans and providers within plans.
- Patients should have choice of providers so they can access plan providers within a reasonable length of time, and women should have direct access to their OB/GYNs without having to go through a gatekeeping mechanism (patients who are pregnant or chronically ill should be able to keep their physician for three months if they have to switch health plans involuntarily).
- Patient complaints regarding the provision or payment of service should have access to appeal to an independent review panel.
- Legitimate emergency care should be paid for by plans, regardless of circumstances.
- Physicians and patients should have the right to discuss alternative treatment options, regardless of cost.
- In marketing and enrollment decisions, plans should not be allowed to discriminate against eligible patients based on such factors as race, ethnicity, or mental or physical disability.
- Medical record information, although generally confidential, under certain circumstances in the public's interest may be released to investigate healthcare fraud or to protect the public's health.

During 2000, both houses of Congress passed "patients' bill of rights" aimed at perceived managed care abuses of patients' rights. The two bills included provisions that were so different that the two parties were never able to agree on a compromise version (Scott 2001).

In addition to addressing consumer protection concerns, anti–managed care legislation addresses antitrust concerns. As the healthcare marketplace has consolidated, fears have grown regarding the creation of oligopolies that may lessen competition. However, most economists believe that as long as two players remain in the major markets, competition will remain. Another antitrust concern is that exclusive arrangements between managed care organizations and providers may lessen competition and inhibit new providers from entering the marketplace. However, the preponderance of point-of-service plans in most markets negates this concern (Zelman 1996).

The second trend that will have an important affect on the healthcare industry is entitlement reform (Nowicki 1996b). In today's entitlement world, everybody seems to feel that they have a right to an award based on a class-action grievance against the government. Claimants include farmers, unions, defense contractors, civil servants, military and social security retirees, savings and loan depositors, home owners—the list goes on and on. This right seems to be based on two beliefs. The first belief is that the government owes claimants the entitlement based on past oppressions that claimants are attempting to overcome. This is the primary argument for welfare, farm subsidies, savings and loan bail-outs, home mortgage interest deductions, and so on. The second belief is that the claimants have a contractual right to the entitlement. This is the primary argument for social security, Medicare, military and other government pensions, and so on.

Regarding the belief that Americans have contractual rights to entitlements, James Peterson (1993), who served as President Nixon's Secretary of Commerce and cofounded the Concord Coalition with Senators Paul Tsongas and Warren Rudman, points out that the U.S. Supreme Court has repeatedly ruled that workers do not retain rights, contractual or otherwise, over taxes paid into entitlement programs like Social Security. Furthermore, valid contracts require a meeting of the minds between the two parties: those who pay and those who receive. The government funds the vast majority of entitlement payments through current tax revenues and the hope for future tax revenues (deficit spending that increases the national debt).[5] Peterson argues that much of the economic burden for funding today's entitlements will fall to future generations, who have not been party to the contract. The Comptroller General of the United States, David M. Walker, quantified that burden in a 2003 speech entitled "Truth and Transparency: The Federal Government's Financial Condition and Fiscal Outlook".

> Let me start by reviewing the federal government's current financial condition. The federal government's fiscal 2002 annual financial report says a lot but not enough. The good news is that as of September 30, 2002, we had about $1 trillion in reported assets. The bad news is that we had almost $8 trillion in reported liabilities. According to my math, that left us with an approximate $7 trillion

accumulated deficit, or a little over $24,000 for every man, woman, and child in the United States. In fiscal 2002, the federal government reported a net operating deficit of $365 billion. . . . The picture is not good and getting worse. For example, the Congressional Budget Office (CBO) estimates that the unified budget deficits in fiscal years 2003 and 2004 will be $401 billion and $480 billion, respectively. These numbers are up significantly from fiscal 2002. Interestingly, CBO estimates that we will incur about $157 billion in interest on publicly held federal debt in fiscal 2003 even though current interest rates are low on a relative basis. Furthermore, CBO estimates that, excluding Social Security surpluses, the total deficit for fiscal years 2003 and 2004 will be $562 billion and $644 billion, respectively. If all these numbers are making your head spin, don't worry; just remember that they are all big, and they are all bad!

Importantly, while we are starting off in a financial hole we don't really have a very good picture of how deep it is. Specifically, there are a number of very significant items that are not currently included as liabilities in the federal government's financial statements; for example, several trillion dollars in non-marketable government securities in so-called "Trust Funds." In the case of Social Security and Medicare Trust Funds, the federal government took in taxpayer money, spent it on other items and replaced it with an IOU. Given this fact, why aren't the amounts attributed to such activities shown as a "liability" of the U.S. Government? At the present time, they are not! Does this make sense, especially when the government continues to tell Social Security and Medicare beneficiaries that they can count on the bonds in these "Trust Funds"? Is the federal government trying to have its cake and eat it too?

The current U.S. government liability figures also do not adequately consider veterans' healthcare benefit costs provided through the Department of Veteran's Affairs nor do they include the difference between future promised and funded benefits in connection with the Social Security and Medicare programs. These additional amounts total tens of trillions of dollars in discounted present value terms. Stated differently, they are likely to exceed $100,000 in additional [tax] burden for every man, woman, and child in America today, and these amounts are growing every day. (Walker 2003)

Proponents of such entitlement programs argue the government is authorized on behalf of future generations to enter into the contract. Most courts would no doubt rule that if this is the case, the contract is unenforceable. Past generations have funded programs similar to entitlement programs with taxes resulting in the motto *tax and spend* so prevalent in the 50s and early 60s. Unfortunately, tax and spend has been replaced with *borrow and spend*, which may make the American Dream an American Nightmare for future generations. Both real median household income and real disposable income per capita, two accepted measures of the standard of living, continue to decline for most Americans. Especially hard hit, however, are the young. The real median income for families with heads of household under 30 declined over 28 percent from 1973 to 1990.

Most economists argue that some entitlement programs, and the growth of entitlement spending over the last 30 years, must be cut, but few are willing to sacrifice their own programs. While some attempts to justify entitlement programs seem real, many attempts turn out to be ill-founded rationalizations based on myths. Peterson (1993) helps separate fact from fiction.

Myth #1—Entitlement spending is not the big and growing problem that many make it out to be

Entitlement spending has grown from $26 billion, or 26.8 percent of the federal budget in 1960, to $807 billion, or 53.5 percent of the federal budget in 1993. Only 22 percent of this increase is attributable to inflation and population increases.

Myth #2—Most entitlement spending goes to the poor

Only about 12 percent of entitlement spending goes to those living in poverty. Fifty percent of entitlement spending goes to households with annual incomes over $30,000, and 25 percent goes to households with annual incomes over $50,000.

Myth #3—As a group, the elderly are poorer than younger Americans and therefore need entitlements to survive

The elderly receive a lion's share of entitlement spending. In 1990, 63 percent of all entitlement spending went to the 13 percent of Americans over age 65. However, only 6.2 percent of the elderly are living in poverty compared to 13.6 percent of Americans ages 18 to 24 and 14.9 percent of Americans under age 18.

Myth #4—Recipients have earned Social Security and Medicare benefits by contributing to those funds through taxes, and are only getting back what they paid in

Americans currently drawing Social Security benefits will draw two to five times more than they paid in after accounting for interest earned. Medicare recipients will draw five to twenty times more than they paid in after accounting for interest. The demographic explanations for these facts are obvious. Average life expectancy at birth in 1935 when the Social Security Act became law was 63. Average life expectancy at birth in 1965 when the Medicare Act became law was 68. Both programs established contributions accordingly. Average life expectancy at birth in 1995 was about 78. Furthermore, the proportion of our over 65 population will grow from the current 13 percent to over 18 percent by the year 2020 when most baby boomers will be turning 65 (see Dychtwald 1989 for a discussion of these demographic changes).

Myth #5—Federal and military retirement benefits, although generous, are deserved because either the base pay was too low or the duty was especially hazardous

Federal and military retirement benefits are indeed generous, the value of which surpasses the average Fortune 500 retirements benefits by 159 percent and 111 percent, respectively (the Fortune 500 average includes only those that receive pensions, over half do not). The difference in the average retirement age and the age when retirement benefits become available explains most of this significant difference. The average retirement age in the private sector is 63; it is 58 for civil service, 46 for military officers, and 42 for military enlisted men. Employees pay part of the cost of private-sector retirement plans, but employees of the military pay nothing toward their retirement. Furthermore, the federal government, unlike the private sector, exempts itself from funding this liability. If the federal government was required to fund this liability, or save for existing employees' future retirements, the federal government would need to fund about $145 billion a year.

The other argument for generous retirement benefits is that the benefits make up for low pay while serving in the military. However, base pays have risen dramatically in recent years. The test of comparable worth might be relevant here. After accounting for the full value of the base pay, life-long benefits like health insurance and retirement, would a person in the military be paid a comparable value in the private sector?

Myth #6—Social Security, Medicare, and federal and military retirement benefits are sacred cows and can't, or won't, be cut by the federal government

These four programs represent over 75 percent of all federal entitlement spending and account for virtually all the historic growth in entitlement spending. The current committed but unfunded liability for these four programs is $14 trillion, or about $140,00 for every American household.

Myth #7—Indirect entitlements like tax breaks for health insurance and home mortgage interest deductions benefit people who could not otherwise afford health insurance and promotes home ownership and stimulates the economy, respectively

Tax breaks for health insurance benefit mostly employers, not employees, and represent approximately $75 billion in lost revenue to the federal government.

Many people who cannot afford health insurance would not be in the financial position to take advantage of such a tax break.

Home mortgage interest deductions represent approximately $46 billion in lost revenue, 80 percent of which will go to households with incomes over $50,000. The main effect of the home mortgage interest deduction is not additional homes, but bigger homes, while diverting investments away from more economically productive sectors of the economy.

It should be clear that entitlement programs will not and cannot continue in the future as they have in the past. While President Clinton introduced the popular proposal for lowering the eligibility age for Medicare benefits to 62, Senator Moynihan (D-NY), protector of Medicare since its inception, disagreed. He admitted that raising the eligibility age to 68 or 70 and means testing, or limiting Medicare to those who cannot afford health insurance, may be the only ways of keeping the program solvent into the next century. The healthcare industry will be hard hit and managers should be preparing now for bigger cuts in federal and state healthcare spending in the future, making financial management more important now than ever before.

The Economy and Healthcare

Russ Coile (2000, 2001), healthcare futurist and author, agrees that the economic condition of the country will determine health policy for the next ten years. Coile has developed three scenarios for healthcare, each dependent on the economy.

Scenario #1—Booming Business

In the first scenario, the economy continues strong and America is willing to invest an increasing share, perhaps as much as 20 percent, of the gross national product on healthcare. Health inflation runs 6 to 10 percent per year. Consumers demand access to costly, new, genetically engineered drugs and treatments. Excess capacity in the healthcare industry is subsidized so consumers can have on-demand access. Managed care organizations function as claims payers in a primarily fee-for-service market. Alternative medicine is an option in most health plans, and most complimentary medicine is paid out-of-pocket. Government health policy expands Medicare benefits to meet the demands of the politically powerful baby boomers. The uninsured are not fully subsidized, although new consumer protection legislation is enacted.

Scenario #2—Market-Driven Reengineering

In the second scenario, economic growth is mixed and health inflation runs 3 to 6 percent per year. Recognizing that America cannot afford to double its $1 trillion health expenditures brings calls for reform from major employers and business coalitions. Managed care is resurrected with multi-year contracts, incentives for improvements in health, and prices locked in at moderate annual increases with increased capitation. Healthcare organizations focus on centers of excellence and excess capacity is reduced. Internet-competent consumers and information-savvy health providers create more efficient processes of care. Consumers have multiple health plan options. Employers convert to defined contribution benefit policies leaving consumers to spend their money for services such as alternative medicine.

Scenario #3—Single Payer Solution

In the third scenario, the economy slips into a recession and health inflation runs 1 to 2 percent per year. Many for-profit managed care organizations fail, including many Medicare and Medicaid managed care plans. Realizing that market-based reforms have also failed, employers and abandoned consumers turn to the government for help. A new, national single-payer plan, which administers a comprehensive but minimal health benefits package, is enacted by Congress. A federal commission sets prices and approves all new capital expenditures. Many healthcare organizations fail quickly, reducing excess capacity. Access to genetically engineered drugs and treatments is closely controlled by the federal government. A small insurance industry offers supplemental health insurance policies to those who can afford them.

Baby Boomers Change Healthcare

Baby boomers—the 80 million Americans born between 1946 and 1964 representing 30 percent of the population—are moving into the 50+ age group. As they increasingly experience acute episodes of what will become chronic illnesses, the boomers will make unprecedented demands on the healthcare industry. For instance, once their illnesses have been diagnosed, boomers will use the Internet to not only find information on their illnesses, but also to find the best doctors and hospitals to treat their illnesses. A panel of experts predicted that by 2004, more than half of the baby boomers will use the Internet to check on the quality of their hospital, physician, and prescription drugs (Coile 2001). All organizations must understand the unique and demanding nature of the boomer generation, a generation that significantly changed every industry and social institution it has passed through (Dychtwald 2000). Organizations might consider appointing a chief baby-boomer officer to identify and attempt to meet the needs of the boomers as they begin demanding more healthcare services.

Notes

1. Growth in the number of physicians in relation to the population should increase competition and lower prices. However, the federal government did not take into account the effects of supplier-induced demand, which is the degree to which physicians can control the demand for their services. Several studies during the 1970s reported that higher physician

density had little effect on physician income. Three hypotheses have been forwarded to explain this contradiction to the law of supply and demand. The first suggests that an increase in physician density results in an increase in service to previously unserved populations and stable physician incomes. The second suggests that new demand is physician generated. The third suggests that in the face of increasing competition, physicians simply increase fees in a fee-for-service environment.

2. The law attempts to make insurance coverage more accessible to the self-employed and small businesses by forcing insurance companies that offer such coverage to be less selective. However, the unintended consequence may be insurance companies eliminating coverage to the self-employed and small businesses altogether.

3. The patient's freedom of choice for providers may be more of an emotional issue than an economic one. The Rand Health Insurance experiment concluded that patient loyalty to their physicians had a minimal price—patients were willing to change physicians for a small reduction in premiums (patient loyalty to OB/GYN physicians had a somewhat high price). In point-of-service managed care plans, only 16 percent of the enrollees use the out-of-network option, reflecting a relatively high satisfaction level with network physicians (Gabel et al. 1994, in Zelman)

4. Representative Charles Norwood (R-GA) introduced the "Patient Access to Responsible Care Act of 1997" which quickly added 190 cosponsors in the House. Senator Alfonse D'Amato (R-NY) sponsored the Senate version. The idea behind Norwood's bill seems well suited for Republican ideology—it guarantees individual freedoms in the form of choice. However, Republicans are somewhat fragmented in determining the identity of the individual, patient, or even the managed care organization (Scott 1998b).

5. While President Bush and legislative leaders argue the best ways to spend the budget surplus, most economists warn that the budget surplus is illusionary. Virtually the entire surplus involves the Social Security retirement and disability funds—funds that are earmarked for future retirees and should be accounted for separately from the general fund. When those surpluses were added, the fiscal 1997 budget deficit was only $22.6 billion; when subtracted those surpluses result in a fiscal 1997 budget deficit of $103.9 billion (Sloan 1998).

Appendix 15.1
Clinton Healthcare Plan

President Clinton's plan, the American Health Security Act of 1993, addressed the problems with access and cost in the prevailing healthcare system. Clinton's plan attacked the access problem by:

- guaranteeing the provision of coverage to everyone;
- reforming insurance practices (specifically the practices of excluding coverage because of preexisting illness and limiting or eliminating coverage because of illness);
- protecting small businesses from high costs by requiring insurance companies to offer group coverage to small businesses;
- expanding community-based prevention programs;
- guaranteeing health insurance coverage to AIDS patients and increasing funding for AIDS research;
- improving healthcare to women by increasing funding for the delivery of care and research of illnesses inherent to women; and
- diversifying long-term care from institutionalization to alternative delivery mechanisms.

Clinton's plan attacked the cost problem by:

- establishing global budgets, which limit total expenditures for healthcare;
- creating managed competition based on both cost and quality;
- establishing health networks of providers;
- streamlining the billing system;
- containing drug prices; and
- reforming state malpractice and federal antitrust laws.

Clinton's plan would work by:

1. grouping all Americans into giant buying groups, called health alliances, either by large employers or by geographic regions;
2. requiring all health alliances to offer identical basic coverage (which was extensive). Employers would be required to pay at least 80 percent of the premium with no more than 20 percent paid by the employee.
3. providing enrollees a choice of three delivery plans, the latter two with increasing cost to the enrollee: HMO; hybrid (HMO with some choices of providers); and fee-for-service. Varying premiums for the three delivery plans were based only on the following four criteria: single individuals; couples without children; single-parent households; and two-parent households.
4. accommodating several different coverage situations:
   - Part-time employees would pay premiums inversely proportional to the hours worked.
   - Self-employed would pay both the employer share and employee share, but would be able to deduct 100 percent of the cost on income tax returns.

- Retirees could opt to stay in employer's health alliance or go with Medicare coverage, which would ultimately become a health alliance. Early retirees would be subsidized by the federal government.
- Employees in transition would be subsidized by the federal government.
- Low-income families would be subsidized by the federal government.
- Chronically unemployed would be subsidized by the federal government.
- Small businesses would be subsidized by the federal government.

In October, 1993, the White House announced that the plan's five-year cost would be $389 billion, financed through federal revenue gains resulting from growth in the economy, federal government savings resulting from the downsizing initiative headed by Vice President Gore, federal government savings in the Medicare and Medicaid programs, and an increased tobacco tax.

On February 9, 1994, the Congressional Budget Office released its analysis of the Clinton plan.

- The Congressional Budget Office predicted a 1.2 million job loss by businesses encouraging employees to take early retirement at the federal government's expense.
- Also predicted was a 1.2 million job loss by small businesses who could not afford the mandated coverage, even though it was subsidized by the federal government.
- The five-year expense budget projection was understated by $132 billion, which was mostly paid in federal government subsidies.
- As an unfunded mandate on business, and state and local governments, the cost to business should be treated as a government receipt similar to a tax.

While the Clinton plan was debated during late 1993 and early 1994, business support for the plan had eroded based on the widely held belief that the plan would further increase—not decrease—healthcare costs. A large number of businesses turned to managed care organizations to reduce costs. As a result, managed care enrollments grew dramatically in the mid-1990s. At the same time, hospitals, physicians, and other providers were consolidating into larger, integrated, and organized delivery systems. These large delivery systems could lower costs and bid successfully for health alliance dollars in the event the Clinton plan became law, or bid for managed care organization premium dollars in the event the Clinton plan failed.

According to Walter A. Zelman, who served as senior health policy adviser to the Clinton administration and who also participated on Hillary Clinton's task force, the Clinton plan was dead by late summer, 1994 (Zelman 1996). Zelman attributes the plan's failure to the following core reasons that gave the public the perception that the plan represented the very worst in "big government:"

- To provide the level and competitive field that was necessary for competition on cost and quality to take place, the plan called for significant insurance reform, which many perceived as unnecessary government intrusion into the private sector.
- The Clinton administration pushed the idea of health alliances (i.e., purchasing cooperatives) too aggressively, which allowed critics to dub the plan "socialized medicine."
- The administration's goal of universal coverage required an unending list of insurance rules, legislative demands, and federal government subsidies that in the end, could not guarantee universal coverage.
- Given the deficit concerns, the administration could not sell what many believed to be an open-ended entitlement. Congressional budget rules, deficit projections, and political forces all demanded a guarantee that costs would not rise above projections. To provide that guarantee, more legislation, particularly in the insurance industry, would be required and would be vigorously opposed. To not provide that guarantee would risk the administration's core theme of health security for every American.
- Clinton's plan went well beyond solving problems with access and cost, and sought to regulate the very relationships that patients had with their healthcare providers (Zelman 1996). It was the freedom of choice, and the accompanying increase in costs, that inspired Clinton's pursuit of the plan in the first place. Patients in prevailing fee-for-service plans could get whatever care they wished from any providers they wished who could prescribe and charge whatever they wished. Insurance companies paid the claims without question and passed the cost in the form of insurance premiums to the employers. Ironically, managed care, the private sector's answer to the Clinton plan, has generated the same complaints about provider choice (Kilborn 1998).

References

Berman, H. J., S. F. Kukla, and L. E. Weeks. 1994. *The Financial Management of Hospitals, 8th ed.* Chicago: Health Administration Press.

Brink, S. 1998. "HMOs Were the Right Rx." *U.S. News and World Report* March 9, 47–50.

Centers for Medicare and Medicaid Services, Office of the Actuary, 2004. [Online retrieval, 02/16/04]. http://www.cms.hhs.gov/statistics/nhe/projections.htm.

Cher, D. J., and L. A. Lenert. 1997. "Method of Medicare Reimbursement and the Rate of Potentially Ineffective Care of Critically Ill Patients." *Journal of the American Medical Association* 278 (12): 1001–1007.

Coile, R. C. 2001. *Futurescan 2001: A Millennium Forecast of Healthcare Trends 2001–2005.* Chicago: Health Administration Press.

———. 2000. *New Century Healthcare: Strategies for Providers, Purchasers, and Plans.* Chicago: Health Administration Press.

Dychtwald, K. 2000. *Age Power: How the 21st Century Will Be Ruled by the New Old.* New York: J.P. Tarcher.

———. 1989. *Age Wave.* New York: St. Martin's Press.

Eastaugh, S. R. 1987. *Financing Health Care: Economic Efficiency and Equity.* Dover, MA: Auburn House.

Feldor, F. P. 1998. "Advisory Opinions Help Clarify Fraud and Abuse Laws." *Healthcare Financial Management* 52 (4): 70–72.

Healthcare Financial Management Association. 2001. "Industry Scan." *Healthcare Financial Management* 55 (1):21.

Healthcare Financing Administration, Office of the Actuary. 2001. "Health Spending Projections Through 2010." [Online retrieval, 02/28/01]. http://www.hcfa.gov/stats/NHE-Proj/proj1996/tables/Table1.htm.

Heffler, S., S. Smith, S. Keehan, M. R. Clemens, M. Zezza, and C. Truffer. 2004. "Trends: Health Spending Projections Through 2013." *Health Affairs*—Web Exclusive. [Online retrieval, 03/16/04]. http://content.healthaffairs.org/webexclusives/index.dt/?year=2004.

Kilborn, P. T. 1998. "Managed Care: Looking Back at Jackson Hole." *New York Times,* March 22.

Nowicki, M. 1996a. "New Economics of Hospital and Ambulatory Care in Urban Areas." Presented at the annual meeting of the Texas Hospital Association, San Antonio, 2–4 January.

———. 1996b. "The Entitlement Ethic." *Journal of Healthcare Resource Management* 14 (1): 29–31.

———. 1994. "Hospital Strategies in Response to Healthcare Reform." Presented at the quarterly meeting of the MidTexas Chapter of the American College of Healthcare Executives, Temple, 21 May.

Pear, R. 2003. "Medigap Insurance Barred." *New York Times,* December 7, F71.

Peterson, P. G. 1993. *Facing Up: How to Rescue the Economy from Crushing Debt and Restore the American Dream.* New York: Simon and Schuster Publishers.

Poisal, J.S., and Murray, L. 2001. "Growing Differences Between Medicare Beneficiaries With and Without Drug Coverage." *Health Affairs* 20 (2): 74–85.

Scalise, D., and T. H. Thrall. 2002. "American's Uninsured: Rethinking the Problem That Won't Go Away." Hospitals and Health Networks 76 (11): 31–40.

Scott, J. S. 2001. "Partisan Politics Spells Trouble for Health Care." *Healthcare Financial Management* 55 (1): 26–27.

———. 1998a. "ClintonCare II: The Revenge." *Healthcare Financial Management* 52 (1): 24–25.

———. 1998b. "Managing Managed Care: A Battle for Citizens' Hearts and Minds." *Healthcare Financial Management* 52 (3): 25–26.

Sloan, A. 1998. "The Surplus Shell Game." *Newsweek,* January 19: 28.

Smith, S., M. Freeland, S. Heffler, and D. McKusick. 1998. "The Next Ten Years of Health Spending: What Does the Future Hold?" *Health Affairs* 17 (5): 128–140.

Starr, P. 1982. *The Social Transformation of American Medicine.* New York: Basic Books.

U.S. Department of Health and Human Services. 2001. "Healthy People 2010." [Online retrieval, 02/28/01]. http://www.health.gov/healthypeople.

————. 1990. *Healthy People 2000: National Health Promotion and Disease Prevention Objectives.* Washington, DC: DHHS.

Walker, D. M. 2003. "Truth and Transparency: The Federal Government's Financial Condition and Fiscal Outlook." Speech to the National Press Club, Washington, DC, 17 September.

Zelman, W. A. 1996. *The Changing Health Care Marketplace.* San Francisco: Jossey-Bass Publishers.

Recommended Readings — Part VI

Coile, R. C. 2000. *New Century Healthcare: Strategies for Providers, Purchasers, and Plans.* Chicago: Health Administration Press.

Dychtwald, K. 2000. *Age Power: How the 21st Century Will Be Ruled by the New Old.* New York: J.P. Tarcher.

———. 1989. *Age Wave.* New York: St. Martin's Press.

Eastaugh, S. R. 1994. *Facing Tough Choices: Balancing Fiscal and Social Deficits.* Westport, CT: Praeger Press.

Healthcare Financial Management (ed). 2001. "*Healthcare Financial Management's* Healthcare Outlook". *2001 Resource Guide*: 7–11.

Helms, R. B. (ed.). 1993. *American Health Policy: Critical Issues for Reform.* Washington, DC: The AEI Press.

Modern Healthcare (ed.). 1999. "Bringing the Future into Focus: Envisioning Healthcare 20 Years into the New Millennium. A supplement to *Modern Healthcare*, 29 (39): 1–32.

Peterson, P. G. 1996. *Will America Grow Up Before It Grows Old?* New York: Random House.

Zelman, W. A. 1996. *The Changing Health Care Marketplace.* San Francisco: Jossey-Bass Publishers.

LIST OF ACRONYMS

ACEHSA	Accrediting Commission on Education for Health Services Administration
ACHE	American College of Healthcare Executives
AFDC	Aid to Families with Dependent Children
AHA	American Hospital Association
AHIMA	American Health Information Management Association
AICPA	American Institute of Certified Public Accountants
ALOS	average length of stay
AMA	American Medical Association
APC	ambulatory payment classification
ASC	ambulatory surgical center
AUPHA	Association of University Programs in Health Administration
BBA	Balanced Budget Act of 1997
BBRA	Balanced Budget Refinement Act of 1999
BIPA	Medicare, Medicaid, and SCHIP Benefits Improvement & Protection Act of 2000
CAH	critical access hospital
CCO	corporate compliance officer
CEO	chief executive officer
CEP	coordinated examination program
CFO	chief financial officer
CHE	Certified Healthcare Executive
CHFP	Certified Healthcare Financial Professional
CHIPS	Center for Healthcare Industry Performance Studies
CHSO	cooperative hospital service organization
CIA	Corporate Integrity Agreement (or CI)
CIO	chief information officer
CMP	civil monetary penalty
CMS	Centers for Medicare & Medicaid Services
CPA	certified public accountant
COBRA	Consolidated Omnibus Budget Reconciliation Act
CON	certificate of need
COO	chief operating officer
CPT	current procedural terminology
CSG	clinical service group
CT	computed tomography

DEFRA	Deficit Reduction Act
DHEW	Department of Health, Education, and Welfare
DME	durable medical equipment
DRG	diagnostic-related grouping
DSH	disproportionate share hospital
EDI	electronic data interchange
EIN	Employer Identification Number
EOQ	economic order quantity (also Q_e)
EPSDTS	early and periodic screening, diagnosis, and treatment services
ERISA	Employee Retirement Income Security Act of 1974
ESC	evidence of standard compliance
FACHE	Fellow of the American College of Healthcare Executives
FASB	Financial Accounting Standards Board
FHFMA	Fellow of the Healthcare Financial Management Association
FIFO	first-in, first-out
FMR	focused medical review
FTE	full-time equivalent personnel
FV	future value
GAAP	generally accepted accounting principles
GASB	governmental accounting standards board
GAO	Government Accounting Office
GCD	greatest common denominator
GNP	gross national product
HFMA	Healthcare Financial Management Association
HHS	U.S. Department of Health and Human Services
HI	hospital insurance
HIM	health information management
HIPAA	Health Insurance Portability and Accountability Act
HMO	health maintenance organization
HSA	health savings accounts
ICF	intermediate care facility
IDFS	integrated delivery and financing system
IOM	Institute of Medicine
IPA	independent practice association
IRR	internal rate of return
IRS	Internal Revenue Service
JCAHO	Joint Commission on Accreditation of Healthcare Organizations
JIT	just-in-time inventory
LIFO	last-in, first-out
MAAC	maximum allowable actual charge
MBO	management by objectives

MMA	Medicare Prescription Drug, Improvement, and Modernization Act of 2003
MOS	measures of success
MRS	medical record system
MSA	medical savings account
NPSG	national patient safety goals
NPV	net present value
NF	nursing care facility
NR	departments that do not generate revenue
OB/GYN	obstetrician/gynecologist
OBRA	Omnibus Budget Reconciliation Act
OIG	Office of the Inspector General
ODS	organized delivery system
PAR	Participating Physician and Supplies Program
PBS	patient billing system
PERT	program evaluation and review technique
PFA	priority focus area
PFP	priority focus process
PHI	protected health information
PHO	physician-hospital organization
PILOT	payment in lieu of taxes
PMC	patient management categories
POS	point-of-service plan
PPO	preferred provider organization
PPR	periodic performance review
PPS	prospective payment system
PRO	Peer Review Organization
ProPAC	Prospective Payment Assessment Commission
PSO	provider-sponsored organization
PSRO	Professional Standards Review Organization
PV	present value
Q_e	economic order quantity (also EOQ)
RBRVS	Resource-Based Relative Value System
RCC	ratio of cost to charges
RVU	relative value unit
SCH	sole community hospital
SCHIP	State Children's Health Insurance Program
SNF	skilled nursing facility
SOI	severity of illness
SMI	supplemental medical insurance
SMSA	standard metropolitan statistical area
SSI	Supplemental Security Income
SWOT	strengths, weaknesses, opportunities, and threats

TEFRA	Tax Equity and Fiscal Responsibility Act of 1982
THA	Texas Hospital Association
TQM	total quality management
UPL	upper payment limit
UBI	unrelated business income

GLOSSARY

2–10, net 30. Organization receives a 2-percent discount on bill if the bill is paid within 10 days.

501(c)(3) corporation. Federal Internal Revenue Service (IRS) designation for not-for-profit corporations operated exclusively for religious, charitable, scientific, testing for public safety, literary, or educational purposes; whose net earnings do not go to the private benefit of any stockholder or individual; and whose activities in no way attempt to influence legislation or participate in political campaigns.

ABC inventory method. Classifying inventory by cost or by nature of the supply.

Abuse. Unintentional misrepresentation of fact.

Accounting system. System that accurately and promptly assigns costs and charges to the appropriate cost centers and revenue centers.

Accounts payable. Current liability that includes moneys owed, but not yet paid, to vendors for supplies already received.

Accounts receivable. Monies due to the organization from patients and insurers for services that the organization has already provided.

Accrediting Commission on Education for Health Services Administration (ACEHSA). Primary accrediting body for graduate programs in health administration.

Accrued wages payable. Current liability that includes moneys owed, but not yet paid, to employees for work already performed.

Activity-based costing. Method of determining product cost by using cost drivers to assign indirect costs to products or services.

Actual costs. Historic costs incurred.

Add-on interest loan, or installment loan. Borrower receives the principal and repays the principal plus interest in monthly installments.

Adverse opinion. One of four possible opinion paragraphs in an audit report, the adverse opinion means that the financial statements do not fairly present the financial position, results of operations, and/or cash flows of the organization in conformance with GAAP. Auditors use an additional paragraph(s) after the opinion to describe the reasons for an adverse opinion.

Agenda for Change. Joint Commission strategic direction initiated by Joint Commission president Dr. Dennis O'Leary in 1986 with the dual purpose of accrediting healthcare organizations and implementing a national performance measurement database.

American College of Healthcare Executives (ACHE). Primary professional society for healthcare executives that provides professional certification at two levels: diplomate and fellow. ACHE has approximately 30,000 members with 5,000 certified as Diplomates (Certified Healthcare Executive or CHE) and 3,000 certified as Fellows (FACHE).

American Institute of Certified Public Accountants (AICPA). Governs and publishes prescribed formats for financial accounting information.

Anti-Kickback Act. Federal legislation that mandates civil liability for kickbacks, which can result in fines of $10,000 plus two times the total amount of the kickback.

Anti–managed care laws. Laws designed to control the growth and decision-making authority of managed care organizations.

Any-willing-provider laws. Anti–managed care laws that allow patients to receive care from providers outside the network.

Association of University Programs in Health Administration (AUPHA). Primary membership association for university programs in health administration at undergraduate and graduate levels. AUPHA provides panel reviews (accreditation-equivalent) for undergraduate programs to gain full membership.

Assignment. Insurance term that means that providers must accept what the insurance company pays as full payment.

Authority. Characteristic of the management function of organizing that defines the amount of power to delegate to employees so that they can perform their assigned tasks.

Average costs. Full costs that are divided by the number of products or services.

Baby-boomer population. Very large generation of Americans born between 1946 and 1964 that reflects approximately one-third of the existing U.S. population.

Bad debt. Accounting term used when the provider bills and expects payment from a patient or third party who pays less than the full amount expected by the provider. Bad debt amounts should be recorded based on charges, not costs.

Balance billing. Billing term meaning that providers cannot bill the patient for amounts over the fee schedules agreed to with the service plan.

Balanced Budget Act of 1997. Federal legislation signed by President Clinton that reduced Medicare reimbursement to providers by $115 billion over five years.

Billings for teaching physicians. HHS rule that prohibits a hospital from billing Medicare for teaching physician services when the teaching physician is not actually present at the time of service.

Bill collection. Step in the billing process where the organization makes additional steps to collect the bill before turning the account over to a collection agency.

Bill cutoffs. Step in the billing process during which the organization determines the bill is complete and ready for submission.

Bill print. Step in the billing process during which a claim form is completed.

Bill resolution. Step in the billing process during which the organization makes a final decision about an uncollected account.

Bill submission. Step in the billing process during which a claim for payment leaves the organization.

Book overdraft. Process of transferring money from an interest-bearing account to the checking account as the money is drawn.

Break-even point. Volume in units at which the total revenue equals the total cost.

Capitation. Method of reimbursement in which the payer pays the provider a prospective, fixed amount called a premium for providing care to a defined population.

Carrying costs. Associated with accounts receivable, carrying costs are the costs incurred by the organization related to extending credit.

Carrying costs. Associated with inventory, carrying costs are the costs of holding an inventory of items.

Case mix. Mix of patients treated in a particular organization. Mix can be defined by age or payer, but usually refers to severity of illness.

Cash. Money on hand and money to which the organization has immediate access.

Cash budget. Predicts the timing and amount of cash flows and systematically examines the cost implications with each alternative.

Cash conversion cycle. Process of converting resources represented by cash outflows into services and products represented by cash inflows.

Cash equivalents. Often reported as cash and include investments with maturities of three months or less.

Cash flow. Difference between cash receipts and cash disbursements for a given period.

Centers for Medicare and Medicaid Services (CMS). Financing branch of the U.S. Department of Health and Human Services (HHS) that has administrative responsibility for Medicare. Formerly known as the Health Care Financing Administration.

Charge capture assessment. Ensures that providers are not losing charges in the organization.

Charge masters. List of items for which providers generate charges.

Charge master enrichment. Ensures that providers are charging for items that third-party payers are recognizing as legitimate.

Charge-based patients. Patients who pay providers' full charges.

Charges. Method of reimbursement in which the payer reimburses the provider the price or rate set by the provider.

Charges minus a discount. Method of reimbursement in which the payer reimburses the provider the charge set by the provider minus a negotiated discount.

Charging analysis. Ensures that the charge set for each item maximizes reimbursement in relation to payer classification.

Charitable organization. Organization whose primary purpose is charitable in nature.

Charity care. Accounting term used when the provider delivers care to a patient that at time of service the provider knows is unable to pay.

Chart of accounts. Listing of cost and revenue centers.

Chief executive officer (CEO). Formal position with authority and responsibility for the organization—reports to the governing body.

Chief financial officer (CFO). Formal position with authority and responsibility for the organization's financial departments and functions—reports to the chief executive officer (CEO).

Chief operating officer (COO). Formal position of authority and responsibility for the organization's operations—reports to the chief executive officer (CEO).

Clean claims. Bills that have no defect, impropriety, or special circumstances.

Closed panel HMOs. A type of HMO that exerts maximum control over physician providers by contracting with or employing the physicians to provide care to enrollees.

Code jamming. Coding by nonphysician personnel for procedures that the ordering physician had omitted.

Coding compliance plan. Policies, procedures, and practices that ensure correct coding.

Collection period. Number of days between the time of service, or the time the medical record is completed, and the time of payment.

Commercial indemnity plans. Method of financing and delivering healthcare in which employers/employees pay insurance companies that reimburse providers chosen by employees.

Community benefit standard. Established by IRS Ruling 69-545 in 1969, which expanded the financial ability standard to organizations that promoted health.

Community rating. A method of determining insurance premiums that results in everyone paying essentially the same premium.

Competition-driven charging. Method of setting prices to dominate market share.

Compounding. Process used to determine how much money an investment will make.

Concurrent review. Utilization review that occurs while care is delivered.

Conflict of interest. Owing duties to two or more parties, but in which meeting a duty to one party somehow harms the other party.

Consensus-driven charging. Healthcare providers set charges consistent with other providers in the community.

Consolidated Omnibus Budget Reconciliation Act (COBRA) of 1985. Federal legislation signed by President Reagan that made Medicare coverage mandatory for state and local government employees hired after 1985; also directed the Secretary of HHS to develop prospective payment reimbursement for physicians.

Contractual allowances. Accounting term for the difference in the amount of billed charges and the amount the payer has agreed in advance to pay.

Contribution margin. Expressed in either dollars or percentage, the contribution margin is the amount a product contributes to fixed costs or profit.

Controllable costs. Costs under the manager's influence.

Controller. Formal position with authority over and responsibility for the organization's accounting functions—the controller reports to the chief financial officer (CFO).

Coordinated examination program (CEP). IRS audit program that includes multidisciplinary audit terms that examine not-for-profit healthcare organizations.

Coordination of benefits. Step in the billing process during which the order of insurance company liability is identified for accounts that have multiple insurance companies.

Corporate compliance officer. High-level employee who is charged with overseeing the corporate compliance program.

Corporate compliance program. Voluntary programs in healthcare organizations designed to prevent and detect violations of Medicare fraud and abuse statutes.

Corporate restructuring. Legal strategy to maximize the economic position of the organization by developing new corporations.

Corporations. Legal entity status granted to organizations by the state.

Cost. The amount spent to acquire an asset.

Cost accounting. A field of accounting that studies costs including methods for identifying, classifying, and allocating costs.

Cost allocation. Process of allocating direct and indirect costs from non-revenue generating departments to departments that generate revenue.

Cost-based reimbursement. Method of reimbursement in which the payer reimburses the provider the cost of services provided, which are usually determined with a cost report, after the provider has provided the services.

Cost cutting. Practice of cutting costs, instead of increasing charges, to offset losses from patients.

Cost drivers. Activity measures used to determine product cost in activity-based costing.

Cost plus a percentage for growth. Method of reimbursement in which the payer reimburses the provider the cost of services provided, usually determined with a cost report, plus a negotiated percentage for growth.

Cost sharing. Transfer of healthcare costs to patients by the insurance company or employer, typically through such mechanisms as deductibles, co-insurance, and increased share of premiums.

Cost shifting. Practice of shifting costs to some patients to offset losses from other patients.

Credentialing. A review process to determine a healthcare professional's qualifications.

Current assets. Cash and other short-term assets that the organization expects to convert to cash within one year.

Current liabilities. Obligations or claims on assets that will come due within one year.

Deemed status. Medicare designation for providers accredited by the Joint Commission on the Accreditation of Healthcare Organizations.

Deficit Reduction Act (DEFRA) of 1984. Federal legislation signed by President Reagan that froze physician fees to the Medicare program and initiated the Physician and Supplies Program (PAR), which encouraged physicians to accept assignment by expediting assigned billing and listing PAR physicians in a federal PAR directory.

Defined benefit plan. Employee benefit plan that provides a specific benefit package—variability resides in the premiums.

Defined contribution plan. Employee benefit plan that provides a fixed contribution on the part of the employer and the employee selects benefits and pays for any excess cost.

Delinquency costs. Associated with accounts receivable, delinquency costs are the costs incurred by the organization that are related to patients and their insurance companies not paying on time.

Deontologic view of ethics. The underlying premise is that the rightness or wrongness of an act or decision is determined by duties owed to one another, and is independent of the end result. The view is characterized by the theory of reversibility: "Do unto others as you would have them do unto you."

Department of Health and Human Services. Federal cabinet-level department with overall responsibility for the Medicare program.

Departmentalization. Characteristic of the management function of organizing which divides employees into groups or teams that have similar responsibilities.

Diagnostic-related grouping (DRG). Methodology developed by John Thompson at Yale University to compare similar diagnoses for research purposes. Used by the federal government to reimburse hospitals under prospective payment based on the rationale that similar diagnoses should require similar resource consumption. The DRGs are determined by 92 data elements coded by ICD-9 codes; primary determining factors include primary diagnosis (what occasioned the admission after study), secondary diagnosis, age, sex, principal procedures, and discharge status.

Differential costing. Method of assembling costs, and sometimes revenues, of alternative decisions.

Differential costs, or incremental costs. Cost differences between two or more alternative decisions.

Direct apportionment. Cost allocation method that involves a one-time allocation of all cost centers of departments that do not generate revenue to the revenue centers of departments that do generate revenue.

Direct contract model. A type of open panel HMO that contracts with individual physicians to provide care to enrollees in the physicians' own offices.

Direct contracting. The practice of large employers contracting directly with providers to provide healthcare to employees.

Direct costs. Costs that can be traced directly to a department, product, or service.

Directionality. Statistical property for numbers that always improve in one direction and always worsen in the other direction.

Direct measures of quality. Measures—goal-based, responsive, decision-making, and connoisseurship—of quality that assume that quality can be defined and measured.

Direct service plans. Method of financing and delivering healthcare in which employers prepay the providers for healthcare coverage for their employees.

Discharged, not final billed. Step in the billing process during which the medical record is transferred from the clinicians to the medical records department.

Disclaimer of opinion. One of four possible opinion paragraphs in an audit report, the disclaimer of opinion means that the auditor does not express an opinion on the financial statements usually because the scope of the audit was insufficient for the auditor to render an opinion.

Discount interest loan. Borrower receives the principal minus the interest at the beginning of the loan period.

Disproportionate share hospitals. Federal designation for hospitals that treat a disproportionately high share of Medicaid patients and as a result receive high Medicaid reimbursement.

Dividends. Distributions of earning paid to stockholders based on the number of shares of stock owned.

Double apportionment. Cost allocation method that involves a one-time allocation of all costs from cost centers of departments that do not generate revenue to other cost centers of departments that do not generate revenue, and a simultaneous one-time allocation of costs centers that do generate revenue to cost centers of departments that do generate revenue before a final allocation of costs to the patient.

Downsizing. Reduction of resources to meet reduced demand.

DRG payment window. HHS rule which prohibits a hospital from billing Medicare for outpatient services provided within 72 hours of an admission.

Dual eligible. Persons eligible for both Medicare and Medicaid.

Dunning notices. Step in the billing process during which billing reminders are sent to patients and their insurers who have failed to reimburse the provider.

Economic order quantity (EOQ or QA). Inventory term and formula that derives the number of items to order each time that will result in minimizing total inventory costs associated with the item.

Effective charges. Charges minus negotiated discounts.

Electronic data interchange (EDI). Process by which payers can wire the organization's receipts directly to the bank where the receipts are deposited.

Excess benefit transaction. Unreasonable compensation or any other transaction in which payment or benefit exceeds the value of the transaction.

Expense. Amount spent consuming an asset.

Experience rating. Method of determining insurance premiums based on the past experience of population subgroups.

Explanatory paragraph. Part of the audit report that is included only if GAAP was not used in preparing the financial statements or if any uncertainty exists regarding how the financial statements were prepared.

Factor. Process of selling accounts receivable to a bank or other agent.

Factoring. Accounts receivable term for selling receivables.

Fair Credit Reporting Act. Federal legislation that governs the permissible uses of credit reports.

Fair Debt Collection Practices Act. Federal legislation that applies only to third-party collection agencies and governs the following collection practices: skiptracing, collector communication, harassment, and deceptive and false representation.

False Claims Act. Federal legislation that mandates civil liability for false claims that can result in fines of $10,000 for each false claim plus three times the total amount of the loss.

Federal safe harbors. Payment practices to physicians that are safe from federal prosecution under the Anti-Kickback Act.

Fiduciary. Person in a position of great trust and confidence.

Finance. A subset of the field of financial management that includes the analysis of the information provided by managerial accounting using techniques such as ratio and capital analyses.

Financial ability standard. Established by IRS Ruling 56-185 in 1956, it required that healthcare organizations provide care to those unable to pay to retain tax-exempt status. It was expanded to community benefit standard by IRS Ruling 69-545.

Financial accounting. A field of accounting that provides to external users accounting information in prescribed formats that is generally historic in nature.

Financial accounting (accounting) costs. Measurements, in monetary terms, of the amount of resources used for a purpose.

Financial analysis. Methods used by investors, creditors, and management to evaluate past, present, and future financial performance.

Financial counseling. Step in the billing process during which credit is extended to self-pay patients.

Financial expediency–driven charging. Practice of setting charges based on the financial needs of the provider.

Financial statement analysis. Methods used by investors, creditors, and management to evaluate past, present, and future financial performance by focusing on information provided in the financial statements.

First-in, first out (FIFO). Method of valuing inventory that places the cost of inventory at the price paid for the newest items placed in inventory.

Fiscal intermediaries. Organizations that have contracted with Medicare to process and pay Medicare claims.

Fixed costs. Costs that remain constant in relation to changes in volume.

Float period. Time difference between the day checks are written and the day checks are presented to the bank for payment.

Focused medical reviews (FMRs). Reviews by fiscal intermediaries designed to detect coding errors in submitted claims.

Follower pricing. Practice of pricing products and services relative to the market leader.

Fraud. Intentional misrepresentation designed to induce reliance by another.

Fraud and False Statements Act. Federal legislation that mandates criminal liability including fines and imprisonment for fraudulent billing practices.

Full costing. Method of assembling direct costs and an allocated share of indirect costs to a product or service.

Full costs. Costs that include both direct costs and indirect costs.

Future value. Future amount of money in investment decisions.

Generally accepted accounting principles (GAAP). Accounting standards, conventions, and rules established by an authoritative body recognized by the AICPA Council that accountants follow in recording and reporting accounting transactions.

Graying of America. Descriptor for the increasing proportion of the total population age 65 and older.

Great Society. President Lyndon Johnson's legislative program designed to eradicate poverty in the United States.

Group model HMO. A type of closed panel HMO that contracts with a multi-specialty group of physicians to provide all physician care to enrollees.

Healthcare Financial Management Association (HFMA). Primary professional society for healthcare financial executives that provides certification at two levels: healthcare financial professional with an emphasis in accounting and finance, patient financial services, managed care, or financial management of physician practices; and fellow. HFMA has approximately 30,400 members with 513 certified as Certified Healthcare Financial Professionals (CHFP) and 1,678 certified as Fellows (FHFMA).

Health Care Financing Administration (HCFA). Financing branch of the U.S. Department of Health and Human Services (HHS) that has administrative responsibility for Medicare. HCFA changed its name to the Centers for Medicare and Medicaid Services (CMS) in 2002.

HCFA Resource-Based Relative Value System (RBRVS). Federal regulations that changed the Medicare method of reimbursement for physicians from reasonable and customary charges to a prospective, flat fee per visit.

Health information management. Nomenclature for departments that process medical records.

Health Insurance Portability and Accountability Act (HIPAA) of 1996. Federal legislation signed by President Clinton that introduced significant insurance reform.

Holding cost. Costs of storing, securing, and insuring items in inventory.

Horizontal analysis. Financial analysis method that evaluates the trend in line items by focusing on the percentage change over time.

Horizontal integration. Expansion of a product or service line at the same point in the production process (e.g., nursing homes integrating with other nursing homes).

Hospital Survey and Construction Act of 1946 (Hill-Burton). Federal legislation that provided significant funding for hospital construction and renovation.

Hospital transfers. HHS rule that prohibits hospitals from billing Medicare for hospital discharges when the patient has been transferred.

Incremental costs, or differential costs. Cost differences between two or more alternative decisions.

Independent practice association (IPA). A type of open panel HMO that contracts with associations of physicians to provide care to enrollees in the physicians' offices.

Indirect (overhead) costs. Costs that cannot be traced directly to a department, product, or service.

Indirect measures of quality. Measures of quality that assume that quality cannot be defined and measured, but that the results of which can be identified and measured as resource, outcome, reputation, and value-added measures.

Integrated delivery system. A system of healthcare providers capable of accepting financial responsibility for and delivering a full range of clinical services to an enrolled population.

Intensity of services. Number and kinds of services per patient.

Internal auditor. Employee of the organization who, working independently of the finance and accounting departments, checks on adherence to management policies, existence of proper internal controls, and misappropriation of funds.

Internal control. Accounting systems and supporting procedures that provide systematic and automatic safeguards to protect the integrity of the accounting information.

Introductory paragraph. Part of the audit report that identifies the financial statements audited, identifies management's responsibilities in preparing the financial statements, and identifies the auditor's responsibilities in expressing the audit opinion.

Inventories. Value of supplies on hand at a given time.

Inventory. Items that have an expected useful life of less than 12 months.

Inventory management. Control of items that have an expected useful life of less than 12 months.

Inventory turnover ratio. Financial analysis ratio that measures the number of times an organization turns over its inventory relative to operating revenue and other income.

Investment policy. Directs the chief financial officer (CFO) or controller in making short-term investment decisions.

Job order costing. Method of determining product cost by sampling the product's actual direct costs.

Joint Commission on Accreditation of Healthcare Organizations (JCAHO). Primary accrediting body for healthcare organizations.

Joint venture. A relationship between two business entities entered into for a specific purpose and point of time.

Just-in-time (JIT) inventory method. Inventory method in which supply items are delivered immediately prior to use.

Kids Care. Program in the Balanced Budget Act of 1997 that effectively extends Medicaid coverage to children whose parents' income is too high to qualify for Medicaid but too low to make private health insurance affordable.

Laffer curve. Hypothetical relationship between tax revenues (or tax receipts by the federal government) and individual marginal tax rates.

Lag time. Inventory management term that defines the time between ordering and receiving a supply item.

Last-in, first-out (LIFO). Method of valuing inventory that places the cost of inventory at the price paid for the oldest items placed in inventory.

Length-of-stay laws. Anti–managed care laws that mandate minimum length of stays for certain diagnoses.

Line relationship. Also called line authority, the manager or employee is directly responsible for organizational resources such as employees and supplies.

Liquidity. Ability of a current asset to be consumed or converted to cash.

Lock box. Mechanism to expedite patient payment in which patients and their insurers mail payment directly to a bank that deposits the payment directly into the provider's account.

Loss-leader pricing. Practice of pricing products and services low to attract customers to complementary products and services.

Managed care organizations. Umbrella term used to describe organizations that manage the cost, quality, and delivery of care.

Management functions. Universal actions of managers that include planning, organizing, staffing, influencing, and controlling.

Management processes. Universal actions of managers that are inherent in each management function: decision making; coordinating; and communicating.

Managerial accounting. Field of accounting that provides to internal users accounting information that is both historic and prospective in nature. There are no prescribed formats for managerial accounting information.

Managerial accounting costs, or financial costs. Measurements in monetary terms of present and future costs that help management make better decisions.

Marginal costs. Changes in costs related to changes in volume.

Medicaid. Federal and state program established by the Social Security Amendments of 1965 that provides health insurance to the poor.

Medical-industrial complex. Term attributed to Arnold Relman in 1980 that characterizes a "large and growing network of private corporations engaged in the business of supplying health-care services to patients for profit."

Medically indigent. Individuals who can afford normal living expenses but cannot afford healthcare expenses.

Medical record system. Automated system that records clinical information.

Medical savings accounts. Insurance accounts for the self-employed and employees of small employers that allow the beneficiaries substantial rebates if utilization is low.

Medicare. Federal program established by the Social Security Amendments of 1965 that provides health insurance to the elderly.

Medicare Integrity Program. HHS program that permits HHS to contract with private organizations to decrease fraud and abuse.

Modality. A segment of time used for treatment and billing purposes.

Multiple (algebraic) apportionment. Method of cost allocation that involves a two-step allocation, but takes into account multiple simultaneous apportionments during the first step.

National Health Planning and Resource Development Act of 1974. Federal legislation signed by President Ford that established planning mechanisms including certificate-of-need programs.

National Patient Safety Goals (NPSG). Patient safety goals of specific concern to JCAHO.

Nature of relationships. Characteristic of the management function of organizing that defines whether managers and/or employees have a line or staff relationship in the organization.

Net assets. Difference between assets and liabilities in a not-for-profit organization.

Net income. Difference between collected revenue and expenses also reported as excess of revenues to expenses.

Network HMO. A type of HMO that exerts moderate to maximum control over physician providers because they contract with physician groups to provide care for enrollees.

Net working capital. Difference between current assets and current liabilities.

Nonoperating costs. Costs associated with supporting the production of a product or service.

Nonproductive asset. Assets that do not produce revenue or increase in value.

Omnibus Budget Reconciliation Act (OBRA) of 1980. Federal legislation signed by President Reagan that eliminated the prior hospitalization requirement for home health services visits, and eliminated the limitation on the total number of home health visits.

Omnibus Budget Reconciliation Act (OBRA) of 1981. Federal legislation signed by President Reagan that increased Medicare deductibles for Parts A and B.

Omnibus Budget Reconciliation Act (OBRA) of 1986. Federal legislation signed by President Reagan that expanded Medicaid eligibility for low-income pregnant women, children, and infants by eliminating the requirement to be enrolled in the state's Aid to Families with Dependent Children (AFDC) first.

Omnibus Budget Reconciliation Act (OBRA) of 1989. Federal legislation that established a physician fee schedule for Medicare and limited the amount physician's charges could exceed the fee schedule, thus limiting the amount physicians who had rejected assignment could balance bill Medicare beneficiaries.

Omnibus Budget Reconciliation Act (OBRA) of 1990. Federal legislation that folded capital costs into the DRG formula over a 10-year period. These costs had previously been reimbursed by cost.

Omnibus Budget Reconciliation Act (OBRA) of 1993. Federal legislation signed by President Clinton that removed the cap on wages subject to the Medicare Part A payroll tax and introduced a new tax on social security benefits above certain incomes.

Open panel HMO. A type of HMO that exerts moderate control over physician providers because the organization contracts with physicians to take care of enrollees in the physicians' offices.

Operating costs. Costs associated with producing a product or service.

Operation Restore Trust. HHS program designed to detect and punish Medicare fraud and abuse.

Opinion paragraph. Part of the audit report that includes the auditor's statement about whether the financial statements are correct as to accounting format.

Opportunity costs. Costs foregone by rejecting an alternative.

Ordering cost. Administrative costs associated with placing a single order for an inventory item.

Organizational chart. Identifies who is responsible per functional unit or department.

Out of network. Term referring to providers not covered, or partially covered, by a particular managed care organization.

Out-of-pocket costs. Healthcare costs that the patient pays directly to the provider and includes deductibles and copays.

Overstock costs. Costs associated with having more than enough inventory to meet demand.

Parent holding corporation. One of four possible corporate structures, the parent holding corporation is used to protect present and future assets.

Part A. Hospital insurance under Medicare that covers hospital services, outpatient diagnostic services, home health agency services after hospitalization, and extended care facility services after hospitalization.

Part B. Supplemental medical insurance under Medicare that covers physician and other medical services, outpatient therapeutic services, home health agency services, certain preventive services, and hospice services.

Patient billing system (PBS). Automated system designed to bill patients in a prompt and efficient manner.

Patient dumping. Practice of denying treatment to patients or transferring patients based on their inability to pay.

Payment cycle. Step in the billing process at which the medical record has been completed and payment is expected.

Peer Review Organization (PRO). Established under the TEFRA legislation, PROs review Medicare discharges to determine appropriateness of care.

Per diagnosis. Methods of reimbursement in which the payer reimburses the provider a prospective, flat rate based on the patient's diagnosis that has been negotiated in advance.

Per diem. Methods of reimbursement in which the payer reimburses the provider a prospective, flat rate per day.

Permanent working capital. Minimum amount of working capital always on hand.

Personal Responsibility and Work Opportunity Reconciliation Act of 1996. Federal legislation signed by President Clinton that made restrictive changes to welfare eligibility and that in turn restricted eligibility to Medicaid.

Phase-out pricing. Practice of pricing products and services high to eliminate poor quality or under-usage.

Phillips Curve. Relationship, thought to be inverse, between unemployment rate and inflation rate.

Physician-hospital organization (PHO). Joint ventures between hospitals and medical staffs designed to position the organization for managed care contracting.

Pledge. Accounts receivable term for using receivables as collateral for a loan.

Point-of-service plan (POS). A type of managed care organization that exerts little to no control over their providers because the organization allows enrollees to seek care from providers not on contract.

Predatory pricing. Practice of pricing products and services low in the short-term to gain market share.

Preemptive pricing. Practice of pricing products and services low to discourage new entrants in the market.

Preferred provider organization (PPO). A type of managed care organization that provides discounted provider services to insurance carriers and employers.

Prepaid expense. Money paid in one accounting period for value consumed in subsequent accounting periods.

Present value. Present amount of money in investment decisions.

Price-driven costing. Practice of determining effective charges and then cutting costs to break even.

Prime rate. A bank's lowest rate of interest on loans afforded to customers with low credit risk.

Process costing. Method of determining product cost during a given accounting period.

Product costing. Method of assembling costs by product or service.

Professional Standards Review Organization (PSRO). Federal legislation signed by President Nixon to establish and fund review organizations to review appropriateness and quality of care delivered to Medicare beneficiaries.

Prospective payment. Method of reimbursement to providers established by payers before the service is provided to patients. Prospective payment is usually a flat amount per head or per diagnosis.

Purchasing cost. Total cost paid to vendors for a specific item during an accounting period.

Qualified opinion. One of four possible opinion paragraphs in an audit report, the qualified opinion means that the financial statements present fairly, in all material respects, the financial position, results of operations, and cash flows of the organization in conformance with GAAP, except for matters identified in additional paragraphs of the report. Auditors use qualified opinions when there is insufficient evidential matter, when the organization has placed restrictions on the scope of the audit, or when the financial statements depart in a material, though not substantial, manner from GAAP.

Quasi-independent sister corporation. One of four possible corporate structures, quasi-independent sister corporation is used to maximize patient care and other operating revenues.

Qui Tam Provisions. Fraud and abuse provisions that protect and reward (15 to 25 percent of the total recovery) whistleblowers who identify instances of fraud and abuse to the federal government.

Rate-based indicators. Process measures that allow for an error rate and require case review only if the error rate is exceeded.

Ratio analysis. Financial analysis method that evaluates financial performance by computing relationships of important line items found in financial statements.

Ratio of costs to charges. Method of determining product cost by relating its cost to its charge.

Reengineering. Fundamental rethinking and radical redesign of work processes to achieve improvements.

Relative value unit (RVU). A sample of resources that each product or service consumes.

Relevant costs. Future costs that will differ between alternatives.

Reorder point. Inventory management term that defines the number of units used or number of days necessary between ordering an item and receiving an item.

Responsibility. Characteristic of the management function of organizing that defines the obligation necessary to perform assigned tasks.

Responsibility accounting. Process of holding managers responsible for their revenue centers and cost centers.

Responsibility costing. Method of assembling costs by responsibility center or cost center.

Retrospective payment. Methods of reimbursement that determine the amount reimbursed after the delivery of services and products.

Retrospective review. Utilization review that occurs after care is delivered.

Revolving credit agreement. Formal line of credit with a commercial bank.

Risk management. The process of identifying, preventing, controlling, and financing all types of risks to patients, employees, visitors, equipment, and plant.

Routine credit-and-collection costs. Associated with accounts receivable, credit-and-collection costs are the costs incurred by the organization related to credit-and-collection efforts during the organization's average payment cycle.

Scope paragraph. Part of the audit report that describes the criteria used in the audit (e.g., GAAP or GASB).

Second-party payment. Term which describes a direct financial relationship between the patient and the provider.

Segment pricing. Practice of pricing products and services high in relation to their "snob appeal."

Semi-variable costs. Costs that vary incrementally with changes in volume.

Sentinel indicators. Process measures of significant importance that require case review and reporting to the Joint Commission for every occurrence.

Shareholders equity. Difference between assets and liabilities in for-profit organizations.

Short-term securities. Investments with a maturity of less than one year.

Simple interest loan. Loan for which the borrower receives the principal and repays the principal plus interest at the end of the loan period.

Skill mix. Varying levels of specialization of workforce.

Skim pricing. Practice of pricing products and services high because of high quality or low availability in the market.

Skiptracing. Provisions of the Fair Debt Collections Practices Act that governs who collection agencies can communicate with other than the consumer owing the debt and how the agency can communicate with those people.

Slash pricing. Practice of pricing products and services low in the long-term by making fundamental changes in the product.

Slide-down pricing. Practice of pricing products and services at different rates for different customers.

Socialized medicine. Political term used to describe health insurance and/or healthcare financed and delivered by the federal government.

Social Security Act of 1935. Federal legislation signed by President Roosevelt that initiated the social security program for the elderly (early drafts included compulsory health insurance).

Social Security Amendments of 1965. Federal legislation signed by President Johnson that initiated both the Medicare and Medicaid programs.

Social Security Amendments of 1972. Federal legislation signed by President Nixon authorizing price controls to control inflation in the economy.

Social Security Amendments of 1983. Federal legislation signed by President Reagan that included provisions for Medicare prospective payment.

Span of management. Characteristic of the management function of organizing that defines the optimum number of employees that a manager can manage based on the nature of the tasks and the background of the employees.

Specialization. Characteristic of the management function of organizing that divides tasks into manageable categories and assigns the categories to employees in the organization with the appropriate skills.

Specific identification. Method of valuing inventory that places the cost of inventory at the actual price paid for each item in inventory.

Staff model HMO. A type of closed panel HMO that employs individual physicians to provide all physician care to enrollees.

Staff relationship. Also called staff authority. The manager or employee acts in an advisory capacity without direct responsibility for organizational resources such as employees and supplies.

Standard costing. A method of establishing benchmark costs, usually budget costs, for the purpose of comparing actual costs.

Standard costs. Estimated or budgeted costs used for comparison purposes.

Step-down apportionment. Cost allocation method which involves a two-time allocation.

Stock-out. Inventory management term that means that an inventory item is out of stock.

Stock-out costs. Costs associated with having insufficient inventory to meet demand.

Subscriber. Member of an enrolled population covered by a managed care agreement that reimburses providers on a per capita basis.

Sunk costs. Costs that have already been incurred and thus will not be affected by present or future decisions.

Tax capacity. A measure of the amount individuals can pay in taxes, usually defined as median household income.

Tax Equity and Fiscal Responsibility Act of 1982 (TEFRA). Federal legislation signed by President Reagan that included significant tax changes, and significant Medicare reimbursement reform in the form of cost limits per case and per year.

Tax price. A measure of the median voter's share of unit cost of providing additional unit of public service.

Temporary working capital. Additional working capital needed to respond to increases in business that are the result of seasonal fluctuations.

Third-party payers. Agents of the patient who contract with providers to pay all or part of the patient's bill.

Total cost. Inventory formula that produces the minimum costs associated with keeping a specific item in inventory for a period of one year.

Trade credit. A method of financing working capital by "borrowing" money from a vendor that the organization already owes money to. This is done by delaying payment to the vendor and accepting a late fee or finance charge.

Treasurer. Formal position with authority and responsibility for the organization's finance functions including the management of working capital and the investment portfolio, and the financing of capital expenditures.

True costs. Hypothetical costs that represent the most accurate representation of full costs.

Truth in Lending Act. Federal legislation that establishes disclosure rules for consumer credit sales.

Uncompensated care. Term that includes the provision of care to both indigent patients and bad-debt patients.

Uncontrollable costs. Costs that cannot be influenced by the manager.

Unity of command. Characteristic of the management function of organizing that defines one manager who is responsible for a group of employees.

Unrelated business income (UBI). Income from business activities that is unrelated to the organization's tax-exempt purposes and therefore must be reported as taxable income.

Unqualified opinion. One of four possible opinion paragraphs in an audit report, the unqualified opinion means that the financial statements present fairly, in all material respects, the financial position, results of operations, and cash flows of the organization in conformance with GAAP.

Utilitarian view of ethics. Also known as consequentialism or teleologic view. The underlying premise is that the rightness or wrongness of an act is determined by the relative amount of good the act or decision produces. The view is characterized by the saying, "the greatest good for the greatest number."

Utilization review. A review process that can be prospective, concurrent, or retrospective and that determines whether professional care was appropriate or properly delivered.

Variance. Difference between standard costs and actual costs.

Variable costs. Costs that vary directly and proportionately to changes in volume.

Vertical analysis. Financial analysis method that evaluates the internal structure of the organization by focusing on a base number and showing percentages of important line items to the base year.

Vertical integration. Expansion of a product or service line at more than one point in the production process (e.g., hospitals integrating with nursing homes).

Vision. Strategic planning term that means the view of the future that a particular organization has that will best enable the organization to accomplish its mission.

Voluntary disclosure. Fraud and abuse provisions that limit liability for healthcare organizations that discover, identify to the federal government, and correct billing errors and other fraudulent and abusive practices.

Weighted average. Method of valuing inventory that places the cost of inventory at the average price paid for the items placed in inventory multiplied by the number of units in inventory.

Wholly controlled subsidiary corporation. One of four possible corporate structures, a wholly controlled subsidiary corporation is used to facilitate the development of a new service.

Wholly independent corporation. One of four possible corporate structures, wholly independent corporation is used to attract additional funds through philanthropy.

Working capital. Total current assets.

Working capital policy. Sources and methods used to finance working capital, as well as the quantity of working capital to be maintained.

Workload statistic. Unit of measure used to reflect workload (e.g., patient days, procedures, RVUs, etc.).

INDEX

For-profit corporations: annual reports, 289–290; community benefit standard and, 47–50, 58; income statement, 277; not-for-profit entities, relationships with, 52, 54, 267; tax status, 45; working capital sources, 178–179

Fraud and abuse: civil actions, 122–126; collections practices, 201; compliance programs, 126–127, 129, 198; criminal actions, 126–128; government initiatives on, 119–120; HIPAA reforms, 131, 319 (*See also* Medicare Integrity Program); implicit certification theory, 124–125; Medicare/Medicaid, 95, 117–129, 196; safe harbors, 113–114, 118–122, 126

Fraud and False Statements Act, 117

FTEs. *See* Full-time equivalents

Full costs, 146, 150

Full-time equivalents, 288

Future trends, healthcare management, 309–334

Future value, 184–186, 257

FV. *See* Future value

GAAP. *See* Generally accepted accounting principles

Gains: net realized, 280–281; unrealized, 280–281

Generally accepted accounting principles, 39

Gifts. *See* Philanthropy

Goals: quality measures, 9; setting, 221, 227–228

Governing bodies, 30–41; budgeting role, 245–246; credit-and-collection policy, 192–193, 198–200; investment policy, 184; not-for-profit corporations, 54; strategic planning role, 224–227, 232–233

Government, health role of, 312–315. *See also* Medicaid; Medicare

Group practices, investments in, 122

Group purchasing organizations, payments to, 121

Healthcare expenditure statistics, 94–97, 314–315

Healthcare financial management. *See* Financial management overview

Healthcare Financial Management Association, 5

Healthcare management, objective of, 3–4

Healthcare reform, 314–321

Health information management, 196–198

Health information privacy. *See* Patient information, privacy of

Health Insurance Portability and Accountability Act, 106–113, 119, 130–132, 309, 318–319; administrative simplification standards, 107–113; civil monetary penalty authority, 109, 113–114; privacy and security requirements, 38–39,

112–113, 131–132; revenue cycle performance, 200, 203

Health maintenance organizations, 69, 71–72, 292, 293. *See also* Managed care organizations; legislation to facilitate, 316; Medicare+Choice, 89

Health professionals, healthcare role of, 312. *See also* Physicians

Health professional shortage areas, 122

Healthy People 2010: Healthy People in Healthy Communities, 310–313

HFMA. *See* Healthcare Financial Management Association

HHS. *See* U. S. Department of Health and Human Services

HI. *See* Hospital insurance

HIM. *See* Health information management

HIPAA. *See* Health Insurance Portability and Accountability Act

HMOs. *See* Health maintenance organizations

Home health agencies, 132, 138, 140; Medicaid payments to, 98; Medicare and, 88, 92, 93, 134–135; Medicare/Medicaid fraud and abuse controls, 127

Horizontal analysis, 186–187, 273–274

Hospital insurance, 88, 90–91, 131

Hospital outpatient lab project, 120

Hospitals: Medicaid payments to, 98, 100; Medicare/Medicaid fraud and abuse controls, 127; Medicare payments to, 88, 90–93; rural, 91, 93, 128, 136, 226; teaching, 91, 136–137, 226; urban, 91, 93, 128

Hourly rate charging method, 166

HPSAs. *See* Health professional shortage areas

ICFs. *See* Intermediate care facilities

IDFSs. *See* Integrated delivery and finance systems

Incentives, financial, 72, 77, 91

Income. *See also* Revenue: generation, 6; operating, 279, 284–286; other, 279, 285, 286; statement, 277

Incremental budgeting, 237

Incremental planning, 222

Independent auditor, 39–41

Independent contractors, 55

Independent corporations, 41–42

Independent practice associations, 72

Indigents. *See also* Charity care: legal duty to, 191, 203; Medicaid eligibility, 97–98

Indirect costs, 146–147, 238

Industry comparisons, 187, 274, 302

Influencing. *See* Directing function

Installment loan, 181, 189

Insurance. *See also* Malpractice insurance; Managed care organizations; Uninsured persons: consumer-driven plans, 70–71; coordination of benefits, 199; defined-contribution and defined-benefit plans, 73; direct contracting (self-insuring), 68,